Respiratory Medicine

Series Editor:
Sharon I.S. Rounds

For further volumes:
http://www.springer.com/series/7665

Ran D. Anbar
Editor

Functional Respiratory Disorders

When Respiratory Symptoms Do Not Respond to Pulmonary Treatment

Humana Press

Editor
Ran D. Anbar
Department of Pediatrics
SUNY Upstate Medical University
Syracuse, NY, USA
anbarr@upstate.edu

For videos, please see link:
http://www.springerimages.com/videos/978-1-61779-856-6

ISBN 978-1-61779-856-6 e-ISBN 978-1-61779-857-3
DOI 10.1007/978-1-61779-857-3
Springer New York Heidelberg Dordrecht London

Library of Congress Control Number: 2012937650

Printed on acid-free paper

Humana Press is a brand of Springer
Springer is part of Springer Science+Business Media (www.springer.com)

This book is dedicated to my beloved parents: To my father, Michael Anbar, Ph.D., who encouraged me throughout my life to make major contributions to the human endeavor, and to my mother, Ada Anbar, Ph.D., who taught me about the importance of compassion and altruism.

Preface

Many patients with pulmonary complaints fail to improve despite physicians' best efforts. Sometimes, we ascribe this failure to lack of adherence to therapy or to the severity of the condition. What we often fail to appreciate, however, is that sometimes the lack of improvement can be explained by the patients' psychological states. For example, some patients with asthma can experience shortness of breath as a result of anxiety rather than a physical exacerbation of their asthma. Treating the symptom by ratcheting up pharmacological asthma therapies is of little use and can be harmful. Thus, the first section of this book will help clinicians recognize functional respiratory symptoms that can arise in association with both organic and psychological causes.

Another group of patients have respiratory complaints that many clinicians recognize as functional in nature, such as vocal cord dysfunction, habit cough, anxiety-related dyspnea, and stress-related chest pain. Further, treatment of patients with sleep disorders often involves addressing functional issues that complicate their management, e.g., learning to accept continuous positive airway pressure (CPAP) therapy or psychosocial stressors that can underlie development of parasomnia. Thus, the second section of this book provides detailed discussions of such disorders, links to video examples of laryngoscopic evaluation of patients with vocal cord issues, case studies, and quizzes. The examples and exercises should strengthen the clinician's confidence in identifying and treating these functional conditions.

Finally, even when clinicians are comfortable in identifying patients with functional respiratory disorders, planning a treatment program can be challenging. Some patients may be reluctant to see mental health providers, even when such competent providers are available. For this reason, the third section of the book will help clinicians differentiate patients for whom referral to a mental health provider is necessary from those for whom other approaches may be useful. For the latter group, the book can teach clinicians to empower themselves by learning how to incorporate various nonpharmacological therapeutic modalities for functional disorders into their practice, including biofeedback, breathing techniques, elements of basic cognitive behavioral therapy, hypnosis, speech therapy, acupressure, and meditation. Links are provided to instructive video examples of biofeedback, hypnosis, and speech therapy.

Information regarding how one might receive training in these modalities is provided in the Appendix. Rare instances in which functional respiratory disorders might be treated with pharmacologic agents also are discussed. Helpful case studies and quizzes are provided in this section as well.

The intended audience for this book includes pediatricians, family practitioners, internists, pulmonologists, sleep specialists, psychiatrists, psychologists, and other mental health-care providers. Students, residents, and fellows in medical and behavioral sciences also should find the book of significant interest, as it may help shape their approach to patients throughout their careers.

We are fortunate to have benefited from the expertise of the internationally renowned authors who contributed to this book, including pulmonologists, sleep medicine specialists, family practitioners, pediatricians, psychiatrists, psychologists, speech therapists, and experts in complementary and alternative medicine. It is our hope that the book will help clinicians consider the possible impact of functional contributions to the clinical presentation of every patient with respiratory symptoms and identified respiratory disease.

Syracuse, NY Ran D. Anbar

Acknowledgments

The concept for this book arose following presentation of a short course entitled "Functional Contributions to Respiratory Disorders in Children and Adults," which was offered at the 2010 American Thoracic Society conference in New Orleans, LA. I was approached by Amanda Quinn, an editor at Springer, who proposed the possibility of covering the topic in a book. I enthusiastically accepted this opportunity given the importance of alerting clinicians regarding the large and often unrecognized impact of functional respiratory disorders in clinical practice.

I would like to thank all of my coauthors, Devang Doshi, Reinhild Draeger-Muenke, Courtney DuMond, Adam Elias, Juliet Foster, Howard Hall, Charles Harris, Heather Hodges, Douglas Homnick, Christine Jenkins, David Johnson, Paul Lehrer, Dewey Meyers, Maximilian Muenke, Dilip Patel, Zafer Soultan, Brett Toelle, Miles Weinberger, and Joseph Zastrow, who worked diligently on their contributions to the book. Many of them helped review and provided invaluable feedback regarding some chapters in the book that were written by our coauthors.

This book has been enriched with videos that accompany some of the chapters. I would like to acknowledge the following individuals who helped produce the videos: Steven Garlock, Steve Marks, and Eric Willmarth.

Many others deserve a grateful acknowledgment for their help with development of the concept of this book and review of some of the chapters including Ralph Berberich, Julie Bergquist, Fiona Miniter Briggs, William Doheney, Pamela Duger, Jenica Harmon, Robert Kaslovsky, Lewis Kass, Colin King, Daniel Kohen, Julie Linden, Richard Moss, Thomas Schwartz, Laurence Sugarman, Paul Taylor, Fredrick Wamboldt, and Thomas Welch.

My editor, Michael D. Sova, deserves a special thank you for his essential and calm guidance throughout the process of preparing this book.

Finally, I would like to acknowledge my dear wife, Hannah, and my children Josh, Rebecca, Ellie, and Yoni for their support and understanding throughout the process of writing this book, which all too frequently necessitated my absence from family activities.

Now, it's time for a family vacation!

Contents

Contributors

Ran D. Anbar Department of Pediatrics, SUNY Upstate Medical University, Syracuse, NY, USA

Devang R. Doshi William Beaumont School of Medicine, Oakland University, Bloomfield, MI, USA

Reinhild Draeger-Muenke Independent Private Practice, Bala Cynwyd, PA, USA

Courtney E. Du Mond Department of Pediatrics, SUNY Upstate Medical University, Syracuse, NY, USA

Adam S. Elias Department of Psychiatry, Cambridge Health Alliance, Cambridge, MA, USA

Juliet M. Foster Respiratory & Environmental Epidemiology Group, Woolcock Institute of Medical Research, Camperdown, NSW, Australia

Howard R. Hall Department of Pediatrics, Case Medical Center, University Hospitals, Rainbow Babies & Children's Hospital, Cleveland, OH, USA

Charles R. Harris Department of Psychiatry, SUNY Upstate University Hospital, Syracuse, NY, USA

Heather L. Hodges Department of Rehabilitation Services, National Jewish Health, Denver, CO, USA

Douglas N. Homnick Department of Pediatrics, Michigan State University, Kalamazoo Center for Medical Studies, Kalamazoo, MI, USA

Christine R. Jenkins Clinical Professor, University of Sydney, Co-operative Research Centre for Asthma and Woolcock Institute of Medical Research, Thoracic Physician, Concord Hospital, Australia

Department of Thoracic Medicine, Concord Hospital, Concord, NSW, Australia

David A. Johnson Adirondack Internal Medicine and Pediatrics, Saranac Lake, NY, USA

Paul M. Lehrer Department of Psychiatry, University of Medicine & Dentistry of New Jersey, Johnson Medical School, Piscataway, NJ, USA

Dewey G. Meyers Clear Mind Body Institute, Syracuse, NY, USA

Maximilian Muenke Medical Acupuncture and Complementary Medicine, Bala Cynwyd, PA, USA

Dilip R. Patel Department of Pediatrics, Michigan State University, Kalamazoo Center for Medical Studies, Kalamazoo, MI, USA

Zafer N. Soultan Department of Pediatrics, SUNY Upstate Medical University, Syracuse, NY, USA

Brett G. Toelle Respiratory & Environmental Epidemiology Group, Woolcock Institute of Medical Research, Glebe, NSW, Australia

Miles M. Weinberger Department of Pediatrics, University of Iowa Hospital, Iowa City, IA, USA

Joseph F. Zastrow Primary Care Associates, Lake Norman, Mooresville, NC, USA

Part I
Recognition of Functional Respiratory Symptoms

Chapter 1
What Is a Functional Respiratory Disorder?

Ran D. Anbar and Howard R. Hall

Abstract Functional respiratory disorders can be characterized as occurring in patients with persisting respiratory symptoms lacking an identifiable organic or physiologic basis, or symptoms in excess of what would be expected from just their physiologic cause. Such functional disorders typically have emotional or psychological associations. Common respiratory conditions that are thought to be functional include dyspnea/hyperventilation, habit cough, paroxysmal sneezing, throat clearing, and vocal cord dysfunction. These occur predominantly in children, adolescents, and young adults. Additionally, a functional component should be entertained as complicating existing diagnosed physical conditions, such as asthma, chronic obstructive pulmonary disease, and cystic fibrosis, which are diseases that affect patients of all ages. Treatment of functional respiratory disorders can include providing reassurance, biofeedback, breathing relaxation techniques, cognitive behavioral therapy, hypnosis, or speech therapy. Pharmacologic therapy for functional respiratory disorders occasionally may be helpful. Patients with functional respiratory disorders benefit from prompt identification and therapy, as this prevents perpetuation of the associated symptoms, development of further complicating sequelae, unnecessary medical investigations, and prescription of ineffective medical therapy that might have harmful side effects.

Keywords Anxiety • Asthma • Dyspnea • Habit cough • Hyperventilation • Somatoform disorders • Vocal cord dysfunction

R.D. Anbar (✉)
Department of Pediatrics, SUNY Upstate Medical University, 750 East Adams St., 13210-1834, Syracuse, NY, USA
e-mail: anbarr@upstate.edu

H.R. Hall
Department of Pediatrics, Case Medical Center, University Hospitals, Rainbow Babies & Children's Hospital, Cleveland, OH, USA

R.D. Anbar (ed.), *Functional Respiratory Disorders: When Respiratory Symptoms Do Not Respond to Pulmonary Treatment*, Respiratory Medicine,
DOI 10.1007/978-1-61779-857-3_1, © Springer Science+Business Media, LLC 2012

Functional respiratory disorders traditionally have been defined as symptoms occurring in the absence of organic pulmonary pathology. Functional disorders have been termed medically unexplained physical symptoms (MUPS), functional somatic symptoms (FSS), abnormal illness behavior, idiopathic symptoms, and somatoform symptoms (physical expression of psychological or psychiatric issues) [1, 2]. Frequently, these are transient phenomena and resolve without specific therapy [2]. At times, however, functional respiratory symptoms can be quite persistent and may require appropriate professional intervention [3]. In this chapter, the term functional respiratory disorder will be used to refer to patients with *persistent* respiratory symptoms in the absence of any identifiable organic or physiologic cause, or symptoms that are in excess of what would be expected from just their physiologic cause. Such functional disorders typically have psychological associations.

This chapter reviews how clinicians can enhance the effectiveness of their care by promptly diagnosing and offering treatment for functional respiratory disorders, including their associated complications such as sleep disturbances. Further, it illustrates how attention to possible psychological triggers of functional respiratory disorders can define or augment the appropriate course of treatment.

Background

A connection between psychological factors and respiratory disorders should not be surprising. Since antiquity, the word for breath has been strongly connected with the spiritual facets of human life. For example, the term for spirit in Hebrew is *ruach,* which also means breath or wind. As described in the Old Testament book of Genesis 2:7, the creation of human life began with God forming man from the dust of the ground and breathing into his nostrils, "the breath of life and man became a living soul." In the New Testament, the Greek term *pneuma* refers to breath, life, and God [4]. Not only does life begin with breath, but life also ends with the cessation of breath. Equivalent terms for this life force can be found in other cultures around the world in words such as *prana* from India, *Qi* and *Chi* from China, and *ki* from Japan [5].

An understanding of the association between psychological and breathing disorders developed in the medical field during the 1930s, when asthma was known as one of the Holy Seven psychosomatic disorders, alongside hypertension, ulcerative colitis, Graves' disease, rheumatoid arthritis, peptic ulcer, and neurodermatitis [6]. According to the prevalent psychoanalytic model, a child's separation from his or her mother caused an emotional conflict leading to anxiety, which underlay the development of asthma. Subsequent research, however, failed to find support for the existence of this specific conflict in individuals with asthma, and more nonspecific stress models began to emerge with the work of Selye and others [6].

Our growing understanding of the interaction between psychological factors and physical conditions was demonstrated through the evolution of the series of diagnostic and statistical manual of mental disorders (DSM) published by the American Psychiatric Association. For example, the DSM-II (1968) appeared to restrict "psychophysiologic disorders" to nine specific types including (305.2) psychophysiologic respiratory disorders such as "bronchial asthma, hyperventilation syndromes, sighing, and hiccoughs in which emotional factors play a causative role" [7]. A major shift in this category had taken place upon publication of the DSM-III (1980), in which specific diseases were no longer listed but instead considered within the general category of (316) "psychological factors affecting physical conditions" [8]. This invited the clinician to more broadly note the contribution of psychological factors to the initiation or exacerbation of any physical disorder. DSM-III also introduced the category of "somatoform disorders," wherein physical symptoms can be associated with psychological factors in the absence of precipitating anatomic or physiologic causes.

Of course, we have long recognized that asthma is not simply a behavioral disease, but there have been major advances in our understanding of how behavioral and psychological factors can exacerbate or ameliorate this particular condition in a major way [9]. For example, stress may be mediated through the autonomic nervous system (ANS), hormonally, or through immune mechanisms, and thereby influence the extent of airway inflammation in patients with asthma [9]. Anxiety disorders, panic symptoms, and depression have been associated with asthma symptoms through indirect effects such as disorganization of self-care behaviors or through direct physiological effects mediated through the ANS or immune system. Yet, given the inconsistent findings and limitations of current published studies, definitive conclusions cannot be drawn regarding the interactions of mood and asthma [9].

Commonly recognized functional respiratory disorders present with dyspnea/hyperventilation, habit cough, paroxysmal sneezing, throat clearing, and vocal cord dysfunction. These occur predominantly in children, adolescents, and young adults [10, 11]. Additionally, functional factors may add to the management complexity of identified respiratory diseases, such as asthma, chronic obstructive pulmonary disease, and cystic fibrosis, which affect patients of all ages. Sleep disturbances frequently accompany respiratory disorders and may impact respiratory symptoms [12]. For example, fatigue and sleep disturbances have been associated with perceptions of poor health in adult patients with chronic obstructive pulmonary disease (COPD). Further, insomnia may arise in the context of school- or work-related worries in patients with functional respiratory disorders such as habit cough or vocal cord dysfunction.

The Wide Spectrum of Functional Respiratory Disorders and Associated Conditions

Functional respiratory disorders are associated with two distinct scenarios:

1. The disorder develops in isolated association with a psychological stressor. A common example is the teenager with no history of asthma, who develops vocal cord dysfunction because of stress arising from participation in competitive

athletics, or a patient who develops anxiety-associated dyspnea as result of concerns about loss of income or job. A frequently unrecognized variant of this scenario is the patient who has been misdiagnosed with an organic disease, thereby receiving a medical diagnosis with potential lifelong ramifications, because he or she presented with functional symptoms consistent with that diagnosis. For example, a patient with habit cough who has been misdiagnosed with asthma may report episodes of anxiety-related dyspnea that are interpreted as representing exacerbations of uncontrolled asthma. In such cases, exploration of possible psychological stressors should be carried out in conjunction with appropriate medical assessment. This may prompt reconsideration of the diagnosis and will allow development of a more effective treatment plan.

2. The disorder develops in association with a diagnosed medical illness or an environmental exposure. Functional manifestations can arise because of fear or anticipation of worsening of symptoms due to a medical illness or threatening environmental exposure. For example, a patient with asthma may hyperventilate because of fear that an asthma exacerbation might become severe. In others, functional respiratory symptoms can be triggered because of anxiety following exposure to an environmental trigger such as a strong odor, even in the absence of documented allergic sensitivity. Similarly, anxiety can trigger noncardiac chest pain in patients with a history of a myocardial infarction or can lead to sensations of chest tightness in patients with early cancer that does not involve the lungs. Another variation of this scenario involves patients whose psychological factors influence treatment of a respiratory condition. For example, a patient with asthma and underlying anxiety may develop dyspnea as the result of school-related experiences such as test taking or bullying. However, in response to the dyspnea, a health-care provider often assumes that the patient's asthma is the trigger, and treats accordingly by modifying the asthma medications. The school-related anxiety, however, will not improve as a result of this medical therapy, and the patient thereafter may be characterized erroneously as having asthma that is difficult to treat.

Scenario 1 encompasses the diagnoses most frequently recognized as representing functional respiratory disorders, including habit cough and vocal cord dysfunction without a history of asthma. However, while frequently unrecognized, Scenario 2 conditions actually are much more common given the high prevalence of chronic respiratory illnesses, cardiac disease, and cancer. In these patients, stress and anxiety can be associated with exacerbations of respiratory symptoms such as chest pain, cough, and dyspnea/hyperventilation. For example, 29% of adult patients with asthma in primary care settings have been reported as having dysfunctional breathing [13]. Further, nearly 50% of pediatric patients with asthma in one study were identified as having clinical anxiety that could affect their medical management [14]. Scenario 2 also applies to patients with vocal cord dysfunction combined with asthma. In such cases, in order to distinguish between vocal cord dysfunction and asthma, clinicians need to probe and differentiate characteristics of the associated respiratory symptoms. For example, breathing difficulties arising during inhalation and reported by patients to cause a feeling of blockage in the neck are more likely to be the result of vocal cord dysfunction. As another Scenario 2 example, the course of COPD appears to be influenced by anxiety and depression, which lead to poorer health quality-of-life measures [12, 15]. In turn, poor quality of health scores has been associated with increased risks for hospital readmission and mortality in adults with COPD [16, 17].

Regardless of the presenting scenario, functional respiratory disorders can cause physical pathology. For example, severe habit cough can lead to the development of tracheal petechiae or rib fractures [18]. Severe vocal cord dysfunction can cause loss of consciousness [19]. Anxiety-induced hyperventilation can trigger bronchospasm in patients with asthma, since air that is inhaled rapidly through the mouth does not get filtered, warmed, and moistened as with nasal inhalation, and thus is more likely to trigger asthma [20, 21]. In turn, an asthma exacerbation can lead to escalation of the anxiety. Chronic fatigue as a result of insomnia can be associated with a number of health complications. It is important that clinicians not confuse the secondary organic changes in such settings as the primary cause of the functional symptoms.

Not only can the development of functional respiratory disorders be the result of psychological factors, but functional disorders can lead to psychological sequelae. For example, anxiety may result from long-standing respiratory symptoms without an identifiable cause. Some patients may grow more resistant to therapy as their functional symptoms and associated psychological issues become more entrenched [22]. The functional symptoms of some patients can be reinforced by medical and family attention provided as a result of the symptoms [23–25]. In such instances, resolution of the symptoms can be facilitated by discontinuing extensive medical interventions and encouraging patients' families to become nonreactive in the face of ongoing symptoms. An unusual circumstance arises when patients receive disability payments as the result of functional symptoms, which can prompt their perpetuation [2]. Finally, patients' lives can be altered significantly as a consequence of persisting functional respiratory symptoms. Participation in athletic activities may cease because of dyspnea or vocal cord dysfunction. Disruptive habit cough and resulting negative interactions with teachers or fellow students can lead to absenteeism and dislike of school. In some instances, such life changes provide the patient with secondary gain as a result of the functional symptom. For example, a patient with academic difficulties may welcome being excused from school as the result of a disruptive habit cough and may prove resistant to its treatment.

Classification of patients with functional respiratory symptoms into one of the two scenarios can be helpful in terms of treatment planning. Most Scenario 1 patients tend to improve with behavioral and psychological therapy directly aimed at resolving the respiratory symptoms. Scenario 2 patients may require attention in tandem for both their psychological and underlying disease factors.

Lack of recognition of a functional component in the presentation of patients with respiratory symptoms can lead to ineffective or potentially harmful therapy. For example, long-term systemic corticosteroids might be prescribed for patients with asthma complicated by functional symptoms [20] or can lead to patients who grow frustrated with the medical system because they are not improving [26].

Furthermore, some patients with unrecognized functional respiratory disorders are classified as being "difficult" either because their disease appears resistant to medical therapy, or it is suspected that their lack improvement is related to their poor adherence to prescribed therapy [27]. Ironically, such patients' rate of adherence to therapy may be compromised because of its seeming ineffectiveness!

Psychiatric Classification of Functional Respiratory Disorders

Functional respiratory disorders can be classified according to the DSM-IV-TR category of (316) psychological factors associated with the initiation, exacerbation, or course of a medical condition [28]. This would include both scenarios described above. Small subsets of functional respiratory disorders are attributable to specific psychiatric disorders (Table 1.1). Most of these can be classified as somatoform (from the Greek *soma* = body), which are defined as physical complaints without identified medical abnormalities.

Somatoform disorders can be subdivided into four types relevant to functional respiratory disorders:

1. Conversion disorder—This relatively rare disorder typically occurs suddenly in association with a very stressful event in a patient's life. The conversion symptoms usually are preceded by a psychological conflict or stressor that involves the development of a protective physical symptom. The medical complaint functions to resolve the psychological dilemma (i.e., converts a psychological conflict into a physical form). The physical symptom may suggest physical disease, but often does not follow a physiologic or anatomically appropriate pattern, such as conversion blindness or pseudoseizures. The conversion disorder serves two

Table 1.1 Psychiatric classification of some functional respiratory disorders

Somatoform disorders
Conversion disorder
Subconscious conversion of a psychological conflict to a physical symptom
Somatization disorder
Symptoms involve many organ systems, causing significant discomfort and distress
Pain disorder
Significant pain in the absence of physical findings
Hypochondriasis
Excessive fear of a serious illness persisting despite lack of medical evidence
Malingering
Pretending to have a significant symptom as an avoidance behavior
Factitious disorder (Munchausen's syndrome)
Manufacturing of evidence that leads to diagnosis of a medical condition
Vocal tic disorders
Vocal or phonic tic may involve coughing, throat clearing, sniffing, grunting, squeaking, screaming, barking, blowing, and sucking sounds

psychological functions. The "primary gain" is to keep the emotional conflict or stressor out of conscious awareness, while the "secondary gain" can help get the person out of a difficult situation and gain sympathy.

An example of a functional respiratory disorder attributable to conversion involves a girl who developed vocal cord dysfunction because she was afraid of possible repercussions of disclosing that she had been abused sexually. Therefore, she subconsciously developed vocal cord dysfunction that made her unable to breathe properly and precluded her from speaking well. A patient suffering from a conversion disorder often appears minimally distressed by the symptom (termed *la belle indifférence*), probably because it solves an issue for him or her [29]. However, as *la belle indifférence* can be expressed by patients with identified medical disease as well, it alone does not reliably identify patients with conversion reactions [30].

2. Somatization disorder—This diagnosis is characterized by patients' reports of multiple symptoms, typically involving many organ systems, and causing significant discomfort and distress. Its respiratory manifestations can include shortness of breath, palpitations, and chest pain. Often, patients have seen multiple health-care providers for their various symptoms and may have been prescribed multiple medications. Thus, a patient with habit cough as a result of somatization disorder also might complain of headaches and recurrent abdominal discomfort [3].
3. Pain disorder—Patients with this condition report significant pain that may even cause disability in the absence of physical findings to explain the extent of the symptom. For example, a patient with asthma might complain of severe debilitating chest pain associated with relatively mild exacerbations of his or her condition.
4. Hypochondriasis—Patients with hypochondria have a fear that they have serious illness such as asthma or lung cancer, even though medical tests show no abnormality. Despite reassurance from their physicians that their symptoms do not indicate serious illness, patients with hypochondria may remain excessively worried and preoccupied with the symptoms. Often, such patients may seek multiple medical opinions in search of a "real" diagnosis. Although not classified as hypochondriasis, some parents of a child with dyspnea without an identifiable medical cause may refuse to accept the diagnosis of a functional disorder. Such parents typically are concerned that serious harm might come to their child if an underlying medical cause remains undiagnosed.

Two rare psychiatric diagnoses that can lead to functional respiratory symptoms and are unrelated to somatoform disorders are:

1. DSM-IV-TR (V65.2) malingering [28]—In which the patient voluntarily produces symptoms to attain some goal. For example, a teenager may lie or exaggerate about development of dyspnea in association with exercise in order to avoid participation in gym class.
2. DSM-IV-TR (300.19) factitious disorder (Munchausen's syndrome) [28]—In this unusual situation, patients seek medical attention to such a degree that they manufacture evidence that would lead to diagnosis of a medical condition. For

example, a patient might inhale an irritating substance in order to induce coughing. (Munchausen's by proxy involves a caretaker who manufactures evidence that leads to an erroneous medical diagnosis in their child.)

It should be noted that persistent malingering with respiratory symptoms may be uncommon and factitious disorder in this setting is rare [2].

DSM-IV-R (307) tic disorders [28] is another diagnostic category associated with respiratory conditions:

1. Chronic vocal tic disorder—Vocal or phonic tics may involve coughing, throat clearing, sniffing, grunting, squeaking, screaming, barking, blowing, and sucking sounds [31]. The duration of chronic tic disorder is defined as longer than 1 year.
2. Transient tic disorder—Duration less than 12 consecutive months.
3. Tourette's disorder—This disorder involves multiple motor and vocal tics. Given that it appears to have some genetic basis, patients with tics related to Tourette's disorder should not be classified as having a functional respiratory disorder.

In cases involving psychiatric disorders, patients should be referred to providers specializing in mental health care.

Diagnosis of Functional Respiratory Disorders

An evaluation for functional respiratory disorders should include a thorough medical history, including a review of symptoms suggestive of functional respiratory disorders, as listed in Table 1.2. When inquiring whether patients are symptomatic during sleep, it is important for clinicians to keep in mind that while functional respiratory symptoms usually (but not invariably) resolve during sleep, they frequently worsen when the patient is lying awake in bed. Patients who report that their respiratory symptoms only are triggered in certain circumstances are more likely to have a functional respiratory problem. For example, vocal cord dysfunction is more likely to occur in competitive athletic situations rather than during athletic practice.

Following physical examination, and measurement of hemoglobin saturation with pulse oximetry, pulmonary function testing should be performed, if the patient is capable of cooperating. Additional diagnostic procedures might be appropriate including a chest x-ray (e.g., to exclude the possibility of foreign body aspiration or other pulmonary abnormality), blood gas analysis (e.g., to check for evidence of hypocapnia as a marker of hyperventilation), exercise or cold-air bronchoprovocation testing (e.g., to assess for asthma or vocal cord dysfunction), pertussis serological titers (e.g., to check for a cause of harsh prolonged cough), and flexible bronchoscopy (e.g., to check for vocal cord dysfunction, foreign body, or tracheomalacia) [11, 24]. Assessment for psychological issues such as panic, depression, and family disorganization also may be very helpful for managing asthma and other respiratory conditions with possible functional components [9].

Clinicians should keep in mind that identified abnormalities, such as may be discovered during bronchoprovocation testing, might not be the cause of a presenting

Table 1.2 Symptoms suggestive of functional respiratory disorders

Respiratory symptoms
Chest pain in the absence of cardiac or gastrointestinal disease
Difficulty with inspiration[a]
Disruptive cough[b]
Dyspnea despite normal lung function[c]
Hyperventilation (which patients may term breathing too fast)
Inspiratory noise (e.g., stridor, gasping, rasping, or squeak)[a]
Localization of breathing problem to the neck or upper chest[a, c]
Sighing[c]
Other symptoms
Anxious appearance
Dizziness[c]
Feeling something is stuck in the throat
Lifted shoulders
Palpitations
Paresthesias[c]
Shakiness[c]
Tics[b]
Weakness
Symptom characteristics
Absence during sleep or when patient is distracted
Associated with a particular location or activity
Emotional response to symptoms
Emotional trigger of symptoms
Exposure to traumatic life event
Incomplete response to medications

[a]Suggestive of vocal cord dysfunction
[b]Suggestive of habit cough
[c]Suggestive of functional dyspnea/hyperventilation

Adapted from Anbar RD, Geisler SC. Identification of children who may benefit from self-hypnosis at a pediatric pulmonary center. BMC Pediatrics 2005; 5: 6, with permission

functional symptom. For example, some patients with anxiety-induced dyspnea have been diagnosed erroneously as having asthma-associated dyspnea solely on the basis of their abnormal bronchoprovocation test results. In such situations, the clinician should consider the possibility of a functional component when patients fail to respond to asthma therapy.

Habit cough and vocal cord dysfunction can be diagnosed based on characteristic symptoms, as discussed in Chaps. 5 and 6. However, when functional respiratory disorders occur in association with organic disease (Scenario 2), some of the symptoms can be attributed to either psychological or organic causes. For example, vocal cord dysfunction can be triggered by psychosocial stressors, gastroesophageal reflux to the level of the larynx, or postnasal drip associated with chronic sinusitis. Clinicians should be alert for any symptoms suggestive of a functional etiology as part of the initial assessment of patients presenting with pulmonary complaints. When such symptoms are identified, patients benefit from receiving concurrent assessment and treatment for organic and functional disease. In this way, they are likely to improve more readily. Further, a prompt, complete, and comprehensive diagnostic approach may avoid extensive testing that frequently is undertaken when the diagnosis of a functional respiratory disorder is considered one of exclusion. Such testing can cause patients to feel more certain that they have a serious medical condition and thus less receptive to therapy for what turns out to be a functional disorder [24].

It should be kept in mind that airway behavior varies across the life span [32]. A complex interaction exists involving gender differences, sociocultural influences, and biologic factors such as lung size and immunological and hormonal factors since all may have an impact on airway behavior. Thus, stages of child development also play a role in the presenting characteristics of patients with functional respiratory disorders. For example, habit cough has been described primarily in pediatric and adolescent populations and as occurring much less commonly in adults [31]. Patients with habit cough are more likely to present with barking or honking cough during childhood, as compared to when they are older [31, 33].

Treatment of Functional Respiratory Disorders

Treatment of functional respiratory disorders requires acknowledgement of its existence by the patients, families, and the health-care staff. Some patients may be resistant to the idea that there is a psychological trigger of their symptoms because they feel that this means the clinicians do not believe their symptoms are real. The patients may think that the clinicians believe, "it's all in my head," think they are mentally disturbed, or that they are purposely causing their symptoms. When the possibility of a functional disorder is raised in such situations, patients feel disbelieved or dismissed, as if they are being given the functional diagnosis merely because the clinician is incapable of ascertaining the true medical cause. When this occurs, at minimum, rapport is disturbed, and frequently patients choose not to return for follow-up. When patients feel repeatedly disbelieved by medical practitioners, they may end up seeking care from nonmedical providers who might be unhelpful or unscrupulous [2]. Some patients may demonstrate an escalation of their symptom as a way of convincing the clinician that something is "truly" wrong [1].

Other patients reject the idea that they might have control over their symptoms because they do not feel strong enough emotionally to cope with the responsibility of taking care of themselves. Also, they may fear that they will be blamed if their symptoms fail to improve. Yet others may not want their symptoms to resolve because they benefit from secondary gain.

In situations when patients seem nonreceptive to the diagnosis of a functional disorder, clinicians should help the patients clarify their thoughts and feelings through a careful interview process, offer the patients reassurance that their thoughts are valid, and review various options regarding how their symptoms might be addressed [34]. For example, clinicians might begin by reassuring the patients that

Table 1.3 Treatment of functional respiratory disorders

	Acute	Chronic
Origin	Often minor stressors	Often major or multiple stressors
Treatment	Reassurance	Refer to mental health professional
Options	Address underlying organic disease Self-regulation strategies Pharmacologic therapy	Address psychological stressor Address psychiatric diagnosis Pharmacologic therapy

their symptoms are real, even if they are subjective. It can be emphasized that the functional nature of the symptoms provides an opportunity for utilization of self-regulatory therapies that give patients control, and gives them a chance to help themselves without the need for medications with their associated risk of side effects. The clinicians should state clearly that a patient's ability to help symptoms resolve does not mean that the symptoms are not real or caused by the patient. An analogy that might be useful in this setting is reminding the patients of how they felt while learning how to ride a bicycle. While the patients did not cause themselves to fall off their bicycle on purpose, ultimately they learned to ride a bicycle by learning how to think differently. In some cases, referral to a respiratory specialist can help reinforce the functional diagnosis and help assure the patient that serious pathology is unlikely. When patients are receptive, mental health professionals can serve as a therapeutic bridge between their medical provider and functional symptoms.

The health-care staff may grow impatient and frustrated with providing care for patients with functional respiratory disorders because medical causes of the symptoms often cannot be identified, and even when the symptoms are associated with medical illness, they do not improve readily with standard therapy. Under such circumstances, patients and their families often are blamed for the lack of improvement. The medical staff also may be inclined to provide further therapeutic interventions based upon their frustration because the patient who is suffering with a functional disorder is not improving. Thus, it is important to review with health-care staff the nature of functional respiratory symptoms and appropriate approaches to patients with these symptoms.

Therapeutic approaches differ for acute and chronic functional respiratory disorders (Table 1.3):

1. Acute—These patients account for the majority of those with functional respiratory disorders. Their symptoms often are associated with acute stressors, such as vocal cord dysfunction that occurs in association with an athlete's desire to excel during a competition, or habit cough that arises following an upper respiratory infection.

   Acute symptoms sometimes resolve with reassurance alone, which can be provided through physician disclosure of benign medical findings [24]. It can be important for reassurance to be accompanied by an explanation of how the functional respiratory disorder may have arisen as a result of physiologic or neurologic dysregulation. When a patient is told, instead, that there is no disease, he or she may feel as if the clinician has not undertaken sufficient investigations. For example, a patient with habit cough might be told that the cough was caused by discomfort in the throat as a result of an upper respiratory infection, and that ongoing coughing perpetuated the throat discomfort that led to the persistence of the cough; or a patient with vocal cord dysfunction might be told that the condition occurred as the body's way of saying the patient was stressed.

Some acute functional symptoms that are triggered by an identified disease (Scenario 2) simply resolve with its successful treatment. (For example, when uncontrolled asthma causes anxiety with associated dyspnea, treatment of the asthma often helps relieve the anxiety.)

If acute symptoms do not improve with the aforementioned approaches, they usually resolve readily shortly after patients are taught self-regulation techniques such as biofeedback (Chap. 10), breathing relaxation techniques (Chap. 11), hypnosis (Chap. 12), or speech therapy (Chap. 13). Importantly, these therapies typically also help the patient cope better with any psychological stressor that may have triggered the acute symptoms, and can even help patients when they encounter future life stressors. For example, the breathing relaxation techniques used to prevent vocal cord dysfunction recurrence in a competitive athlete can also help calm the athlete's psychological reactivity to competitive challenges. Pharmacologic treatment of exercise-induced vocal cord dysfunction with the inhaled anticholinergic ipratropium bromide may be therapeutic in this setting because the symptom is triggered through cholinergic stimulation that is mediated through the vagus nerve (Chap. 6). If acute symptoms do not resolve readily, then referral to a mental health specialist should be encouraged [34].

2. Chronic—Some patients develop chronic, persistent functional respiratory disorders, related to a significant psychological disturbance. For example, a patient might develop habit cough following a parent's death, or vocal cord dysfunction because of sexual abuse. In this setting, the functional symptom may act as an answer to the patient's dilemma. For example, development of dyspnea is a face-saving solution for a patient who does not want to participate in a sport despite parental urging. Another patient might develop habit cough as a way of expressing her worry about her father's smoking of cigarettes. As previously discussed, conversion disorder represents the classic diagnosis in which a symptom serves as a solution to an emotional conflict.

   In patients with chronic symptoms, the underlying psychological issue needs to be explored and treated in order for symptoms to improve or resolve. A primary care provider may be in the position of helping some of these patients when sufficient time is allotted for a discussion of their psychosocial stressors and with application of appropriate cognitive behavioral techniques (Chap. 9). However, patients with psychiatric symptoms such as anxiety or depression should be referred to a mental health-care provider [34]. In rare instances, pharmacotherapy, especially with antidepressants, has been helpful in the treatment of persistent functional disorders (Chap. 14) [35].

The choice of therapy for a functional respiratory disorder primarily is based on the needs of the patient as well as on the clinician's expertise. In the third section of this book, "Treatment of Functional Respiratory Disorders," different treatment modalities for patients with functional respiratory disorders are described. Some of these therapies can be offered by primary care providers or pulmonologists who have the time and expertise to employ them. Qualification for providing such treatment may require clinicians to receive additional training.

Caveats

When functional manifestations of illness are treated without regard to potential underlying psychological issues, the physical symptoms may persist because they serve an important psychological function for the patient who is concurrently dealing with emotional stressors. On the other hand, when functional symptoms improve or resolve, patients may need to find another way of expressing their psychological issues. Rarely, improvement of functional symptoms may result in symptom substitution [36], wherein a new symptom arises that does not necessarily involve the respiratory system. For example, a child who had vocal cord dysfunction may subsequently develop hyperventilation with associated panic disorder, while another child with long-standing habit cough that resolved with hypnosis may later develop chronic headaches. In other situations, the patient may experience increased mental distress following resolution of a functional symptom.

Misdiagnosis of an organic disease as being attributable to a functional cause can delay the appropriate medical treatment. In one study, approximately a quarter of patients referred for hypnosis for a suspected functional disorder had an unrecognized biologic basis for their symptoms [37]. Thus, through close follow-up, clinicians should be prepared constantly to reevaluate their diagnoses if symptoms fail to improve. Even if the symptoms improve, clinicians should continue to monitor their patients for recurrence of the same or other symptoms that might reflect medically treatable disease, analogous to follow-up provided when patients are treated with medications for other conditions.

Conclusions

Patients with functional respiratory disorders benefit from prompt identification and therapy, which prevents perpetuation of the associated symptoms, development of sequelae, unnecessary medical investigations, and prescription of ineffective medical therapy that might have harmful side effects.

References

1. Fink P, Rosendal M. Recent developments in the understanding and management of functional somatic symptoms in primary care. Curr Opin Psychiatry. 2008;21(2):182–8.
2. Mayou R, Farmer A. ABC of psychological medicine: Functional somatic symptoms and syndromes. BMJ. 2002;325(7358):265–8.
3. Anbar RD, Hall HR. Childhood habit cough treated with self-hypnosis. J Pediatr. 2004;144(2):213–7.
4. Martin WC. The Layman's Bible encyclopedia. Nashville, TN: The Southwestern Company; 1964.
5. Eisenberg D, Wright TL. Encounters with Qi: Exploring Chinese medicine. New York, NY: W. W. Norton & Company; 1975.
6. Saravay SM. Presidential address: Academy of Psychosomatic Medicine Tucson, AZ November 2006. Psychosomatics. 2008;49(1):3–7.
7. American Psychiatric Association: Diagnostic and statistical manual of mental disorders, 2nd ed. Washington, DC: American Psychiatric Association;1968.
8. American Psychiatric Association: Diagnostic and statistical manual of mental disorders, 3rd ed. Washington, DC: American Psychiatric Association;1968.
9. Lehrer P, Feldman J, Giardino N, Song HS, Schmaling K. Psychological aspects of asthma. J Consult Clin Psychol. 2002;70(3):691–711.
10. Butani L, O'Connell EJ. Functional respiratory disorders. Ann Allergy Asthma Immunol. 1997;79(2):91–9.
11. Niggemann B. How to diagnose psychogenic and functional breathing disorders in children and adolescents. Pediatr Allergy Immunol. 2010;21(6):895–9.
12. Hynninen MJ, Pallesen S, Nordhus IH. Factors affecting health status in COPD patients with co-morbid anxiety or depression. Int J Chron Obstruct Pulmon Dis. 2007;2(3):323–8.
13. Thomas M, McKinley RK, Freeman E, Foy C, Price D. The prevalence of dysfunctional breathing in adults in the community with and without asthma. Prim Care Respir J. 2005;14(2):78–82.
14. Ortega AN, Huertas SE, Canino G, Ramirez R, Rubio-Stipec M. Childhood asthma, chronic illness, and psychiatric disorders. J Nerv Ment Dis. 2002;190(5):275–81.
15. Balcells E, Gea J, Ferrer J, et al. Factors affecting the relationship between psychological status and quality of life in COPD patients. Health Qual Life Outcomes. 2010;8:108.
16. Curtis JR, Patrick DL. The assessment of health status among patients with COPD. Eur Respir J Suppl. 2003;41:36s–45s.
17. Domingo-Salvany A, Lamarca R, Ferrer M, et al. Health-related quality of life and mortality in male patients with chronic obstructive pulmonary disease. Am J Respir Crit Care Med. 2002;166(5):680–5.
18. Lorin MI, Slovis TL, Haller JO. Fracture of ribs in psychogenic cough. NY State J Med. 1978;78(13):2078–9.
19. Anbar RD, Hehir DA. Hypnosis as a diagnostic modality for vocal cord dysfunction. Pediatrics. 2000;106(6):e81.
20. Anbar RD. Self-hypnosis for anxiety associated with severe asthma: A case report. BMC Pediatr. 2003;22:3:7.
21. Gardner WN, Bass C, Moxham J. Recurrent hyperventilation tetany due to mild asthma. Respir Med. 1992;86(4):349–51.
22. Hayes JP, Nolan MT, Brennan N, Fitzgerald MX. Three cases of paradoxical vocal cord adduction followed up over a 10-year period. Chest. 1993;104(3):678–80.
23. Anbar RD. User friendly hypnosis as an adjunct for treatment of habit cough: a case report. Am J Clin Hypn. 2007;50(2):171–5.
24. Niggemann B. Functional symptoms confused with allergic disorders in children and adolescents. Pediatr Allergy Immunol. 2002;13(5):312–8.

25. Elkins GR, Carter BD. Hypnotherapy in the treatment of childhood psychogenic coughing: a case report. Am J Clin Hypn. 1986;29(1):59–63.
26. Hanna DE, Hodgens JB, Daniel Jr WA. Hyperventilation syndrome. Pediatr Ann. 1986;15(10):708–12.
27. Anbar RD, Sachdeva S. Treatment of psychological factors in a child with difficult asthma: a case report. Am J Clin Hypn. 2011;54(1):47–55.
28. American Psychiatric Association: Diagnostic and statistical manual of mental disorders, 4th ed., Text Revision. Washington, DC, American Psychiatric Association, 2000.
29. Anbar RD. Stressors associated with dyspnea in childhood: patients' insights and a case report. Am J Clin Hypn. 2004;47(2):93–101.
30. Stone J, Smyth R, Carson A, Warlow C, Sharpe M. La belle indifférence in conversion symptoms and hysteria: systematic review. Br J Psychiatry. 2006;188(3):204–9.
31. Irwin RS, Glomb WB, Chang AB. Habit cough, tic cough, and psychogenic cough in adult and pediatric populations: ACCP evidence-based clinical practice guidelines. Chest. 2006;129 (1 Suppl):174S–9S.
32. Becklake MR, Kauffmann F. Gender differences in airway behaviour over the human life span. Thorax. 1999;54(12):1119–38.
33. Goetz CG, Tanner CM, Stebbins GT, Leipzig G, Carr WC. Adult tics in Gilles de la Tourette's syndrome: description and risk factors. Neurology. 1992;42(4):784–8.
34. Powell C, Brazier A. Psychological approaches to the management of respiratory symptoms in children and adolescents. Paediatr Respir Rev. 2004;5(3):214–24.
35. Jackson JL, O'Malley PG, Kroenke K. Antidepressants and cognitive-behavioral therapy for symptom syndromes. CNS Spectr. 2006;11(3):212–22.
36. Montgomery GT, Crowder JE. The symptom substitution hypothesis and the evidence. Psychother Theory Res Pract. 1972;9(2):98–102.
37. Olness K, Libbey P. Unrecognized biologic bases of behavioral symptoms in patients referred for hypnotherapy. Am J Clin Hypn. 1987;30(1):1–8.

Chapter 2
Functional Aspects of an Organic Respiratory Disorder: Cystic Fibrosis

Dewey G. Meyers and Ran D. Anbar

Abstract The management of respiratory diseases with organic causes often can be complicated by the emergence of concurrent functional respiratory symptoms. Thus, clinicians must be alert to the possibility that functional symptoms may develop in this setting. For example, anxiety with associated dyspnea can affect the management of many patients with significant respiratory disease such as asthma, chronic obstructive pulmonary disease, and cystic fibrosis (CF). An understanding of functional aspects of respiratory disorders will aid the clinician in identifying the correct cause of symptoms. In turn, this will help guide the application of appropriate therapy, thus preventing unnecessary tests and treatments that may compound an existing medical problem or create a new one. As an example illustrating how clinicians can approach patients with a respiratory disease that can have both organic and functional components, this chapter focuses on patients with CF. Case studies are presented through which the clinician will gain a better appreciation for the interaction of functional and organic causes of symptoms in this setting.

Keywords Adherence • Anxiety • Cystic fibrosis • Depression • Dyspnea • Habit cough • Insomnia

D.G. Meyers
Clear Mind Body Institute, Syracuse, NY, USA
e-mail: clearmindbodyinstitute@gmail.com

R.D. Anbar (✉)
Department of Pediatrics, SUNY Upstate Medical University, 750 East Adams St., 13210-1834, Syracuse, NY, USA
e-mail: anbarr@upstate.edu

R.D. Anbar (ed.), *Functional Respiratory Disorders: When Respiratory Symptoms Do Not Respond to Pulmonary Treatment*, Respiratory Medicine,
DOI 10.1007/978-1-61779-857-3_2, © Springer Science+Business Media, LLC 2012

Background

The management of respiratory diseases with organic causes often can be complicated by the emergence of concurrent functional respiratory symptoms. Thus, clinicians must be alert to the possibility of the development of functional symptoms in this setting. For example, anxiety with associated dyspnea can affect the management of many patients with significant respiratory disease such as asthma, chronic obstructive pulmonary disease, and cystic fibrosis (CF). An understanding of functional aspects of respiratory disorders will aid the clinician in identifying the correct cause of symptoms. In turn, this will help guide application of appropriate therapy, thus preventing unnecessary tests and treatment that may compound an existing medical problem or create a new one.

As an example illustrating how clinicians can approach patients with a respiratory disease that can have both organic and functional components, this chapter focuses on patients with CF.

For readers who are not familiar with CF, the first part of this chapter provides a brief introduction to the clinical presentation of this chronic and eventually fatal illness, with a special focus on symptoms and signs that can overlap with the clinical presentation of functional symptoms.

The second part introduces functional conditions that have been described particularly affecting patients with CF. This part places emphasis regarding symptoms that can arise as a result of these functional conditions that potentially overlap with those caused by the physiological abnormalities encountered in CF.

The third part discusses how clinicians might differentiate functional from organic symptoms in patients with CF and how to effectively balance evaluation and treatment of organic and functional symptoms in this population. Case studies are presented through which the clinician will gain a better appreciation of the interaction of functional and organic symptoms in patients with CF.

Key Organic Features of Cystic Fibrosis [1–11]

General Considerations

CF is the most common, fatal, hereditary disorder of Caucasians. The disorder also is common in Latinos and Native Americans. It is less common in Blacks and Asian Americans. CF affects the exocrine or secretory glands that normally produce mucus, the thin, watery, and slippery substance that coats the lining of the mouth, nose, sinuses, throat, lungs, and gastrointestinal tract. In CF, this mucus is abnormally thick and sticky. Rather than functioning as a protective lubricant, CF mucus builds up and blocks the passage ways of the lungs, pancreas, and reproductive system. This blockage encourages the growth of bacteria associated with chronic infections and inflammation of the lungs, ultimately leading to irreversible lung damage, respiratory failure, and an early death from pulmonary complications in 90% of the patients. Other manifestations include pathognomonically high sweat chloride levels, life-threatening respiratory complications, pancreatic dysfunction, a number of other serious digestive problems, and fertility issues.

Causes and Incidence

CF is an autosomal recessive disorder caused by a mutation of the CF transmembrane conductance regulator (CFTR) protein, which leads to abnormal ion transport. Autosomal recessive inheritance means that in this case, both parents carry a single copy of the CF mutation and each of their children has a 25% chance of receiving a copy from both parents. Having two copies of the CF mutation leads to development of the disease.

CFTR functions as a channel across the membrane of cells that produce mucus, sweat, saliva, tears, and digestive enzymes. The channel transports negatively charged chloride ions into and out of cells. The transport of chloride ions helps control the movement of water in tissues, which is necessary for the production of thin, freely flowing mucus. The CFTR protein also regulates the function of other channels, such as those that transport sodium ions across cell membranes and which are necessary for the normal function of organs such as the lungs and pancreas.

To date, approximately 160 gene mutations have been identified as causing clinical CF. (Most of the approximately 2,000 mutations in the CFTR protein are not thought to cause disease.) Nearly 90% of Americans who have CF carry at least one copy of the delta F508 gene. CF affects approximately 30,000 Americans and an additional 40,000 individuals worldwide. In United States Caucasians, about 1 out of 3,200 individuals has CF.

Clinical Findings [2]

Respiratory tract symptoms include coughing, dyspnea (shortness of breath), increased mucus in sinuses, sinus pain or pressure, sinus polyps (overgrowth of sinus tissue), sputum production from the lungs that can cause lung crackles, recurrent episodes of pneumonia, bronchiectasis (damaged airways), atelectasis (small areas of collapsed lung tissue), hemoptysis (coughing up blood), and pneumothorax (air leak from the lungs that can cause collapse of a large part of a lung).

Gastrointestinal manifestations may include pancreatic insufficiency (90% of patients) that leads to malabsorption (especially of fat) associated with steatorrhea (fat in the stools), pancreatitis, nausea, loss of appetite, weight loss, malnutrition, abdominal pain, bloating, gas, constipation often from distal intestinal obstruction syndrome, and meconium ileus (obstruction of the intestine due to overly thick fecal material) at birth.

Infertility is present in almost all men as result of congenital absence of the vas deferens with azoospermia. Women have thickened cervical mucus that results in a 20% decrease in fertility rate.

Other findings and complications include digital clubbing, delayed puberty, diabetes (which affects 50% of those over 30 years old), osteoporosis, arthritis, biliary cirrhosis, liver failure, gall stones, and rectal prolapse.

Patients with *advanced disease* may present with hypoxemia (low levels of oxygen), hypercapnia (high levels of carbon dioxide), and cor pulmonale (heart dysfunction that arises because of the severe lung disease).

Diagnosis

Newborn screening for CF accounts for most patients who currently are being diagnosed. The diagnosis is confirmed by genetic testing and/or a test of the salt content of the sweat.

Treatment

The goals of pulmonary treatment are to decrease airway mucus viscosity so that it can be coughed out more easily, improve clearance of sputum through provision of chest physiotherapy, decrease airway inflammation, and prevent and treat lung infections. The goals of gastrointestinal treatment are to replace pancreatic enzymes and vitamins and to provide aggressive nutritional support and therapy to prevent liver disease, if indicated.

Commonly Used Medications

- Recombinant human DNase (dornase alpha), nebulized, to thin sputum (thereby acting as a mucolytic)
- Hypertonic saline, nebulized, to increase airway hydration and induce cough
- Inhaled bronchodilators to aid in opening the airways
- Antibiotics to treat airway infection either when needed or preventively
- Pancreatic enzyme replacement to aid the absorption of fats and proteins
- Vitamin supplements, especially of fat soluble vitamins A, D, E, and K

Therapeutic Procedures

- Mechanical interventions to clear lower airway secretions include manual chest physiotherapy consisting of chest percussion and postural drainage, high

frequency chest wall oscillation with a mechanical vest, and use of positive end expiratory pressure.
- High calorie, high fat, and high protein diet.
- Exercise—regular aerobic and strength training.
- Drink plenty of fluids in order to maintain hydration.
- Avoid—smoke, dust, dirt, fumes, household chemicals, mold, and mildew.

Surgery

Some patients require insertion of a gastrostomy feeding tube because of their malnutrition. Lung transplantation is an option for patients with CF who have end-stage lung disease. At this time, the 5-year survival following transplantation is approximately 50%.

Prognosis

Most children remain relatively healthy throughout school and finish college and/or find employment. The mean life span of a CF patient is 38.3 years [4], which is a remarkable improvement over the past few decades and is attributable to the introduction of many new therapies for the disease.

Functional Conditions Associated with Cystic Fibrosis

Many psychiatric and psychosocial factors can develop as patients with CF become older, which affect their clinical presentation and quality of life, as well as the appropriateness and efficacy of their treatment. For example, adolescents with chronic illnesses are at increased risk of developing adjustment problems and internalizing symptoms of depression and anxiety. Thus, patients presenting with CF may exhibit concurrent behavioral problems that cause physical symptoms such as abdominal discomfort, muscle tension, shortness of breath, and/or tremors (e.g., as a result of anxiety). Other behavioral issues can affect adherence to the prescribed medical therapies. While treatment for CF necessarily focuses on the medical condition, the underlying psychological factors should be addressed simultaneously in order to achieve optimal results.

Many primary care or pulmonary specialists fail to consider psychological evaluation of their patients because they are unfamiliar with how to diagnose psychiatric conditions or how to assess the psychosocial impact on their patients' clinical presentations. Further, children and adolescents, who may have difficulty clearly describing their symptoms, may be difficult to diagnose with a psychological disorder. Thus, this section reviews the diagnostic criteria for the psychiatric disorders and psychosocial considerations commonly associated with CF.

Psychiatric Considerations

Psychopathology within the CF community has been reported to be as high as 57% with a diagnosable psychiatric disorder [2]. The current basis for assessment of psychiatric disorders is the Diagnostic and Statistical Manual, fourth edition, Text Revision (DSM-IV-TR) that contains a chapter regarding Mental Disorders Due to General Medical Conditions. The criteria for such disorders include that the disturbance is the result of a physiological consequence of a general medical condition such as CF, is not better accounted for by another mental disorder, and does not occur exclusively during the course of delirium. Indications that a psychiatric disorder may be caused by a medical condition include acute onset without apparent cause; correlation between the onset, exacerbation, and remission of psychiatric symptoms with the course of the medical condition; and atypical features, such as aggression with anxiety.

Notably, DSM-IV-TR also recognizes that psychological factors can affect medical conditions (see Chap. 1). For example, generalized anxiety disorder (GAD) is a diagnosis commonly associated with a chronic respiratory disease such as CF that can affect its clinical presentation. GAD can cause worry, restlessness, fatigue, loss of concentration, irritability, muscle tension, and sleep difficulties. All of these behavioral signs and symptoms should be considered when evaluating a patient for GAD or assessing for other possible mental health disorders.

Although a thorough psychiatric assessment including mental status and neurological examination is ideal, it is rarely practical or immediately necessary, if the clinician has a basic knowledge of behavioral symptoms. For example, a patient might be suspected of having a psychiatric disturbance based on complaints of feelings of worthlessness and fatigue. A diagnosis can be made through consultation with a mental health care professional who is clinically experienced with patients who suffer from medical conditions.

Anxiety

A patient with CF reports experiencing nightly insomnia for 2 months after being discharged following a recent hospitalization for a respiratory exacerbation. He states that at night he develops nightmares about being readmitted to the hospital and during the day he worries about contracting respiratory infections that might trigger yet another exacerbation. Sometimes, when he focuses on his worries, he develops shortness of breath, chest tightness, dizziness, and paresthesia.

The most common mental health diagnosis for children and adolescents with CF is anxiety, which afflicts as many as 35% of school-aged children with CF. Forms of anxiety in CF include separation anxiety disorder (25%) GAD (15%), phobias (7.5%), obsessive compulsive disorder (5%), and panic disorder (4%) [12]. Notably, individual patients may suffer as a result of more than one type of anxiety at the same time.

Anxiety affects 30% of adolescents with CF, which makes it the most common psychiatric disorder in this age group, as well [2]. Anxiety in adolescence often is related to the patients' developmental emphasis on peer bonding, autonomy, conflict, and sexual exploration [13]. Paradoxically, anxiety has been associated with improved adherence to prescribed treatment because of adolescents' preoccupation with the idea that symptoms from their illness may adversely affect their peer relationships [2].

Parents of children with CF have been found to develop anxiety, worry, sadness, and hypervigilance when their children have been diagnosed with CF, even when the diagnosis was made following prenatal screening [14]. Caregivers of pre-schoolers with CF have been documented to have anxiety (16.4%) and depression (33%) associated with their children's sleep, eating, adherence, and mealtime issues [15, 16]. Parents of school-aged children demonstrated increased rates of anxiety (50%) often related to concerns over treatment adherence [16]. Similar issues are evident with parents of adolescents, who may find themselves in conflict with their children's desire for autonomy that can lead to risky behaviors and compromised health care [17].

Importantly, parental anxiety may adversely affect their children's mental health and treatment for CF. For example, sometimes children's anxiety can develop or intensify as a result of their parents' anxiety. Conversely, families who function well, as demonstrated through measures of cohesiveness, expressiveness, and organization, have been associated with psychological well-being in their CF adolescents [18].

Symptoms of anxiety that can overlap with organic issues in CF include dyspnea, chest pain, difficulty with swallowing, abdominal discomfort, tremor, and insomnia.

Depression

An adolescent with CF comes to your office complaining of feeling constantly sad and guilty about the death of her brother, which occurred over a year ago as a result of his CF. She explains that she feels as if she were the one who should have died since he took all of his therapies, while she frequently skipped therapies. As a result of her sad feelings, she reports that she has been unable to focus on her schoolwork and her grades have suffered. She also is concerned because some of her friends have left her because they told her it is no longer fun to be around her. She has experimented on one occasion with snorting cocaine to help her feel better.

The second most common mental health disorder in children and adolescents with CF is depression, which affects as many as 29% of patients in both age groups, as assessed by the children's depression inventory (CDI) [19]. Parents and caregivers of recently diagnosed children with CF have been found to have at least mild depressive symptoms at a frequency as high as 44% in mothers and 33% in fathers using the Beck Depression Inventory (BDI) [20].

Major depression is known to adversely affect cognition, attention, energy, and motivation, which leads to a decrease in task completion, adherence to medical regimens, missed clinic appointments, increased at risk behaviors (smoking and drinking), eating disturbances, poor body image, and decreased quality of life [21, 22]. Depression has been shown to have an impact on the daily functioning of CF patients and their caregivers [23]. Parent and child depression has been shown to correlate with worse adherence to airway clearance in school-aged children and adolescents [24]. Depression in the parent/caregiver has been associated with a decreased adherence to use of pancreatic enzymes in their children, with resultant poor weight gain [25].

Health-related quality of life (HRQOL) measurements on standardized screening tools like the cystic fibrosis questionnaire-revised (CFQ-R) were worse in CF patients with depressive symptoms. Those with moderate to severe lung disease and depression had poorer scores than those with severe lung disease without depression, which supports the hypothesis that depression heightens the effects of chronic illness such as CF [26]. Depressed CF patients also had decreased HRQOL scores on body image scales, eating problems, and emotional functioning [22].

Symptoms of depression that can overlap with organic issues in CF include fatigue, malaise, loss of appetite, weight loss, insomnia, night awakenings, and an increase of any CF-associated symptom as a result of poor adherence to prescribed therapy.

Comorbidity of Anxiety and Depression

A 17-year-old with CF tells you that over the past year, he has felt more breathless, keyed up with muscle tension, and in the past 2 months has had recurrent thoughts of death.

In the general US population, anxiety and depression have been reported as occurring in 25–29% of all children and adolescents [27]. Patients in medical settings have been found to have comorbidities at frequencies as high as 75% [28]. In CF adolescents, strong positive associations have been found between anxiety and depression [29], although there has been scant research on this relationship in CF [29].

No systematic studies have been undertaken to determine what specific effects mental illness has on CF health care outcomes [30]. However, patients with chronic lung diseases and anxiety or depression have been noted to have increased symptoms and functional impairment, including adverse effects on cognition, attention, energy, and motivation that lead to decreased task completion [21, 31].

Evaluation of anxiety and depression may initially be improved by the implementation of annual, routine, standardized screening procedures, such as the Hospital Anxiety and Depression Scale [32], or the Revised Child Anxiety and Depression Scales [33], which are useful with children and adolescents, and the Beck Anxiety and Depression Inventories [34, 35] or the Multidimensional Anxiety Questionnaire [36], which are applicable to adult patients and caregivers [30]. These tests are simple and quick to take and score. Such screening followed by treatment improves outcomes especially when offered at specialized CF centers [23].

Treatment for preschool children with mild to moderate depression is recommended to be family therapy [37]. First-line treatments for school-aged children with anxiety and depression include behavioral interventions such as interpersonal or cognitive behavioral therapy (CBT, Chap. 9) [37–43]. Interpersonal therapy (IPT) is a diagnosis-targeted, time-limited, present-focused treatment that makes a practical link between the patient's mood and disturbing life events (such as bereavement, loss of social support, or life transitions) that either trigger or follow from the onset of a mood disorder [40]. IPT application may be of particular value during the transition from adolescence to adulthood [41]. CBT and family therapy have been shown to help improve short-term knowledge and, combined with behavioral interventions, aid nutrition and growth [42].

Psychopharmacological medication also has been used in patients with anxiety and depression (Chap. 14) [44, 45]. Use of psychotherapy in conjunction with medications may be a more effective treatment than either alone [38].

Mood Disorders

A young adult with CF confides that she has not been adherent to her CF treatment regimen. She reports that she has been feeling much better by staying up all night. She has not been tired during the day for over 2 weeks. She is going to the race track daily in order to bet on the horses with the expectation of winning a large race and then quitting her job.

Mood disorders encompass not only depression but also bipolar, dysthymic, and cyclothymic disorders. The differential diagnosis includes borderline personality disorders and mental disorders due to a general medical condition [46]. Although the initial functional presentation may appear to be related to depression, bipolar disorder should be suspected if the constellation of symptoms includes inflated or irritable mood, decreased need for sleep, pressured speech, inflated self-esteem, and increased psychomotor agitation, lasting a week or more. Such a modification in diagnosis will dramatically change the treatment regimen.

Symptoms of a mood disorder that can overlap with organic issues in CF include irritability, insomnia, and increase of any CF-associated symptom as the result of poor adherence to prescribed therapy.

Somatoform Disorders

Your 32-year-old patient with CF who been stable clinically for a number of years reports that he is concerned he has had increased mucus plugging in his lungs with excruciating associated chest pain, although objective findings including his physical examination, pulmonary function testing, and chest x-ray have not changed in over a year.

Somatoform disorders can be defined as a history of physical complaints without identified medical abnormalities. An overview of somatoform disorders has been presented in Chap. 1 and summarized in Table 1.1.

Somatization disorder should be considered when a patient experiences pain in four or more body areas or functions. Patients with CF often report pain in association with their disease, including 59% of children and 89% of adults [47, 48]. For example, patients frequently report chest pain associated with mucus plugging or recurrent lung infections. In patients with CF, somatization disorder may be associated with repeated hospitalizations due to personal or family issues, poor living conditions, or parental psychiatric conditions [49].

Pain disorder is another somatoform classification in which the patient presents with pain in one or more sites, e.g., chest pain [50]. This pain may or may not be related to a CF-related organic abnormality. For example, pain disorder may occur in the lungs simply due to the phobic anxiety of developing recurrent pneumonia when a minor unrelated chest pain occurs.

Conversion disorder occurs when a patient has a psychologically based motor or sensory symptom or deficit that is unintentionally produced and may be preceded by conflicts or stressors [46].

Hypochondriasis or the preoccupation with fears of having a serious disease despite nonsupportive medical evaluation has been reported in adults with CF [51].

Symptoms of somatoform disorders that can overlap organic issues in CF include cough, stridor, or dyspnea related to conversion symptoms; reports of pain in the lungs, heart, pancreas, and joints; gastrointestinal symptoms such as nausea and vomiting; and loss of libido.

Sleep Disorders

A 24-year-old with CF is transferring to you from another CF center, where he had just been started on albuterol prior to administration of hypertonic saline. He has developed anxiety, tremor, and insomnia and wonders about the origin of these symptoms.

It is well recognized that patients with CF have disrupted sleep histories [52–56]. Contributors to CF sleep abnormalities may include the use of certain medications such as β_2-agonists before sleep [53], vitamin deficiencies [54], chronic anxiety, and depression [55]. Other underlying etiologies of sleep disturbances in CF include nocturnal coughing, obstructive apnea as a result of sinus disease or enlarged tonsils and adenoids, increased work of breathing due to progressive lung disease, and periodic leg movements. By the time they develop end-stage lung disease, patients' sleep also can be disrupted by hypoxemia and hypercapnia [52].

A sleep disturbance in a patient with CF can cause exacerbation of anxiety, depression, irritability, and attention deficit hyperactivity disorder (ADHD), all of which can lead to increased nonadherence to prescribed therapy and poorer medical outcomes.

As a sleep disturbance in CF can be the result of organic and/or psychological factors, both possible etiologies must be evaluated and addressed.

Eating Disorders

An adolescent girl with CF comes to your office complaining of an intolerable stomach ache. You ask her about the regularity of her treatment regimen and she says that she strictly adheres to the treatment guidelines. You notice she is tugging at her slacks and commenting that she is concerned that she is gaining weight. She explains that she wants to remain slim in order to make the cheerleading squad.

Nutritional issues are of concern for patients with CF as they usually require a high calorie, high fat diet. Adherence to this dietary regimen is limited in preschool CF children, 32% of whom have been reported to have eating problems [56]. Nutritional difficulties are of particular concern in the treatment of adolescent girls who tend to have poorer adherence to nutritional recommendations [57] because of their heightened awareness regarding how others perceive their appearance. Notably, there are no reports that CF predisposes to the development of anorexia nervosa or bulimia nervosa [58].

Symptoms of eating disorders that can overlap with organic issues in CF include loss of appetite, nausea, emesis, abdominal discomfort, and weight loss.

Oppositional Defiant Disorder

A 12-year-old with CF has begun smoking cigarettes and refuses to cooperate with airway clearance and nebulized medication treatments. He complains that his treatments take too much time. He continues to smoke and remain noncooperative with his therapies even though he acknowledges the adverse health consequences of his behaviors. He says he is not interested in being rewarded with small financial prizes for improved adherence to his therapies.

Of children 7–12 years old with CF with a parent-reported behavior problem, 62% met the criteria for a DSM diagnosis based on clinical interview. Diagnoses of anxiety and oppositional disorder were most frequent [59] with a prevalence of 22.5% for oppositional defiant disorder [12]. Oppositional problems involve children and adolescents and can progress to conduct disorder, which in adulthood can manifest as antisocial personality disorder.

Patients with CF often oppose the pervasive intrusion into their lives of their demanding treatment regimen. Their extensive prescribed therapies require time out of their daily schedule, remind them that they are different than their peers, and can reveal their condition to others. Opposition to therapy often results in conflicted relationships with parents, especially in combination with the usual child and adolescent drive to separate from parental influence and become increasing reliant on peers [49]. Further, symptoms resulting from CF usually worsen with age, which adds to the burden of therapy and associated conflict regarding its use.

Attention Deficit Hyperactivity Disorder

A teenager with CF becomes distracted easily while doing his therapies and therefore curtails their use regularly. He often forgets to take his pancreatic enzymes, cannot remember where he put his medication containers, and has been unable to follow through on recommendations to organize his medications.

His older young adult sibling, who also has CF, complains about his employer's blatant lack of regard for his medical condition by not allowing him to take breaks in order to follow his treatment regimen. He jumps up and begins pacing and yelling about his mistreatment and the life-altering effects of his condition.

ADHD has been reported as being a common comorbidity in patients with CF [60–62]. This condition can be confused with oppositional defiant disorder as a cause of persistent, angry, resentful behaviors in which patients are easily annoyed by others, lose their temper, and blame others. It has been suggested that stimulant, non-stimulant, and combination ADHD treatments for patients with CF can help improve adherence to their prescribed therapies [61, 62].

This disorder, which was originally considered a child and adolescent condition, is known to carry over into adulthood.

Post-traumatic Stress Disorder

A 30-year-old woman who just was discharged from the ICU following a life-threatening exacerbation of her CF appears distressed in your office. When questioned, she admits to recently avoiding her treatment regimen, even though she has a long history of treatment adherence. She reports recurrent nightmares about her experiences in the ICU, from which she awakens profusely sweating, and is unable to fall back asleep for "hours."

Post-traumatic stress disorder (PTSD) has been shown to occur after extensive or traumatic hospital stays [47, 63, 64]. Risk factors include length of stay in the hospital or ICU and a history of requiring mechanical ventilation or high level sedative medication. Other factors may involve female gender, younger age, past psychiatric history, and the number of traumatic and delusional memories [63]. As many as 50% of patients who have been in the ICU have been diagnosed with PTSD [47]. Having a patient with severe symptoms that require serious treatment, such as delivered in an ICU, should alert the treating clinician that the patient is at risk of developing this condition.

Symptoms of PTSD that can overlap with organic issues in CF include insomnia and an increase of any CF-associated symptom as result of poor adherence to prescribed therapy.

Psychosocial Considerations

Gender

A 15-year-old girl refuses to follow a high calorie diet because she says she wants to remain thin and pretty.

Morbidity and mortality rates are higher in females with CF [65–67]. Girls, 10–21 years old, reported significantly more illness-related concerns, including emotional issues, discouragement about treatment, and lower self-esteem [68]. These issues have been associated with behaviors that have been detrimental to their health including poor adherence to prescribed treatment regimens, engagement in cough suppression, and an inadequate fat and caloric intake. The situation is complicated further because poor adherence can lead to further discouragement regarding the effectiveness of therapy and even lower self-esteem [57, 69]. A sense of isolation due to repeated respiratory exacerbations can lead to a fear of early death, depression [65], PTSD, and possible suicidal ideation [70].

Adherence to Treatment

Recently, one of your 17-year-old CF patients has noticeably lost weight and has had frequent pulmonary exacerbations followed by brief hospitalizations. You are concerned and question why. He says that it is winter and he has been unlucky in catching a series of colds. He appears fatigued and seems indecisive.

Current treatments for CF require extensive, consistent, often tedious, and time-consuming interventions that involve complex pulmonary, nutritional, medication, and exercise regimens [24, 71]. Daily treatments may necessitate 2–3 h or more. The consequences of inadequate adherence to prescribed therapies are considerable and associated with more exacerbations, increased hospital admissions, and increased mortality [72]. Overall, the mean rate of nonadherence in children with CF is reported to be between 30% and 50% or more with a trend of adolescents being less adherent than younger children and adults even less adherent [72, 73].

Factors associated with poor adherence include psychiatric, psychological, and emotional considerations [24]. Depression may follow serious chronic illness and lead to compromised adherence. One study indicated that depressed patients were three times more likely than those not depressed to be nonadherent with medical treatment recommendations [74]. As mentioned earlier, adults with CF and depression are known to have impaired lung function and poorer HRQOL [75]. Anxiety, oppositional disorders, and eating disorders can also impact the level of adherence. Therefore, we recommend that nonadherent CF patients be screened routinely for coexisting psychiatric and psychosocial issues. (For more information about screening tools, see Chap. 8.)

Parental and Family Issues

During an appointment with a family with twin adolescent boys who have CF, you notice that the one boy who gets along well with his parents seems well adjusted and content, whereas the boy with oppositional behavior toward his parents is much less open and conversant. He is wearing a teen club jacket, appears bored and irritated, and complaints bitterly about all the wasted time spent on CF treatments while watching his parents carefully for their reaction. He appears short of breath as he speaks. The parents appear worried and anxious.

For children and adolescents, family life is central to their self-esteem and adherence [76] and thus influences their pulmonary health [24]. Positive family relationships were reported to be associated with greater adherence to airway clearance and aerosolized medications [76].

Parental reaction to a diagnosis of CF in their infant often involves development of stress and guilt that can alter the family structure. Affected parents have demonstrated more controlling, serious, and less encouraging behaviors, and their children were less responsive to parental guidance [77].

Among parents of preschool children, as many as 40% blame themselves for their child's CF. Such self-blame has been associated with poorer emotional adjustment and possible anxiety and depression in children and their parents [78]. Families whose preschool children have CF can develop significant difficulties with interpersonal interactions, setting appropriate behavioral expectations and enforcement, and marital role strain [79].

Adolescents with CF whose parents supervise their treatment time have better adherence [80]. For adolescents, peers provide more emotional and companionship support than do their families, and such support may serve as a cushion for negative family interactions [81].

Peer Relationships and Socialization

The troubled parents of the twin teenage boys with CF indicate that the oppositional twin hangs out with his peers and is rarely home, so they are unaware of his level of adherence. He attempts to hide or deemphasize his CF. He is participating in risky behaviors including smoking and drinking that are adversely affecting his health and quality of life, which ironically makes him even more upset and dependent on his parents.

The importance of peer interactions and socialization increases with age. With children's entrance into school, they begin to compare themselves to peers as a gauge for their identity and sense of social competence. Such comparisons serve to underscore how having CF has made them different from others. Their desire often is to deemphasize the importance of their treatment regimen in order to appear as normal as possible, which often entails keeping their diagnosis of CF as a secret [49]. This may lead to an inability to develop and maintain intimate friendships, which is an essential part of socialization that is necessary for completion of mature development [82].

Adolescence is the time when peers become even more influential as children distance themselves from their parents as part of the process of their identity formation [13].

Teenagers with CF have been found to have a higher rate of risky behaviors as compared to healthy peers [17]. Even given the health hazards, 20% of CF teenagers admitted to having smoked cigarettes [57], as well as 19% of females and 7% of males who revealed self-imposed weight-loss regimens [70].

Differentiation of Functional from Organic Symptoms in CF

As demonstrated in the first two sections of this chapter, many symptoms of patients with CF can be triggered by both organic and functional causes, and often, these occur in the same patient. The question for clinicians is how to tease out organic from functional causes so that the appropriate therapeutic course can be followed.

We believe that as long as organic causes of symptoms are considered and treated, concurrent assessment of their possible functional components can only be of benefit. It should be kept in mind that because of the high frequency of psychological and psychosocial issues in patients with CF, development of functional symptoms should be expected, and therefore, evaluation for such symptoms should be part of routine care for these patients. It should be emphasized that functional symptoms can arise as a result of a primary psychological disorder or as a consequence of the organic illness.

Symptoms that often reflect underlying functional components are listed in Table 1.2. Further, a functional component should be suspected if an organic symptom causes excessive distress or impairment or if the symptom appears to be intentionally produced or feigned.

The following brief case studies demonstrate how functional and organic respiratory symptoms frequently overlap in patients with CF. The reader is invited to reflect on how the cases might have unfolded if the functional contribution to the patients' symptoms had been addressed earlier, as opposed to the possible outcomes if the functional components were not recognized or addressed.

Case 1: 4-Year-Old with Cough [83]

The patient was an almost 5-year-old who was diagnosed with CF following birth with meconium ileus. He developed pneumonia at 3 months of age, and by a year of age, was found to harbor *Pseudomonas aeruginosa* in his airway. Subsequently, he was treated with every-other-month tobramycin by inhalation (TOBI®) and daily dornase alpha. When he was well, he did not cough.

At 4½ years of age, the patient manifested severe coughing after contracting influenza. At that time, he was diagnosed with a second pneumonia and treated with intravenous antibiotics. Two months later, computerized tomography revealed diffuse sinusitis, which was thought to be aggravating his pulmonary disease. Therefore, he underwent sinus surgery. A week after removal of the postsurgical nasal packing, he developed a loud, harsh cough that occurred every other second for hours at a time, while awake. The cough ceased as soon as he fell asleep.

The patient was treated with oral ciprofloxacin and prednisolone in addition to TOBI®, but there was no improvement in his cough. No new abnormalities were documented on his physical examination. His lung function was normal.

Because of the cough, the patient was unable to attend summer camp.

The patient lived with his parents and 6-year-old sister who also had CF. The sister's respiratory status was good, but she had a gastrostomy tube for supplemental feedings.

The family was reassured that the cough would resolve in time. In order to help the cough resolve, it was suggested the patient be told, "Are you sure you need to be coughing?" However, the mother felt ambivalent about this advice because she was aware that coughing is beneficial for patients with CF.

The cough resolved a month later after application of hypnotic imagery, and the mother's reassuring of herself that the patient's cough was not related to his CF and thus its resolution would be safe for her child.

Questions:

1. The differential diagnosis for this patient's persistent cough includes all of the following EXCEPT:

   (a) Chronic sinusitis
   (b) Foreign body in the airway
   (c) Gastroesophageal reflux
   (d) Habit
   (e) Pneumonia

2. All of the following therapies have been reported to be beneficial in the treatment of habit cough EXCEPT:

   (a) Bedsheet wrap technique
   (b) Clonazepam

(c) Hypnosis
(d) Reassurance
(e) Suggestion therapy with inhaled lidocaine

3. How might the mother's attitude regarding the cough affect its persistence?
   (a) The child might have sensed the mother's ambivalence about its resolution and acted accordingly.
   (b) The mother's concern about the cough increased her own anxiety, which affected the child.
   (c) The child might have received additional attention for the cough that helped reinforce it.
   (d) All of the above.
   (e) None of the above.

Answers:

1. (e): Of the listed diagnosis, the most likely is habit cough, given the disruptive nature of the cough and as it resolved when he fell asleep. Cough associated with (a), (b), and (c) typically would occur during sleep as well. Persistent pneumonia is unlikely, as other symptoms likely would have manifested.
2. (b): There is no indication for clonazepam in this setting. Reassurance usually is ineffective. The bedsheet wrap technique involves the patient tightening a bedsheet around his midsection in order to suppress the urge to cough [84]. Suggestion therapy (Chap. 5) and hypnosis (Chap. 12) have been reported as very effective.
3. (d): Habit cough can persist for all of the listed reasons, as well as in association with various psychosocial stressors such as divorce, loss of a significant other, or difficulties in school. Sometimes, the psychosocial stressors must be addressed in order to permit resolution of the cough.

Case 2: 10-Year-Old with Shortness of Breath [85]

The patient was diagnosed with CF at 2 weeks of life, after he was born with meconium ileus. Complications of his disease included recurrent pneumonia necessitating nine hospitalizations, severe gastroesophageal reflux for which he underwent a Nissen fundoplication at 8 years of age, and renal stones. Despite aggressive therapy, by the time he was 9 years old, he was placed on the waiting list for lung transplantation.

As the patient remained on the transplantation list for 13 months, he became increasingly fatigued, with increased coughing, chest tightness, and shortness of breath. His blood concentration of carbon dioxide was mildly elevated. The burden of his treatments included continual administration of oxygen and assisted ventilation with the aid of tight-fitting nasal prongs (BiPAP) for 2 h in the daytime and throughout the night. He received chest physiotherapy for 30 min, 3–4 times a day. He received three nebulized medications each twice daily, in addition to many pills.

The patient complained that his shortness of breath frightened him. He was asked what changes could be made to make his life more tolerable. The patient stated that he had nothing to look forward to, since his lungs did not appear to be forthcoming. The physician asked him what he wished he could do, and the patient replied he would like to go crab fishing on the Atlantic seaboard. The physician thought this was an excellent goal, and the patient became excited by this prospect. Plans were made for the patient and his family to travel 250 miles to the New Jersey shore 3 weeks later. The patient was prescribed an anxiolytic, twice daily, as needed, for difficulty sleeping or feeling scared.

Subsequently, the patient experienced severe respiratory distress following chest physiotherapy, for which he was hospitalized for 4 days. Upon discharge, the patient resumed planning for his trip and reported that his shortness of breath, while present, did not bother him much. He used his anxiolytic medication on only a few occasions.

The patient's lungs became available during his trip, and he underwent successful lung transplantation.

Questions:

1. The differential diagnosis for this patient's dyspnea is likely to include all of the following EXCEPT:

   (a) Anxiety
   (b) Bronchospasm
   (c) End-stage lung disease
   (d) High blood concentration of carbon dioxide
   (e) Side effect of the multiple nebulized medications

2. Which of the following therapies would be most likely to be helpful for control of this patient's dyspnea in a short time frame?

   (a) Breathing into a paper bag
   (b) Cognitive behavioral therapy
   (c) Hypnotherapy
   (d) Speech therapy
   (e) All of the above

3. How might the patient's dyspnea have improved as a result of his planning for his trip and with hypnotherapy?

   (a) It did not improve; the patient just said it did.
   (b) Thinking about the trip distracted him.
   (c) Shifting his mind's focus to pleasant thoughts with use of hypnosis changed the way the patient perceived the sensations that caused him to feel dyspneic.
   (d) The improvement reflected the natural course of his dyspnea that waxed and waned and was unrelated to the interventions.
   (e) None of the above.

Answers:

1. (e): The patient's lung disease had progressed to the point that the patient had developed significant dyspnea, which could have been related to (b), (c), and (d). In such a setting, it is common for anxiety to occur, which can lead to worsening of dyspnea. This symptom occurred despite aggressive medical therapy, which typically serves to relieve (rather than cause) dyspnea in patients who are not as ill as this boy.
2. (c): A year before his transplant, this patient was taught self-hypnosis techniques in one session, which have been reported to decrease anxiety in patients with cystic fibrosis [86]. Just before the patient's trip, use of hypnotic imagery of going crab fishing to calm himself was associated with improvement in his dyspnea. This patient's dyspnea was not the result of hyperventilation given that his blood concentration of carbon dioxide was mildly elevated, and therefore, breathing into a paper bag would have caused harm. Cognitive behavioral and speech therapies typically take a few sessions and would be unlikely to have a rapid effect in this setting. Chronic dyspnea has been shown to improve with use of biofeedback and breathing techniques (see Chaps. 10 and 11).
3. (c): Hypnosis has been shown to change the way the brain processes pain perceptions and thus may have a similar effect in the processing of the sensation of dyspnea. Distraction has not been shown to have the same effects as hypnosis in the control of pain. A controlled study will need to be conducted in patients with end-stage CF in order to demonstrate whether the improvement in dyspnea can be attributed to hypnosis or planning for an exciting event.

Case 3: 13-Year-Old with Recurrent Exacerbations of Her Lung Disease

By the time this patient was 13 years old, her CF-associated lung disease had become very advanced. The patient required frequent hospitalizations and courses of intravenous antibiotics in order to treat her lung disease effectively. The patient's symptoms included a productive cough, dyspnea, occasional episodes of coughing up small amounts of blood (hemoptysis), and recurrent abdominal discomfort. While receiving intravenous antibiotics, the patient required supplemental oxygen via nasal cannula. During hospitalizations, the patient stated that supplemental oxygen was helpful to her even when her hemoglobin saturations were normal in room air (i.e., >97%).

The patient was an only child, whose parents had separated when she was a toddler. The patient lived with her mother and had virtually no contact with her father. Because of difficulties with the economy, and in being a single parent of a child with a severe chronic illness, the mother had lost jobs on four occasions. The mother had established and broken off relationships with a number of boyfriends during the patient's life. While not formally assessed, the mother often reported being distressed and anxious about the patient's poor health condition and prognosis.

The patient's CF care team noted that the patient tended to report that she was more symptomatic beginning in September (when school started) and when her mother had broken off a relationship or lost her job.

Questions:

1. All of the following of this patient's symptoms could have a functional component EXCEPT:
   (a) Cough
   (b) Dyspnea
   (c) Hemoptysis
   (d) Abdominal discomfort
   (e) Need for supplemental oxygen
2. Possible reasons that the patient's lung disease exacerbations tended to coincide with crises in her mother's life likely include all of the following EXCEPT:
   (a) The mother paid less attention to the patient when she was preoccupied with her own issues, and therefore, the patient received insufficient therapy at those times.
   (b) The patient drew attention to herself when she became more symptomatic, and she wanted increased attention when her mother was preoccupied.
   (c) The patient wanted to feel sicker so that she could share in her mother's misery.
   (d) The mother felt better when the patient was receiving aggressive care, which was important especially when the mother felt poorly as a result of her own issues. Therefore, the mother was more likely to complain of the patient's symptoms in such circumstances.
   (e) By drawing the mother's attention to the patient's symptoms, the patient was distracting her mother from thinking about the mother's issues.
3. The mother's anxiety about the patient's health could have contributed to the patient's reported development of exacerbations through all of the following means EXCEPT:
   (a) The mother became too nervous to assess the patient properly, which led her to ignore some of the patient's symptoms until they became severe enough to require hospitalization.
   (b) The anxiety led the mother to be hypervigilant and therefore more likely to interpret the patient's symptoms as necessitating medical evaluation.
   (c) The patient became anxious as a result of the mother's anxiety, which led to intensification of her symptoms.
   (d) The anxiety caused the mother to doubt her own capability to assess and deal with the patient properly, and therefore, the mother was more likely to seek medical intervention for the patient.
   (e) The anxiety led the mother to think of the worst possible outcomes when the patient reported symptoms and therefore caused her to believe that the patient was in danger.

4. Given that the mother's anxiety may have contributed to the difficulties in managing this patient, appropriate interventions for the mother included all of the following EXCEPT:

   (a) Counseling for the mother
   (b) Family therapy
   (c) Anxiolytic therapy for both mother and patient
   (d) Hypnotherapy for both mother and patient
   (e) Reassurance

Answers:

1. (c): There is no known functional cause of hemoptysis, which typically occurs in patients with CF as a result of erosion of a bronchial artery by airway inflammation. Cough, dyspnea, and abdominal discomfort can all occur as a result of physiologic issues in CF but also can present as functional symptoms. The patient's need for supplemental oxygen despite her normal hemoglobin saturations probably was related to anxiety.
2. (c): All of the other options can help perpetuate functional symptoms. Options (b) and (e) represent examples of secondary gain that tend to perpetuate functional symptoms. Options (a) and (d) demonstrate how parents' reactions to their children's illness may affect its actual or reported severity. Patients do not usually want to feel more ill, as suggested in option (c).
3. (a): Anxious individuals tend to be hypervigilant, and thus, it is unlikely that the patient's mother would tend to ignore symptoms as a result of anxiety.
4. (c): While reassurance may not have been sufficient to address this mother's anxiety, it is an appropriate first course of action. Counseling, family therapy, and hypnotherapy could all have helped with anxiety reduction. Anxiolytic therapy by itself for the mother is unlikely to have worked as it would not have addressed her concerns regarding the patient's health. Furthermore, anxiolytic therapy is not indicated for the patient if her anxiety arose as a reaction to her mother's anxiety.

Case 4: 19-Year-Old with Chest Pain

The patient was a 19-year-old with CF who emigrated with his mother and older brother from an Eastern European country to the United States at the age of 8 years in order to join his father who already had been in America for 2 years. The patient had received only oral antibiotics sporadically for his CF-related lung disease and pancreatic enzyme supplementation. Upon arrival, he was found to be malnourished and to have moderate lung disease. The father left the family shortly after their arrival.

The patient was started on standard therapy for CF including dornase alpha, chest physiotherapy with a high frequency chest wall oscillating vest, pancreatic enzymes, and vitamins. Within a year, his lung function had improved markedly, but he continued to be malnourished despite oral nutritional supplements. Insertion of a gastrostomy feeding tube was recommended when the patient was 10 years old, but because they hoped he could eat enough on his own, his family did not consent to its placement until he was 13 years old. He gained weight rapidly thereafter with the use of nighttime feedings.

The patient did well from a pulmonary and nutritional perspective for the subsequent 5 years. However, he complained that he had no appetite during the days, which was attributed to his being fed overnight. In his later adolescence, the patient reported spending many hours a day fantasizing that he was powerfully built. He reported that he awaked frequently at night and was tired in the daytime. He became very focused on building muscles; however, he was unable to maintain motivation to lift weights on a regular basis. He lost interest in other activities outside of his home.

The patient asked that his CF center physician arrange for him to have a personal trainer, but this was not possible. The patient became increasingly noncommunicative with his physician over the subsequent few months. He began complaining of significant chest pain that made it hard for him to cough. He denied shortness of breath. He denied episodes of regurgitation or emesis. On examination of his chest, his pain was elicited when his mid-sternum was pressed. He also complained of pain when his costochondral joints were pressed bilaterally. His lungs were clear. His pulmonary function was normal. His chest x-ray revealed mild upper lobe bronchiectasis that had not changed in appearance over the past 2 years. The patient reported that use of ibuprofen and acetaminophen did not help with his pain.

The chest pain persisted for the subsequent 6 months. During this time, the patient removed his gastrostomy tube against medical advice and stopped taking his therapies. His appetite remained poor. He began losing weight rapidly and his pulmonary function declined. He refused admission to the hospital or referral to a psychiatrist.

Questions:

1. The differential diagnosis for this patient's chest pain includes all of the following EXCEPT:

   (a) Asthma
   (b) Costochondritis (inflammation and associated tenderness of the cartilage that attaches the front of the ribs to the breastbone)
   (c) Gastroesophageal reflux
   (d) Pneumothorax
   (e) Somatoform disorder

2. All of the following complaints were suggestive of depression EXCEPT:
   (a) Lack of appetite
   (b) Loss of interest in activities
   (c) Sleep disturbance
   (d) Preoccupation with body image
   (e) Lack of adherence to his therapies
3. Referral to all of the following services would be appropriate for treatment of this patient's chest pain EXCEPT:
   (a) Cognitive behavioral therapy
   (b) Hypnotherapy
   (c) Pain clinic for appropriate management of narcotic therapy
   (d) Psychiatry
   (e) Psychology

Answers:

1. (d): The patient is unlikely to have a pneumothorax given the absence of shortness of breath, decreased breath sounds, or x-ray evidence of this condition. Bronchospasm associated with asthma can cause chest pain. Costochondritis was suggested given that the pain was elicited with pressure applied during the physical examination. While the patient did not have symptoms suggestive of gastroesophageal reflux, his nighttime gastrostomy tube feedings placed him at increased risk for this condition. The likelihood of somatoform disorder as a diagnosis was increased given the patient's multiple psychological and family issues.
2. (d): Preoccupation with body image is common in an adolescent. While poor sleep hygiene and lack of adherence to therapies also are typical for adolescents, the extent of these behaviors in this patient was extreme. Loss of interest in favorite activities is common for patients with depression. This patient might have developed his lack of appetite as a result of his gastrostomy tube feedings, but this was unlikely as his appetite did not improve when he did not use the tube. Patients with advanced CF lung disease often lose their appetite, but this patient had only mild lung disease.
3. (c): Given this patient's complex psychosocial difficulties, it is unlikely that the chest pain would resolve with an intervention that mostly targets the symptom, as opposed to the underlying depression.

Case 5: 20-Year-Old with Insomnia [87]

The patient was a 20-year-old young man with advanced cystic fibrosis who had suffered a nearly fatal episode of hemoptysis, for which he necessitated being placed on a ventilator for 6 days, followed by prolonged rehabilitation. Two months later, he reported recurrent nightmares about hemoptysis, which awakened him approximately five times a night. The patient explained that he was concerned about again suffering from massive hemoptysis and that this thought prevented him from falling asleep easily. Also, he was worried about being too physically active in case this might trigger further bleeding. Occasionally, when the patient tasted a small amount of blood, such as a result of a nosebleed, he has had flashbacks to his near fatal episode. He said that even thinking about the possibility of hemoptysis caused his chest to tighten and his heart to beat more strongly.

The patient had been taught how to use self-hypnosis for relaxation 2 years prior to his development of anxiety and nightmares about bleeding. It was suggested that the patient could view his beating heart as a metronome that was sending a wave of relaxation with each beat. When the patient applied this imagery, he reported that he no longer felt his heart was beating too strongly. Also, it was suggested that whenever the patient tasted blood that he might reaffirm his life by telling himself, "I am bleeding; therefore, I am alive."

To help with his nightmares, the patient was instructed to go into hypnosis and to allow his subconscious to show him a dream representative of those that woke him up. After a 3-min hypnosis session, the patient reported he had dreamed he was having another massive hemoptysis episode, which caused him to be very fearful. When he continued to dream, he perceived two possible endings to the dream: In one, he survived, and in the other, he died. The patient concluded that his most important realization was that no matter what happened, he would be "all right" and that the discomfort of the hemoptysis episode would be short-lived.

During the subsequent month, the patient reported having only two further nightmares, which he was able to "work through" while remaining asleep.

Questions:

1. The adverse effect of the patient's concerns about recurrent hemoptysis could have included all of the following EXCEPT:

   (a) He could have interpreted the associated chest tightness as indicating that he was physically ill, which could have led to the need for medical attention and increased anxiety.
   (b) His concerns about his level of activity could have translated into a more sedentary lifestyle that would have decreased his pulmonary toilet.
   (c) His sleep disruption as a result of his nightmares affected his quality of life.
   (d) When he had flashbacks to the hemoptysis, he imagined tasting blood, which is consistent with post-traumatic stress disorder leading to the development of gustatory hallucinations.
   (e) His concerns might have led him to be less adherent to his prescribed inhaled therapies, for fear that they might trigger recurrent hemoptysis.

2. All of the following referrals or therapies would be appropriate for this patient EXCEPT:
   (a) Cognitive behavioral therapy
   (b) Diphenhydramine, oral
   (c) Hypnosis
   (d) Mindful meditation
   (e) Sleep study
3. In addition to use of hypnosis, what other form of psychological therapy was this patient given?
   (a) Cognitive behavioral therapy
   (b) Meditation
   (c) Play therapy
   (d) Sleep hygiene education
   (e) None of the above

Answers:

1. (d): There is no reason to suspect that this patient imagined blood, as he pointed out that he suffers from epistaxis. The potential adverse events that could have arisen as a result of the patient's anxiety about recurrent hemoptysis illustrate the importance of addressing this issue effectively.
2. (b): Use of diphenhydramine could help the patient fall asleep but would not address his anxiety. A sleep study could help define whether there was an organic cause for the patient's sleep disturbance, such as obstructive sleep apnea. The other options could have helped improve his anxiety.
3. (a): By helping the patient identify the fear that was underlying his nightmares, he was able to resolve it. Sleep hygiene education includes establishing a consistent sleep schedule and bedtime routine and modification of the bedroom environment and food intake.

Conclusions

The detailed discussion provided in this chapter of the potential impact of functional symptoms on patients with CF serves as a model for a comprehensive approach to patients with chronic pulmonary diseases. For example, psychiatric and psychosocial factors are well-recognized as affecting patients with asthma and chronic obstructive pulmonary disease [88–91].

Thus, clinicians providing care for patients with chronic pulmonary disease should consider the possible impact of a functional contribution to the clinical presentation of every patient and offer treatment for this relatively early in the therapeutic algorithm. Treatment strategies for functional respiratory symptoms are discussed in the third section of this book, "Treatment of Functional Respiratory Disorders." Such an approach will lead to more efficient and effective management of patients with chronic pulmonary disease.

References

1. Orenstein DM, Winnie GB, Altman H. Cystic fibrosis: A 2002 update. J Pediatr. 2002;140(2): 156–64.
2. White T, Miller J, Smith GL, McMahon WM. Adherence and psychopathology in children and adolescents with cystic fibrosis. Eur Child Adolesc Psychiatry. 2009;18(2):96–104.
3. Parad RB. Buccal cell DNA mutation analysis for cystic fibrosis in newborns and infants inaccessible to sweat chloride measurements. Pediatrics. 1998;101(5):851–5.
4. Cystic Fibrosis Foundation. Patient registry 2010 annual data report. Accessed November 2011.
5. Armstrong DS, Grimwood K, Carlin JB, et al. Lower airway inflammation in infants and young children with cystic fibrosis. Am J Pespir Crit Care Med. 1997;156(4 pt 1):1197–204.
6. Papadakis MA, McPhee SJ, Seiger RF. Cystic fibrosis. Current Consult Medicine 2007. Lange Publications.
7. Flume PA, Mogayzel Jr PJ, Robinson KA, Rosenblatt RL, Quittell L, Marshall BC. Clinical practice guidelines for pulmonary therapies committee; Cystic Fibrosis Foundation Pulmonary Therapies Committee. Cystic fibrosis pulmonary guidelines: Pulmonary complications: Hemoptysis and pneumothorax. Am J Respir Crit Care Med. 2010;182(3):298–306.
8. Farrell FM, Rosenstein BJ, White TB, et al. Guidelines for diagnosis of cystic fibrosis in newborns through older adults: Cystic fibrosis consensus report. J Pediatr. 2008;153(2):S4–S14.
9. Stallings VA, Stark LF, Robinson KA, Feranchak AP, Quinton H. Evidence-based practice recommendations for nutrition-related management of children and adults with cystic fibrosis and pancreatic insufficiency: results of a systematic review. J Am Diet Assoc. 2008;108(5): 832–9.
10. Mogayzel Jr PJ, Flume PA. Update in cystic fibrosis 2009. Am J Respir Crit Care Med. 2010;181(6):539–44.
11. Borowitz D, Robinson KA, Rosenfeld M, et al. Cystic Fibrosis Foundation evidence-based guidelines for management of infants with cystic fibrosis. J Pediatr. 2009;155(6 Suppl): S73–93.
12. Thompson RJ, Gustafson KE, Gil KM, et al. Illness specific patterns of psychological adjustment and cognitive adaptational processes in children with cystic fibrosis and sickle cell disease. J Clin Psychol. 1998;54:121–8.
13. Smetana JG, Campione-Barr N, Metzger A. Adolescent development in interpersonal and societal contexts. Annu Rev Psychiol. 2006;57:255–84.
14. Tluczek A, Koscik RL, Farrell PM, et al. Psychosocial risk associated with newborn screening for cystic fibrosis: Parents' experience while awaiting the sweat-test appointment. Pediatrics. 2005;115(6):1692–703.
15. Bayer JK, Nicholson JM. Problems with sleep, eating, and adherence to therapy are common among children with cystic fibrosis. J Pediatrics. 2009;155(5):759–60.
16. Driscool KA, Maontag-leifling K, Acton JD, et al. Relations between depressive and anxious symptoms and quality of life in caregivers of children with cystic fibrosis. Pediatr Pulmonol. 2009;44(8):784–92.
17. Suris JC, Michaud PA, Akre C, et al. Health risk behaviors in adolescents with chronic conditions. Pediatrics. 2008;122(5):e111–8.
18. Szyndler JE, Towns SJ, van Asperen PP, McKay KO. Psychological and family functioning and quality of life in adolescents with cystic fibrosis. J Cyst Fibros. 2005;4(2):135–44.

19. Smith BA, Modi AC, Quittner AL, Wood BL. Depressive symptoms in children with cystic fibrosis and parents and its effects on adherence to airway clearance. Pediatr Pulmonol. 2010;49(8):756–63.
20. Glasscoe C, Lancaster GA, Smyth RL, Hill J. Parental depression following early diagnosis of cystic fibrosis: a matched, prospective study. J Pediatr. 2007;150(2):185–91.
21. Katon W, Ciechanowske P. Impact of major depression on chronic medical illness. J Psychosom Res. 2002;53(4):859–63.
22. Havermans T, Colpaert K, Dupont LJ. Quality of life in patients with cystic fibrosis: association with anxiety and depression. J Cyst Fibros. 2008;7(6):581–4.
23. Quittner AL, Baker DH, Snell C, et al. Prevalence and impact of depression in cystic fibrosis. Curr Opin Pulm Med. 2008;14(6):582–8.
24. Smith BA, Wood BL. Psychological factors affecting disease activity in children and adolescents with cystic fibrosis: medical adherence as a mediator. Curr Opin Pediatr. 2007;19(5): 553–8.
25. Quittner AL, Baker DH, Geller D, et al. Effects of maternal depression on electronically monitored enzyme adherence and changes in weight for children with CF. J Cyst Fibros. 2007;6(1):77.
26. Quittner AL, Buu A, Messer MA, et al. Development and validation of the Cystic Fibrosis Questionnaire in the United States: a health-related quality-of-life measure for cystic fibrosis. Chest. 2005;128(4):2347–54.
27. Kessler RC, Nelson CB, McGonagle KA, et al. Comorbidity of DSM-III major depressive disorder in the general population: results from the US National Comorbidity Survey. Br J Psychiatry Suppl. 1996 Jun;30:17–30.
28. Costello EJ, Mustillo S, Erkanli A, et al. Prevalence and development of psychiatric disorders in childhood and adolescence. Arch Gen Psychiatry. 2003;60(8):837–44.
29. Casier A, Goubert L, Huse D, et al. The role of acceptance in psychological functioning in adolescents with cystic fibrosis: a preliminary study. Psychol Health. 2008;23:629–38.
30. Cruz MS, Marciel KK, Quittner AL, Schechter MS. Anxiety and depression in cystic fibrosis. Semin Respir Crit Care Med. 2009;30(5):569–78.
31. James A, Soler A, Weatherall R. Cognitive behavioral therapy for anxiety disorders in children and adolescents. Cochrane Database Syst Rev 2005;4:CD004690.
32. Zigmond AS, Snaith RP. The hospital anxiety and depression scale. Acta Psychiatr Scand. 1983;67(6):361–70.
33. Chorpita BF, Yim L, Moffitt C, et al. Assessment of symptoms of DSM-IV anxiety and depression in children: A revised child anxiety and depression scale. Behav Res Ther. 2000;38(8): 835–55.
34. Osman A, Kopper BA, Carrios FX, Osman JR, Wade T. The Beck Anxiety Inventory: Reexamination of factor structure and psychometric properties. J Clin Psychol. 1977;53(1): 7–14.
35. Beck AT, Steer RA, Brown GK. BDI-II, Beck depression inventory: Manual. 2nd ed. Boston: Harcourt Brace; 1996.
36. Reynolds WM. Multidimensional anxiety questionnaire. Lutz FL: Psychological Assessment Resources; 2003.
37. Kapornai K, Vetro A. Depression in children. Curr Opin Psychiatry. 2008;21(1):1–7.
38. Birmaher B, Ryan ND, Williamson DE. Depression in children and adolescents: clinical features and pathogenesis. In: Shulman KI, Tohen M, Kutcher S, editors. Mood disorders across the life span. New York: Wiley-Liss; 1996. p. 51–82.
39. Rapee RM, Schniering CA, Hudson JL. Anxiety disorders during childhood and adolescence: origins and treatment. Annu Rev Clin Psychol. 2009;5:311–41.
40. Markowitz JC, Weissman MM. Interpersonal psychotherapy: principles and applications. World Psychiatry. 2004;3:136–9.
41. Caron A, Weissman MM. Interpersonal psychotherapy in the treatment of depression in medical patients. Prim Psychiatry. 2006;13:43–50.

42. Duff AJ. Psychological interventions in cystic fibrosis and asthma. Paediatr Respir Rev. 2001;2(4):350–7.
43. Glasscoe CA, Quittner AL. Psychological interventions for people with cystic fibrosis and their families. Cochrane Database Syst Rev. 2008;3:CD003148.
44. Kirkwood CK, Hayes PE. Anxiety disorders. In: Dipiro JT, Talvert RL, Yee GC, et al., editors. Psychotherapy: a pathophysiologic approach. Stamford: Appleton & Lange; 2005. p. 1443–62.
45. de Matt SM, Dekker J, Schoevers RA, de Jongh F. Relative efficacy of psychotherapy and combined therapy in the treatment of depression: A meta-analysis. Eur Psychiatry. 2007;22(1):1–8.
46. Diagnostic and Statistical Manuel of Mental Disorders, 4th edn. Text revision, Washington, DC, American Psychiatric Association, 2000.
47. Weinert C. Epidemiology and treatment of psychiatric conditions that develop after critical illness. Curr Opin Crit Care. 2005;11(4):376–80.
48. Kelly AF, Hewso PH. Factors associated with recurrent hospitalizations in chronically ill children and adolescents. J Paediatr Child Health. 2000;36(1):13–8.
49. Ernst MM, Johnson MC, Stark LJ. Developmental and psychological issues in cystic fibrosis. Child Adolesc Psych Clin N Am. 2010;19(2):263–83.
50. Thompson WL, Thompson TL. Psychiatric disorders complicating the treatment of patients with pulmonary disease. New Dir Ment Health Serv. 1993;57:117–30.
51. Anderson DL, Flume PA, Hardy KK. Psychological functioning in adults with cystic fibrosis. Chest. 2001;119(4):1079–84.
52. Jankelowitz L, Reid KJ, Wolfe L, et al. Cystic fibrosis patients have poor sleep quality despite normal sleep latency and efficiency. Chest. 2005;27(5):1593–9.
53. Mattewal AS, Subramanian S. Sleep disturbances in cystic fibrosis. Curr Resp Med Rev. 2009; 5(4):230–2.
54. Williams DC. Periodic limb movements of sleep and the restless legs syndrome. Va Med Q. 1996;123(4):260–5.
55. Thase ME. Depression, sleep, and antidepressants. J Clin Psychiatry. 1998;59(suppl):55–6.
56. Ward CM, Massie J, Glazber J, et al. Problem behaviors and parenting preschool children with cystic fibrosis. Arch Dis Child. 2009;94(5):341–7.
57. Patterson JM, Wall M, Berge J, Milla C. Associations of psychological factors with health outcomes among youth with cystic fibrosis. Pediatr Pulmonol. 2009;44(1):46–53.
58. Pumariega AJ, Pursell J, Spock A, Jones JD. Eating disorders in adolescents with cystic fibrosis. J Am Acad Child Adolesc Psychiatr. 1986;25(2):269–75.
59. Thompson RJ, Gustafson KE, Hamlett KW, Spock A. Psychological adjustment of children with children with cystic fibrosis: The role of child cognitive processes and maternal adjustment. J Pediatr Psychol. 1992;17(6):741–55.
60. Modi AC, Quittner AL. Barriers to treatment adherence for children with cystic fibrosis and asthma: what gets in the way? J Pediatr Psychol. 2006;31(8):846–58.
61. Georgiopoules AM. Prevalence, impact and treatment of ADHD in cystic fibrosis. Pediatr Pulmonol. 2011;4(Suppl):161–2.
62. Georgiopoules AM, Hua LL. The diagnosis and treatment of Attention Deficit Hyperactivity Disorder in children and adolescents with cystic fibrosis: a retrospective study. Psychosom. 2011;52(2):160–6.
63. Kelly AF, Hewson PH. Factors associated with recurrent hospitalization in chronically ill children and adolescents. J Paediatr Child Health. 2000;36(1):13–8.
64. Jackson JC, Hart RP, Gordon SM, et al. PTSD and PTSD symptoms following critical illness in medical intensive care unit patients: assessing the magnitude of the problem. Crit Care. 2007;11(1):R27.
65. Hegarty M, Macdonald J, Watter P, et al. Quality of life in young people with cystic fibrosis: Effects of hospitalization, age and gender and differences in parent/child perceptions. Child Care Health Dev. 2009;35(4):462–8.
66. Iles N, Lowton K. Young people with cystic fibrosis' concerns for the future: when and how should concerns be addressed and by whom? J Inter Prof Care. 2008;22(4):336–8.

67. Arias Liorente RP, Bousono Garcia C, Diaz Martin JJ. Treatment compliance in children and adults with cystic fibrosis. J Cyst Fibros. 2008;7(5):359–67.
68. Patterson JM, Wall M, Berge J, Milla C. Gender differences in treatment adherence among youth with cystic fibrosis: development of a new questionnaire. J Cyst Fibros. 2008;7(2):154–64.
69. Prasad SA, Cerny FJ. Factors that influence adherence to exercise and their effectiveness: application to cystic fibrosis. Pediatr Pulmonol. 2002;34(1):66–72.
70. Barnes AJ, Eisenberg ME, Resnick MD. Suicide and self-injury among children and youth with chronic health conditions. Pediatrics. 2010 May;125(5):1064–5.
71. Kettler LJ, Sawyer SM, Winefield HR, Greville HW. Determinants of adherence in adults with cystic fibrosis. Thorax. 2002;57(5):459–64.
72. DiMatteo MR, Giodani PJ, Lepper HS, Croghan TW. Patient adherence to medical treatment outcomes: a meta-analysis. Med Care. 2002;40(9):794–811.
73. Modi AC, Lim CS, Yu N, et al. A multi-method assessment of treatment adherence for children with cystic fibrosis. J Cystic Fibros. 2006;5(3):177–85.
74. DiMatteo MR, Lepper HS, Croghan TW. Depression is a risk factor for noncompliance with medical treatment: meta-analysis of effects of anxiety and depression on patient adherence. Arch Intern Med. 2000;160(14):2101–7.
75. Riekert KA, Bartlett SJ, Boyle MP, et al. The association between depression, lung function, and health-related quality of life among adults with cystic fibrosis. Chest. 2007;132(1): 231–7.
76. DeLambo KE, levers-Landis CE, Drotar D, Quittner AL. Association of the observed family relationship quality and problem-solving skills with treatment adherence in older children and adolescents with cystic fibrosis. J Pediatr Psychol. 2004;29(5):343–53.
77. Solomon C, Breton J. Early warning signals in relationships between parents and young children with cystic fibrosis. Child Heath Care. 1999;28(3):221–40.
78. Wong MG, Heriot SA. Parents of children with cystic fibrosis: how they hope, cope and despair. Child Care Health Dev. 2008;34(3):344–54.
79. Quittner AL, Opipari LC, Espelage DL, et al. Role strain in couples with and without a child with a chronic illness: associations with marital satisfaction, intimacy and daily mood. Health Psychol. 1998;17(2):112–24.
80. Modi AC, Marciel KK, Slater SK, et al. The influence of parental supervision on medical adherence in adolescents with cystic fibrosis: developmental shifts from pre to late adolescents. Children's Health Care. 2007;37(1):78–92.
81. Herzer M, Umfress K, Aljadeff G, et al. Interactions with parents and friends among chronically ill children: examining social networks. J Dev Behav Pediatr. 2009;30(6):499–508.
82. Berlin KS, Sass DA, Hobart Davies W, et al. Cystic fibrosis disclosure may minimize risk of negative peer evaluations. J Cystic Fibros. 2005;4(3):169–74.
83. Anbar RD. Childhood habit cough treated with consultation by telephone: a case report. Cough. 2009;5:2.
84. Cohlan SQ, Stone SM. The cough and the bedsheet. Pediatrics. 1984;74(1):11–5.
85. Anbar RD, Murthy VV. Reestablishment of hope as an intervention for a patient with cystic fibrosis awaiting lung transplantation. J Alter Complem Med. 2010;16(9):1007–10.
86. Anbar RD. Self-hypnosis for patients with cystic fibrosis. Pediatr Pulmonol. 2000;30(6): 461–5.
87. Linden JH, Bhardwaj A, Anbar RD. Hypnotically enhanced dreaming to achieve symptom reduction: a case study of 11 children and adolescents. Am J Clin Hypnosis. 2006;48(4): 279–89.
88. Peters TE, Fritz GK. Psychological considerations of the child with asthma. Child Adolesc Psychiatr Clin N Am. 2010;19(2):319–33.
89. Di Marco F, Santus P, Centanni S. Anxiety and depression in asthma. Curr Opin Pulm Med. 2011;17(1):39–44.
90. Xu W, Collet JP, Shapiro S, et al. Independent effect of depression and anxiety on chronic obstructive pulmonary disease exacerbations and hospitalizations. Am J Respir Crit Care Med. 2008;178(9):913–20.
91. Kaptein AA, Scharloo M, Fischer MJ, et al. Fifty years of psychological research on patients with COPD – road to ruin or highway to heaven? Respir Med. 2009;103(1):3–11.

Part II
Common Functional Respiratory and Related Conditions

Chapter 3
Chest Pain

Dilip R. Patel

Abstract Chest pain is a common complaint in children, adolescents, and adults. Although, most children with chest pain do not present in severe distress with serious underlying condition, all need a very careful evaluation to rule of such a disorder. Chest pain in a child can cause significant anxiety for the parents. In adults, chest pain is often a sign of serious underlying cardiac or noncardiac disease, and a prompt and thorough evaluation is important before making a diagnosis of functional chest pain. However, when a complete medical evaluation reveals no serious cause, persistence of chest pain can still be a source for ongoing concern and anxiety. A thorough history and physical examination are key elements of a diagnostic evaluation. In addition to organic causes of chest pain, psychological factors must be carefully considered in all patients who present with chest pain. This chapter reviews diagnostic approach and psychological factors in pediatric and adult chest pain.

Keywords Anxiety • Chest pain • Noncardiac chest pain • Panic attack • Somatoform disorder • Stress

Background

Chest pain is reported in 0.3–0.6% of visits to pediatric emergency medicine departments [1, 2]. Few children present with severe chest pain requiring immediate emergency management; most children and adolescents who present with pain are stable and not in significant distress. Driscoll et al., based on their prospective study of chest pain in children with a mean age of 12 years, reported that cardiac disease as

D.R. Patel (✉)
Department of Pediatrics, Michigan State University, Kalamazoo Center for Medical Studies, Kalamazoo, MI, USA
e-mail: patel@kcms.msu.edu

R.D. Anbar (ed.), *Functional Respiratory Disorders: When Respiratory Symptoms Do Not Respond to Pulmonary Treatment*, Respiratory Medicine,
DOI 10.1007/978-1-61779-857-3_3,

a cause of chest pain in children was uncommon [3]. Their study reported nearly half cases were idiopathic (45%), followed by costochondritis (23%). On the other hand, a recent analysis of pediatric chest pain studies by Eslick et al. reported that cardiac cause for chest pain in children is more common than previously thought and may account for 9.5% of all causes for chest pain in children and adolescents [2].

Hambrook et al. analyzed data from 2002 to 2006 National Hospital Ambulatory Medical Care Survey (NHAMCS) for emergency department visits with chief complaint of chest pain in patients less than 19 years of age [4]. The most common cause of chest pain in their study was chest pain not otherwise specified (37%), followed by infection, musculoskeletal trauma, respiratory, gastrointestinal, cardiovascular, psychiatric, and hematologic. Selbst et al. in a systemic review reported the following causes for chest pain in children: idiopathic chest pain was most prevalent (36%), followed by musculoskeletal (20%), then psychological (16%), gastrointestinal (10%), cardiac (10%), and respiratory (8%) conditions as the primary cause of presentation [5].

The main limitations of studies for pediatric chest pain include small sample sizes, low rates of follow-up, and shorter follow-up periods [2].

Adults presenting with acute chest pain present the immediate possibility of acute life-threatening disease and should be thoroughly and promptly evaluated. In the primary care setting, etiology chest pain in adults was found to occur in the following proportions: 16% cardiovascular, 36% musculoskeletal, 5% pulmonary, 19% gastrointestinal, 8% psychogenic, and 16% indeterminant [6]. On the contrary, patients seen in the emergency department often present with more serious disease in the proportions cardiovascular 54%, musculoskeletal 6%, pulmonary 12%, gastrointestinal 3%, psychogenic 9%, and indeterminant 5% [7]. It is interesting that in both settings, the diagnosis of psychogenic or functional chest pain is about equal at just under 10%. As a rule of thumb, any acute chest pain in adults should be evaluated in a setting where emergency evaluation, intervention, and management can be undertaken, especially when associated with respiratory and/or neurological symptoms and of first time onset.

Differential Diagnosis of Chest Pain

Patients who present with chest pain with significant distress need emergent assessment and management in the emergency department setting [8, 9]. The approach to evaluation and diagnosis for most other patients begins with a detailed history to characterize the chest pain, a review of associated symptoms, and a complete physical examination. With no immediate physical cause suspected or detected, psychological factors should be considered as part of the evaluation (Table 3.1). Laboratory and imaging studies are indicated based on findings on history and examination. Clinical features and presentation, however, are the key elements in the diagnosis, and consideration of the patient's age helps define the differential diagnosis.

Table 3.1 Selected psychological factors for chest pain analysis

Pain
Pain characteristics (i.e., frequency, intensity, duration, quality)
Pain antecedents (e.g., exertion, parental separation, interpersonal conflict)
Interoceptive hypersensitivity (i.e., strong emotion, cardiovascular vigilance/attention, pulse checking)
Pain consequences (e.g., pain relief, absenteeism, sick role, attention, secondary gain)
Factors that alleviate pain
Cognitive understanding
Fears (e.g., fear of pain, intolerance of discomfort, serious illness, heart attack)
Beliefs about illness (i.e., cause of the pain, likelihood of death, losing control)
Behavioral responses
Interoceptive avoidance (i.e., restricted physical engagement, including kinesiophobia)
Situational avoidance
Safety behaviors (e.g., pulse checking, lucky charms, experiential states)
Medication use
Social effects
Quality of life (e.g., caregiver role, sibling relationships, family dynamics)
Academic, work, and peer relations

[Adapted from [13]. With permission from Elsevier.]

Children

Numerous conditions should be considered in the differential diagnosis of chest pain in children and adolescents as listed in Table 3.2 [1–4, 10].

Cystic fibrosis (*CF*) is *associated with bronchitis and cough.* Pleuritic pain or sharp pain on deep inspiration is common in CF, especially during acute exacerbations of chronic infection.

Pleuritic pain or pleurisy is also common in both viral respiratory *infections* such as those with coxsackie B virus (epidemic *pleurodynia*) and with bacterial *pneumonia.* Inflammation of the lung and pleura also may lead to effusions and progress to *empyema.* The history often will reveal cough, fever, and increasing dyspnea prior to the onset of chest pain. Chest pain also may be associated with diaphragmatic irritation owing to *subphrenic abscess* or *pancreatitis.*

A history of *foreign-body* aspiration with subsequent fever and chest pain may indicate retention of the foreign body in the airway with subsequent reactive inflammation and infection.

Herpes zoster presents as a vesicular rash located over the chest wall in a pattern to suggest involvement of a dermatome and is both a *neurogenic* and *infectious* cause of chest pain.

Chest discomfort and pain also may occur with *hyperventilation* associated with psychosomatic disease such as panic attack or disorder, although this is more common in teens.

Traumatic causes of chest pain, besides foreign-body aspiration, include a history of chest trauma (e.g., during sports activities) with localized *contusion.* If severe,

Table 3.2 Differential diagnosis of chest pain in children

Cardiac-related causes
Coronary artery disease – ischemia/infarction
Anomalous coronary arteries
Kawasaki disease (coronary arteritis)
Diabetes mellitus (long standing)
Arrhythmia
Supraventricular tachycardia
Ventricular tachycardia
Structural abnormalities of the heart
Hypertrophic cardiomyopathy
Severe pulmonic stenosis
Aortic valve stenosis
Infection
Pericarditis
Myocarditis
Noncardiac-related causes
Musculoskeletal disorders
Chest wall strain
Direct trauma/contusion
Rib fracture
Costochondritis
Respiratory disorders
Severe cough
Asthma
Pneumonia
Pneumothorax/pneumomediastinum
Pulmonary embolism
Psychological disorders
Stress-related pain
Gastrointestinal disorders
Reflux esophagitis
Pill-induced esophagitis
Esophageal foreign body
Miscellaneous disorders
Sickle cell crises
Abdominal aortic aneurysm (Marfan syndrome)
Pleural effusion (collagen vascular disease)
Shingles
Pleurodynia (coxsackievirus)
Breast tenderness (pregnancy, physiologic)
Tietze syndrome
Texidor's twinge/precordial catch syndrome
Chest mass
Idiopathic

[Reprinted from [8]. With permission from Elsevier.]

consider *rib fracture*. *Costochondritis,* or pain over the sternum at the costochondral junction(s), may follow upper body exercise such as weight lifting or any sports activity using the upper body, although a specific cause may not be readily evident.

Spontaneous pneumothorax leads to acute chest pain. The risk increases with diseases such as *cystic fibrosis* and *acute asthma*, but it also may occur in healthy children. Pneumothorax and *hemothorax* may occur after significant chest trauma or thoracic surgical procedures.

Gastroesophageal reflux disease with substernal burning is common in children, and inquiry as to timing of pain to ingestion of meals is important. Inhalation of irritants and smoke also may lead to chest pain or discomfort.

One should seek a history of inhalation of volatile substances such as organic solvents when suspecting *toxins* as an etiology of acute onset of chest pain and dyspnea in an otherwise healthy child.

Congenital causes of chest pain include pleurisy and pneumonitis associated with lung malformations such as *lung cyst*, *cystic adenomatoid malformation*, and *pulmonary sequestration.* A history of recurrence of pneumonia in the same location is a clue to an infected malformation or a retained foreign body.

In patients with sickle cell anemia, acute chest pain associated with crisis or with *acute chest syndrome* occurs commonly. One should ask about prior testing for sickle cell disease and family history of all African-American children presenting with acute chest pain.

Children with pulmonary embolus from lower extremity injury, heart disease, or familial coagulopathy such as *factor V Leiden* deficiency often have acute chest pain associated with other symptoms such as dyspnea, cyanosis, and hemoptysis.

Adolescents

CF as a *metabolic* disease causes chest pain as a common manifestation of acute exacerbations of chronic *pneumonia* or with *pneumothorax*. Pleuritic pain or pain associated with chest muscle strain, accompanying severe cough, also may be present. This and other *infectious* causes of chest pain occur in adolescence as in childhood. *Coxsackie B acute pleurodynia*, as well as pleurisy with other viruses and with bacterial pneumonia, occurs commonly in a teen with increasing cough and respiratory distress.

Subphrenic abscess and *pancreatitis* may manifest as lower chest pain. *Pneumonia* also may present with a history of abdominal pain.

Neurogenic causes of chest pain include *herpes zoster* manifesting as a vesicular rash along a chest wall dermatome. Pain derived from *gastritis* and *esophagitis* owing to *GERD* is neurogenic in origin.

Neoplasia with involvement of the pleura (*mesothelioma* or more often metastases) or with pressure on mediastinal structures may be a cause of chest discomfort and pain. A history of accompanying systemic symptoms such as decreased appetite, dyspepsia, fever, night sweats, and fatigue often accompanies pulmonary and mediastinal neoplasia.

Toxic causes of chest pain include *inhalation injury* and pneumonitis, as in younger children, although inhalation is more often intentional in adolescents (e.g., glue, gasoline, or hydrocarbons). One should seek a careful history of substance inhalation in the case of acute respiratory symptoms, especially without upper respiratory infection symptoms or fever.

Chest wall pain becomes more common in adolescence and in some cases may be *traumatic* (i.e., related to sports injury) but is often *unknown* and likely related to rapid growth. Sometimes, trauma to the abdomen bordering on the chest (e.g., liver and spleen) can cause chest pain.

Adolescents are more likely than younger children to complain of pain associated with *GERD*. *Costochondritis* with pain on palpation over the costochondral junction is common. This often relates to activities such as weight lifting or chest trauma from contact during sports.

Tietze syndrome occurs with a history of painful swelling over the sternal junction. Pain and tenderness over the xiphoid is termed the *xiphoid syndrome.* A history of intermittent costal margin pain often is due to the *slipping rib syndrome.*

Stress fractures of the ribs with localized chest pain and tenderness and a history of chest wall pain on inspiration are common with certain sports activities such as rowing, baseball pitching, and golf.

Particularly in early adolescence, painful nodules of the breasts (*benign gynecomastia*) can be troubling to both male and female adolescents, and mastitis may occur later in adolescent girls.

An unusual syndrome with a history of intermittent acute, sharp chest pain occurring over the precordium and lasting from a few seconds to minutes, sometimes relieved by changing position, occurs commonly in adolescents and is termed the *precordial catch syndrome* (also known as *Texidor's twinge*). The history usually reveals no specific initiating factor. Referred pain from the thoracic spine (e.g., in scoliosis or diskitis) may present as chest wall pain.

Acute chest pain with or without chest wall trauma is a presenting symptom of *pneumothorax* in an otherwise healthy teen.

Pain from *congenital* lesions is less likely at this age. Occasionally, a lung malformation or congenital *neoplasm* will manifest in teens.

Circulatory causes of chest pain are the same as in the childhood years, although, occasionally, *coronary artery disease* and *mitral valve prolapse* may cause pain in this age group. In cases of radiating pain or increasing pain with exercise, cardiology referral is appropriate.

Anterior chest pain or discomfort can occur with chronic cough, and the historical evaluation of *asthma* and *allergy* should uncover this.

Adults

The differential diagnosis of acute chest pain in adults is presented in Table 3.3 [11].

Chronic or chronic recurrent chest pain presents a different diagnostic challenge in the case of the adult presenting for primary care.

Table 3.3 Acute chest pain in adults

Angina
Acute myocardial infarction
Aortic stenosis
Pericarditis
Aortic dissection
Pulmonary embolism
Pulmonary hypertension
Pneumonia
Pleuritis
Spontaneous pneumothorax
Esophageal reflux
Peptic ulcer
Esophageal spasm
Gall bladder disease
Musculoskeletal pain
Herpes zoster
Emotional and psychiatric condition

The most frequent cause of noncardiac chest pain (NCCP) stems from the gastrointestinal tract and includes gastroesophageal reflux disease (GERD), disorders of esophageal motility, and esophageal hypersensitivity (as discussed below). Once pain of cardiac origin is eliminated, pain of gastrointestinal origin is evaluated through both dynamic tests such as esophageal manometry and pH evaluation and provocative tests such as acid infusion or administration of hot or cold foods all in an attempt to reproduce the pain [12]. However, provocative tests have only been found to produce a yield of reproducible pain of 25–50% [13].

Both patients with cardiac pain and with NCCP can experience anxiety and depression. Panic disorder is a common anxiety-driven condition with a well-known correlation with pathophysiologic conditions. Symptoms related to panic as a functional disorder may be difficult to separate from the underlying organic disorder. Examples are presented below.

Psychological and Physiologic Considerations

In addition to a thorough evaluation and consideration for organic causes for chest pain, similar consideration should be given to the psychological factors that may be contributing to the chest pain [10, 14–25]. Although a cause and effect relationship between mitral valve prolapse and panic disorder has not been established, the association of these with nonspecific chest pain has been well described in adults [26]. The cause of chest pain in mitral valve prolapse with panic disorder is not known, but neuroendocrine studies have revealed high adrenergic tone that may be contributing to the symptoms otherwise unexplained on the basis of the valvular abnormality alone [27, 28].

Esophageal and visceral hypersensitivity and hyperalgesia also have been associated with functional chest pain. Although the physiologic mechanism is poorly understood, venlafaxine, a serotonin–norepinephrine reuptake inhibitor, high-dose proton pump inhibitors, and low doses of tricyclic antidepressants have all shown some benefit for symptomatic relief [29–31].

Dyspnea associated with panic attack/disorder is also commonly associated with chest discomfort (see Chap. 4), although the exact mechanism for this phenomenon is unknown.

In organic conditions known to be associated with chest pain, such as chest wall abnormalities, gastroesophageal reflux disease, or costochondritis, consideration of psychological factors is also important in the overall management. This can help the patient and family cope with the condition and facilitate treatment adherence. Depending on the significant and severity of the condition, patients may manifest depression or anxiety. In these cases, also, consultation with a mental health professional is valuable and often essential.

Any chest pain may be perceived by the patient and his or her parents or family as ominous. This is partly a reflection of lay public exposure to easily accessible information in the media regarding the potential serious conditions associated with chest pain [10]. Reports of sudden death of young athletes from previously unidentified heart conditions also heighten the anxiety and sensitivity to serious heart condition as a cause for chest pain [10].

In some children as well as adults, however, no cause for chest pain is found even after a thorough medical evaluation. Pain can persist for a long time, and, even after reassurance, the patient and family may remain quite concerned that a potentially serious condition might have been missed [10]. Parents may unnecessarily become overprotective of the child and may not allow the child to participate in certain activities, and adults may avoid social situations and become isolated. This may result in significant anxiety, stress, and sometimes depression in the child or adolescent, and parents may also experience anxiety and stress [10]. Passive pain-coping strategies such as avoidance, praying, and hoping may be employed in such a setting, in association with decreased self-efficacy that may lead to years of disability from the pain [32].

McDonnell et al. [10] describe a bidirectional relationship between chest pain and emotional distress. They note that children, in addition to feeling pain related to an organic cause, also may experience the bodily sensation of chest pain, tightness, or pressure as part of the psychological arousal that accompanies their emotional experiences. Such emotional distress may increase the severity and occurrence of chest pain. Increased pain then results in increased emotional distress. Intermittent episodes of unexplained chest pain lasting many months or years can cause significant persistent distress and anxiety both in the patient and his or her family.

Anxiety

Anxiety is associated with chest pain in most cases [14]. Conversely, chest pain can be a manifestation of anxiety disorder. A significantly high percentage of patients with unexplained chest pain manifest anxiety symptoms. This finding is also consistent with the association of anxiety symptoms with other unexplained somatic symptoms such as headaches or abdominal pain.

Children may experience anxiety symptoms while being evaluated for chest pain, especially if cardiac cause is being considered [16]. Some investigators suggest that such anxiety symptoms may represent normative response in children; however, these symptoms can occur in association with other somatic symptoms [10, 14, 15]. Somatic symptoms should be evaluated to rule out any underlying organic cause.

McDonnell et al. [10] note that anxiety-related traits may influence a child's experience of chest pain. Thus, perception of bodily sensations may be potentially relevant to child's experience of chest pain. They further note that children and adolescents with noncardiac chest pain tend to have higher anxiety sensitivity. Anxiety sensitivity refers to the trait tendency to fear anxiety-related physiologic sensations [15].

The age and developmental stage of the child are relevant in how he or she interprets chest pain or perceives its significance. Young children may not associate chest pain with serious underlying condition. On the other hand, by early adolescence, the relationship between chest pain and potential serious health condition may be clearer to the adolescent [23].

Somatization

A significant number of children, adolescents, and adults who have unexplained chest pain also report other associated symptoms such as headaches, fatigue, dizziness, or abdominal pain. Children with such multiple somatic symptoms may or may not meet all criteria for somatoform disorder. The exact prevalence of somatization in children with chest pain is not known.

Stress

A psychosocial history is essential in the evaluation of patients who present with chest pain. Psychosocial stressors can be a primary cause or significantly contribute to chest pain. Reported psychosocial stressors in children can range from such events as separation from a parent, new school, or new teacher to more significant events such as death in the family, parental divorce, or death of a pet [10, 14, 16]. Because these events are common, some investigators question the significance of association between chest pain and such events. Not all individuals manifest similar responses to particular stressful events. Their own life experiences, coping mechanisms, and support systems may all influence their response to stressful events [23].

Treatment

Patients with chest pain that is attributable to functional causes can be treated in a number of non-pharmacologic ways including cognitive behavioral therapy (Chap. 9), hypnosis (Chap. 12), acupressure (Chap. 15), or meditation (Chap. 16). Pharmacologic therapy may be indicated on rare occasions (Chap. 14).

Case Studies

Case 1

An 18-year-old otherwise healthy female presents to emergency department with sudden onset of chest pain that is poorly localized and poorly characterized. She also reports her heart pounding, excessive sweating, shortness of breath, and lightheadedness. She thinks she is having a heart attack. Her past, family, personal, and social history is all unremarkable. A review of system is also unremarkable for any additional symptoms. She is alert, oriented, and anxious. Her vital signs are normal. Findings on electrocardiogram and a chest X-ray in the emergency department are normal.

Questions:

1. What is the likely diagnosis of this patient?
   (a) Acute myocardial infarction
   (b) Toxic inhalation
   (c) Panic attack
   (d) Munchausen's syndrome
   (e) None of the above
2. Symptoms in panic attack typically peak
   (a) Immediately after onset
   (b) Within 10 min of onset
   (c) After half an hour of onset
   (d) Gradually over an hour
   (e) Gradually over an extended period for 24 h
3. Symptoms of panic attack often first appear during
   (a) Early childhood
   (b) Early adolescence
   (c) Late adolescence
   (d) Young adulthood
   (e) Middle age

Answers:

1. (c): This patient is having a panic attack. Panic attack is characterized by sudden attacks of terror, usually accompanied by a pounding heart, sweatiness, weakness, faintness, or dizziness [32]. During these attacks, people with panic disorder may flush or feel chilled, their hands may tingle or feel numb, and they may experience nausea, chest pain, or smothering sensations [32]. Panic attacks usually produce a sense of unreality, a fear of impending doom, or a fear of losing control.

   A fear of one's own unexplained physical symptoms also is a symptom of panic attack. People having panic attacks sometimes believe they are having heart attacks, losing their minds, or on the verge of death [33]. They cannot predict when or where an attack will occur, and between episodes, many worry intensely and dread the next attack. Panic attacks can occur at any time, even during sleep.
2. (b): An attack usually peaks within 10 min, but some symptoms may last much longer.
3. (c): Panic attacks often begin in late adolescence or early adulthood. Many people have just one attack and never have another. The tendency to develop panic attacks appears to be inherited. People who have full-blown, repeated panic attacks can become very disabled by their condition and should seek treatment before they start to avoid places or situations where panic attacks have occurred [26]. For example, if a panic attack happened in an elevator, someone with panic disorder may develop a fear of elevators that could affect the choice of a job or an apartment and restrict where that person can seek medical attention or enjoy entertainment [26].

   Some people's lives become so restricted that they avoid normal activities, such as grocery shopping or driving. About one-third become housebound or are able to confront a feared situation only when accompanied by a spouse or other trusted person [26]. When the condition progresses this far, it is called agoraphobia or fear of open spaces.

Case 2

A 16-year-old female is seen again in the office for recurrent chest pain of mild severity, in the "middle of the chest," lasting for few minutes, resolving spontaneously, with no identified modifying factors. Similar episodes have occurred several times over the past 2 years, and she has missed several days of school because of chest pain. Every time she presents, she also reports multiple other different symptoms in addition to chest pain. These include headache, abdominal pain, painful and irregular menstrual periods, back pain, nausea, and feeling of lump in the throat. Because of persistent symptoms and anxiety both in the patient and her mother, over the past 2 years, she has undergone a thorough medical evaluation with all normal findings. She has been treated symptomatically with different medications in the past.

Questions:

1. What is the likely diagnosis of this patient?
   (a) Asthma
   (b) Gastroesophageal reflux
   (c) Reflex sympathetic dystrophy
   (d) Somatization disorder
   (e) Undisclosed history of physical trauma
2. Initial symptoms in somatization disorder are often first seen during
   (a) Early adolescence
   (b) Middle adolescence
   (c) Late adolescence
   (d) Young adulthood
   (e) Mid adulthood
3. Somatization disorder can be seen in what percentage of first degree relatives of women who have somatization disorder?
   (a) Less than 5%
   (b) Between 10% and 20%
   (c) Between 20% and 30%
   (d) Between 30% and 40%
   (e) More than 50%
4. Which of the following statements is true for somatization disorder?
   (a) Every person with a somatization disorder has a history of sexual abuse in childhood.
   (b) Emotional well-being affects the way in which people perceive pain.
   (c) Symptoms typically are mild and do not interfere with daily work or relationships.
   (d) Symptoms are not real, just "in a person's head."
   (e) Somatization disorder has acute onset self-limited course.

Answers:

1. (d): This patient has a somatization disorder. Somatization disorder is a long-term (chronic) condition in which a person has physical symptoms that involve more than one part of the body, but no physical cause can be found [33]. The pain and other symptoms people with this disorder feel are real and are not created or faked on purpose (malingering).
2. (c): Initial symptoms typically present by late adolescence.
3. (b): It is seen in 10–20% of female first-degree relatives of women who have somatization disorder [16].

Table 3.4 Partial list of symptoms that can occur with somatization disorder

• Abdominal pain
• Amnesia
• Back pain
• Bloating
• Chest pain
• Diarrhea
• Difficulty swallowing
• Dizziness
• Headaches
• Impotence
• Joint pain
• Nausea and sometimes vomiting
• Pain during intercourse
• Pain during urination
• Painful menstruation
• Pain in the legs or arms
• Palpitations
• Paralysis or muscle weakness
• Sexual apathy
• Shortness of breath
• Vision changes

4. (b): In the past, this disorder was thought to be related to emotional stress. The pain was dismissed as being "all in their head." However, patients who have a somatization disorder seem to experience pain or other symptoms in a way that increases the level of pain. Pain and worry create a cycle that is hard to break. People who have a history of physical or sexual abuse are more likely to have this disorder [33]. However, not every person with a somatization disorder has a history of abuse. There is more evidence that emotional well-being affects the way in which people perceive pain and other symptoms.

People with this disorder have many physical complaints that last for years. Most often, the complaints involve chronic pain and problems with the digestive system, nervous system, and reproductive system (Table 3.4) [26]. The symptoms often interfere with work and relationships and lead to many visits to different health-care providers. Stress often worsens the symptoms.

Conclusions

When a complete medical evaluation reveals no serious cause, persistence of chest pain can still be a source for ongoing concern and anxiety. A thorough history and physical examination are key elements of a diagnostic evaluation. In addition to organic causes of chest pain, psychological factors must be carefully considered in all patients who present with chest pain.

Acknowledgments The section on diagnosis is adapted with permission from [34].

References

1. Eslick GD. Epidemiology and risk factors of pediatric chest pain: a systematic review. Pediatr Clin North Am. 2010;57:1211–19.
2. Eslick GD. Classification, natural history, epidemiology, and risk factors of noncardiac chest pain. Dis Mon. 2008;54:593–603.
3. Driscoll DJ, Glicklich LB, Gallen WJ. Chest pain in children: a prospective study. Pediatrics. 1976;57:648–51.
4. Hambrook JT, Kimball TR, Khoury P, et al. Disparities exist in the emergency department evaluation of pediatric chest pain. Congenit Heart Dis. 2010;5:285–91.
5. Selbst SM, Ruddy RM, Clark BJ. Chest pain in children follow-up of patients previously reported. Clin Pediatr (Phila). 1990;297:374–7.
6. Ruigomez A, Rodriguez LA, Wallander MA, et al. Chest pain in general: incidence, comorbidity, and mortality. Fam Pract. 2007;8:51.
7. Buntix F, Knockaert D, Bruyninckx R, et al. Chest pain in general practice or in the hospital emergency room. Fam Pract. 2001;18(6):586–9.
8. Selbst SA. Approach to the child with chest pain. Pediatr Clin North Am. 2010;57:1221–34.
9. Cava JR, Sayger PL. Chest pain in children and adolescents. Pediatr Clin North Am. 2004;51:1553–68.
10. Lee TH. Chest pain and palpitations. In: Kasper DL, Braunwald E, Fauci AS, Hauser SL, Longo DL, Jameson JL, editors. Harrison's principles of internal medicine. 16th ed. New York: McGraw Hill Medical; 2005. p. 76–8.
11. Richter JE. Overview of diagnostic testing for chest pain of unknown origin. Am J Med. 1992;92(suppl 5A):41S–5S.
12. Bass C, Wade C. Chest pain with normal coronary arteries: a comparative study of psychiatric and social morbidity. Psychol Med. 1984;14:51–61.
13. McDonnell CJ, White KS. Assessment and treatment of psychological factors in pediatric chest pain. Pediatr Clin North Am. 2010;57:1235–60.
14. American Psychiatric Association. Diagnostic and statistical manual of mental disorders. Washington: American Psychiatric Association; 2000.
15. Martin AL, McGrath PA, Brown SC, et al. Anxiety sensitivity, fear of pain and pain-related disability in children and adolescents with chronic pain. Pain Res Manag. 2007;12:267–72.
16. Delamater A, Jent JF. Cardiovascular disease. In: Roberts MC, Steele RG, editors. Handbook of pediatric psychology. New York: Guilford Press; 2009. p. 381–91.
17. Filho AS, Maciel BC, Martin-Santos R, et al. Does the association between mitral valve prolapse and panic disorder really exist? Prim Care Companion J Clin Psychiatry. 2008;10:38–47.
18. Asnes RS, Santulli R, Bemporad JR. Psychogenic chest pain in children. Clin Pediatr (Phila). 1981;20:788–91.
19. Gilleland J, Blount RL, Campbell RM, et al. Brief report: psychosocial factors and pediatric noncardiac chest pain. J Pediatr Psychol. 2009;34:1170–4.
20. Kislal FM, Kutluk T, Cetin FC, et al. Psychiatric symptoms of adolescents with physical complaints admitted to an adolescence unit. Clin Pediatr. 2005;44:121–30.
21. Lipsitz JD, Masia C, Apfel H, et al. Noncardiac chest pain and psychopathology in children and adolescents. J Psychosom Res. 2005;59:185–8.
22. Lipsitz JD, Masia-Warner C, Apfel H, et al. Anxiety and depressive symptoms and anxiety sensitivity in youngsters with noncardiac chest pain and benign heart murmurs. J Pediatr Psychol. 2004;29:607–12.
23. Muris P, Hoeve I, Meesters C, et al. Children's perception and interpretation of anxiety-related physical symptoms. J Behav Ther Exp Psychiatry. 2004;35:233–44.
24. White KS. Assessment and treatment of psychological causes of chest pain. Med Clin North Am. 2010;94:291–318.
25. Masia-Warner C, Reigada LC, Fisher PH, et al. CBT for anxiety and associated somatic complaints in pediatric medical settings: an open pilot study. J Clin Psychol Med Settings. 2009;16:169–77.

26. Alpert MA, Mukerji V, Sabeti M, Russell JL, Beitman BD. Mitral valve prolapsed, panic disorder, and chest pain. Med Clin North Am. 1991;75:1119–33.
27. Boudoulas H, King BD, Wooley CF. Mitral valve prolapsed: a marker for anxiety or overlapping phenomenon? Psychopathology. 1984;17 suppl 1:98–106.
28. Boudoulas H, Reynolds JC, Mazzaferri E, Wooley CF. Metabolic studies in mitral valve prolapse syndrome. A neuroendocrine-cardiovascular process. Circulation. 1980;61(6):1200–5.
29. Lembo AJ. Visceral hypersensitivity in noncardiac chest pain. Gastroenterol Clin North Am. 2004;33(1):55–60.
30. Chahal PS, Rao SS. Functional chest pain: nociception and visceral hyperalgesia. J Clin Gastroenterol. 2005;39 suppl 3:S204–9.
31. Lee H, Kim JH, Min BH, et al. Efficacy of venlafaxine for symptomatic relief in young adult patients with functional chest pain: a randomized, double-blind, placebo-controlled, crossover trial. Am J Gastroenterol. 2010;105(7):1504–12.
32. Bradley LA, Richter JE, Scarinci IC, Haile JM, Schan CA. Psychological and psychophysical assessments of patients with unexplained chest pain. Am J Med. 1992;92(suppl 5A):65S–73S.
33. National Institutes of Mental Health. Anxiety Disorders. NIH Publication 09 3879. Washington: US Department of Health and Human Services; 2009. http://www.nimh.nih.gov/health/publications/anxiety-disorders/nimhanxiety.pdf
34. Homnick DN. Respiratory system. In: Greydanus DE, Feinberg A, Patel DR, Homnick DN, Reddy V, editors. The pediatric diagnostic examination. New York: McGraw Hill; 2008.

Chapter 4
Dyspnea

Douglas N. Homnick

Abstract Dyspnea, or shortness of breath, frequently accompanies cardiopulmonary disease in both pediatric and adult patients. However, the sensation of breathlessness can also accompany anxiety with somatic symptoms that are troublesome and sometimes disabling. Symptoms are often out of proportion to physical findings, test results often normal, and may decrease substantially when the patient is asleep or distracted. The most common presentations of functional dyspnea include vocal cord dysfunction, hyperventilation, sighing dyspnea, and overbreathing or hyperventilation during exercise. These symptoms are most often confused with poorly controlled asthma resulting in overtreatment with asthma medications, including corticosteroids. After a judicious workup for "organic" cardiopulmonary disease, specific testing may help differentiate these disorders. These include specialized cardiopulmonary testing, provocation tests, and standardized and validated questionnaires. Identification of functional dyspnea can then facilitate short-term intervention and/or psychological evaluation and treatment.

Keywords Dyspnea • Functional respiratory disorders • Hyperventilation • Sighing • Vocal cord dysfunction

Introduction

Dyspnea is defined as difficult or labored breathing or shortness of breath, and patients often complain that "I can't get enough air." The word is derived from the Greek "dys" meaning bad or difficult and "pnoia" meaning breathlessness.

D.N. Homnick (✉)
Department of Pediatrics, Michigan State University, Kalamazoo Center for Medical Studies, 1000 Oakland Drive, Kalamazoo, MI 49008, USA
e-mail: homnick@kcms.msu.edu

R.D. Anbar (ed.), *Functional Respiratory Disorders: When Respiratory Symptoms Do Not Respond to Pulmonary Treatment*, Respiratory Medicine,
DOI 10.1007/978-1-61779-857-3_4,

Dyspnea is often a nonspecific but troubling sensation prompting patients to readily and regularly seek medical help. Dyspnea represents a complex psychophysiologic sensation occurring in a variety of cardiorespiratory and metabolic disorders. It is expected in demonstrable cardiopulmonary disease, or normal with exertion during exercise, but when disproportionate to findings on the physical examination or the level of exertion, should lead the examiner to consider a functional etiology.

A careful history and physical examination and judicious laboratory testing are always indicated to rule out treatable "organic" causes of dyspnea or to rule in those of psychogenic or functional etiologies. The physical examination usually will not reveal specific abnormalities in patients with functional dyspnea except for rapid and deep respirations during an acute episode. Of considerable more difficulty is diagnosing chronic dyspnea as a subtle increase in breathing frequency that may not be as evident (see testing below) and the complaint of the patient may be simply that of air hunger.

Acute, psychogenic, or functional dyspnea usually resolves within minutes without specific therapy, in contrast to that associated with cardiopulmonary or metabolic disease. Functional causes of dyspnea, classified as dysfunctional breathing disorders, are clinically evident with observable deep and rapid respirations, noisy breathing, or are simply perceived by the patient. These include vocal cord dysfunction (VCD), hyperventilation (often associated with panic attack/disorder), and those conditions probably related to hyperventilation, including sighing dyspnea, and some exertional dyspnea [1]. VCD is a common cause of functional dyspnea, particularly in, but not limited to, adolescents. This condition is thoroughly discussed in Chap. 6 and will not be reviewed here. The other conditions are discussed below with illustrative cases.

Hyperventilation

Hyperventilation is defined as respirations in excess of metabolic demands and is often, but not invariable, associated with reduction in arterial pCO_2 ($PaCO_2$) with subsequent increase in pH (alkalosis). It can occur chronically or in response to a provoking stimulus such as sudden fright or other acute stressor. It was originally described associated with tetany in 1922 by Goldman [2] and later as the hyperventilation syndrome associated with anxiety by Kerr [3] in 1937. The exact prevalence of hyperventilation is unknown but thought to occur in 6–10% of adults [4–6]. Even less is known about the prevalence of dyspnea associated with hyperventilation in children; however, the age distribution suggests it is more common in adolescence. Enzer and Walker [7] reviewed the records of 44 children and adolescents admitted to the hospital with symptoms associated with hyperventilation. The majority were greater than 12 years (range 5–16) with a 2:1 female ratio (Fig. 4.1). In another study of children and adolescents with hyperventilation, 53% of patients were between 13 and 15 years with an equal gender distribution [8]. It is most frequently

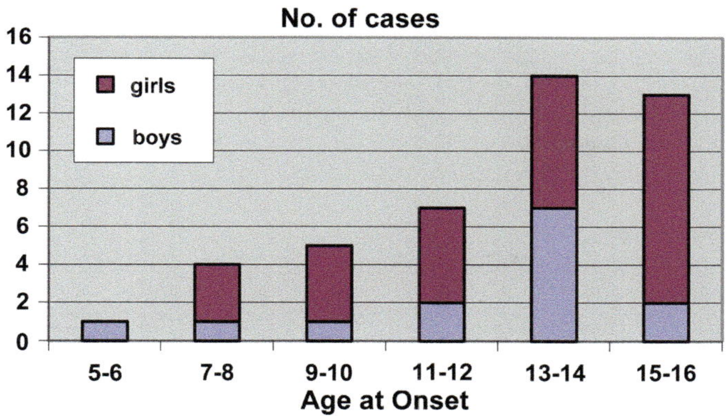

Fig. 4.1 Age and gender distribution of children and youth presenting with hyperventilation Reprinted from [1]. With permission from Elsevier

misdiagnosed as acute or chronic asthma leading to ineffective treatment with asthma medications. However, asthma as a trigger for hyperventilation or vice versa occurs, particularly when mild asthma is undiagnosed [9].

Relationship to Anxiety or Other Psychological Disturbance

The relationship of hyperventilation to psychological states is well established. Of the 44 children and adolescents that Enzer and Walker [7] reviewed, 23 were referred for psychiatric evaluation. Of these, 13 were diagnosed with anxiety disorder, 3 with depression, 1 with psychosis, 4 with conversion reaction, and 2 refused the referral. Issues over sexuality were the most common factors in these conditions. This is also true in adults. In another study, 50% of patients with symptomatic hyperventilation were described as suffering from psychiatric disturbance characterized by anxiety, panic, and phobic symptoms [10]. Hyperventilation has significant overlap rates with known psychiatric conditions. De Ruiter et al. [11] found hyperventilation rates of 48% among patients with panic disorder, 83% for panic disorder with agoraphobia, and 82% with generalized anxiety disorder.

This has spawned debate as to the very existence of the hyperventilation syndrome or whether hyperventilation is a symptom [12–18]. Those believing hyperventilation is a symptom of an underlying psychological disturbance point out the similarity of symptoms to panic attacks (Table 4.1). Also, symptoms of hyperventilation such as chest tightness or discomfort, paresthesias, dizziness, blurred vision, rapid heart rate, sweating, and confusion or feelings of unreality may be reproduced with a stressful mental load without hypocapnia [20]. They also may be reproduced in susceptible individuals during voluntary hyperventilation while maintaining normocapnia. Also patients who experience panic attacks at home show little decrease in transcutaneous CO_2 levels ($tcCO_2$) [15].

Table 4.1 Criteria for panic attack

Note: A panic attack is not a codable disorder. Code the specific diagnosis in which the panic attack occurs (e.g., 300.21 panic disorder with agoraphobia [p. 441])
A discrete period of intense fear or discomfort, in which four (or more) of the following symptoms developed abruptly and reached a peak within 10 min:
(1) Palpitations, pound heart, or accelerated heart rate
(2) Sweating
(3) Trembling or shaking
(4) Sensations of shortness of breath or smothering
(5) Feeling of choking
(6) Chest pain or discomfort
(7) Nausea or abdominal distress
(8) Feeling dizzy, unsteady, light-headed, or faint
(9) Derealization (feelings of unreality) or depersonalization (being detached from oneself)
(10) Fear of losing control or going crazy
(11) Fear of dying
(12) Paresthesias (numbness or tingling sensations)
(13) Chills or hot flashes

Reprinted with permission from [19] (Copyright © 2000)

That is not to say that the symptoms associated with hyperventilation do not have physiological explanations. When hypocapnic alkalosis occurs, the symptom of derealization may be due to hypocapnic-induced decrease in cerebral blood flow and paresthesias can occur as a result of increased neuronal excitability [21, 22]. Chest wall pain and discomfort may be due to hypocapnia-induced chest wall muscle spasm, esophageal spasm, or gastroesophageal reflux disease [23, 24].

Clinical

As dyspnea is a common presenting sign of significant cardiopulmonary or metabolic disease (Table 4.2), the clinician must be cautious in making a diagnosis of functional disease. A complete and careful history can often hone the differential diagnosis and provide for judicious testing. Functional respiratory disorders are often diagnosed as asthma, and overtreatment and ineffective treatment are common. However, dysfunctional breathing and asthma are not mutually exclusive, and, in one study, 29% of adults with asthma screened positively for hyperventilation versus 8% of those without asthma [6]. Niggemann [25] points out several important questions that can help differentiate "organic" from functional respiratory disease (Table 4.3). In a child or teen with a functional respiratory disorder, the possibility of child sexual or physical abuse should always be considered [26].

The physical examination may reveal an anxious and distracted patient and abnormalities in depth of respirations, and breathing frequency and use of accessory

Table 4.2 Causes of dyspnea

Upper airway
• Obstruction foreign body
• Angioedema
• Epiglottitis
• Diphtheria
• Bacterial tracheitis
• Tonsillar abscess
Lower airway
• Asthma
• Pneumonia
• Croup (laryngotracheobronchitis)
• Bronchiolitis
• Pulmonary contusion
• Adult respiratory distress syndrome
• Infant respiratory distress syndrome
• Chronic obstructive pulmonary disease
• Cystic fibrosis
• Pneumoconiosis
• Interstitial lung disease
• Hypersensitivity pneumonitis
• Thermal trauma
Chest
• Pneumothorax
• Pleural effusion, hemothorax, empyema
• Trauma
– Rib fractures
– Flail chest
Congenital thoracic malformations
Diaphragmatic hernia
Cardiac
• Congestive cardiac failure
• Acute pulmonary edema
• Acute myocardial infarction
• Cardiac arrhythmias
Congenital heart disease
Vascular
• Pulmonary embolus
• Pulmonary hypertension
Arteriovenous malformation
Others
• Psychogenic hyperventilation (panic)
• Toxigenic, e.g., carbon monoxide, cyanide, salicylates
• Metabolic acidosis
• Anemia

muscles are important signs. Careful chest and neck examination and auscultation are important, as is the examination of the nose for signs of nasal obstruction. A careful neurologic examination may reveal hyperreflexia associated with anxiety, and skin evaluation can demonstrate hyperhidrosis or self-mutilation.

Table 4.3 History that suggests a functional breathing disorder

Question	Response
How do you exactly characterize your symptoms?	e.g., during inspiration and/or expiration, being out of breath, heavy breathing, dyspnea, pain, etc.; the wording of patients is often consistent, different from organic complaints, and may already allow an assignment
Can any breath sounds be heard during the episodes?	e.g., wheezing, stridor, or no breath sounds at all; can bystanders hear it? Usually, no specific sounds can be heard by the surroundings, except in VCD
Is there a typical time point during the day? Circadian rhythm?	e.g., daytimes or at night, morning, evening, or at any time; usually there is no defined time of the day
Do you awake at night because of the symptoms?	Asking for "symptoms at night" is not exactly enough, because many patients exhibit symptoms when lying in bed but still awake, but not during sleep; this question is one of the most important ones and allows differentiation to at least bronchial hyperreactivity and asthma, which mostly show nocturnal symptoms
Did the symptoms start in the context of a respiratory tract infection? Or after any other event?	Especially psychogenic cough and throat clearing mostly start with a common cold or bronchitis, then patients lower the threshold to cough, and finally they cough without any "reason." Other causes include psychological events such as divorce of parents
What typically acts as a trigger?	e.g., physical exercise—although this can occur both with organic and psychogenic or functional disorders, psychosocial stress, etc., or no typical trigger factors at all
Are sport activities possible or limited?	e.g., usual sport lessons at school, private sporting activities in sporting associations; sport sometimes possible, sometimes not?
How long do episodes last?	e.g., minimum, maximum duration; average in seconds, minutes, or hours; very variable duration?
How long does it take you to recover?	While asthmatic symptoms usually resolve within 10–20 min, psychogenic dyspnea may disappear within only a few minutes
Do you suffer from the symptoms?	e.g., in psychogenic cough, the surrounding (such as teachers, schoolmates, or family) suffers more than the patients; do the surroundings develop even aggressive feelings?
Where is the feeling of breathing difficulty localized?	e.g., let the patient localize with one finger; roughly, psychogenic dyspnea is more often located to the throat than thorax
Did you get any medications for your symptoms? Were they effective? To what extent?	e.g., antiasthmatic therapy in forms of short-acting beta-agonists or inhaled corticosteroids; usually, there is no or only little improvement by drugs, except from the placebo effect strength
Did you ever have clinical signs such as tingling of lips or fingers?	e.g., if hyperventilation is suspected

(continued)

Table 4.3 (continued)

Question	Response
Are there any other tics?	e.g., blinking or throat clearing tic; often, tic disorders occur combined, which strengthen a positive diagnosis if reported or observed
Do parents think they have a healthy or ill child?	In most cases, parents will state that they have a healthy child—if symptoms are absent at present

Adapted from [26]. With permission from John Wiley & Sons, Inc.

The history and physical examination will drive the subsequent laboratory evaluation. Useful laboratory tests include complete pulmonary functions; a metabolic stress test using the bicycle ergometer; bronchoprovocation with methacholine or exercise; an electrocardiogram; metabolic serum analysis including pH, electrolytes, and calcium; thyroid screen; blood glucose; blood gas; and chest X-ray. Referral to a pulmonary specialist can be useful to help efficiently determine, direct, and evaluate the workup as well as reinforce a functional diagnosis. An appropriate workup that is negative can help support reassurance as therapy (see therapy below).

Specific Testing for Hyperventilation

Tests for the presence of hyperventilation are important particularly with the chronic form where symptoms may not be readily apparent and there is a need to corroborate historical information. These tests generally fall into the categories of standardized questionnaires, provocative tests, and specialized pulmonary evaluations. The Nijmegen questionnaire (Table 4.4) is a useful tool with reasonable sensitivity and specificity for diagnosing hyperventilation [28]. It consists of 16 questions concerning symptoms of hyperventilation (and indeed panic attack), each ranging from 0 (never) to 4 (very often). A score of greater than 23/64 indicates a diagnosis of hyperventilation. An 86% concordance was found between a positive score on the Nijmegen questionnaire and symptom reproduction during the hyperventilation provocation test (HVPT).

The HVPT is a test designed to bring out symptoms of hyperventilation in those with intermittent or subclinical symptoms and assumes that these are triggered by the hypocapnia accompanying overbreathing. In the office, the test consists of 3 min of preparatory rest followed by 3 min of forced overbreathing followed by 3 min of rest. The patients are then asked if they experienced the same symptoms encountered in daily life. A more quantitative variation of this measures end-tidal carbon dioxide levels ($ETCO_2$) during the test in order to gain additional physiologic information. Lower $ETCO_2$ values occur at rest during chronic hyperventilation, and there is a delay in recovery of lowered pCO_2 after voluntary overbreathing [27, 29].

Table 4.4 The Nijmegen questionnaire—a score over 23/64 indicates hyperventilation

Symptoms	Never 0	Rarely 1	Sometimes 2	Often 3	Very often 4
Chest pain					
Feeling tense					
Blurred vision					
Dizzy spells					
Feeling confused					
Faster or deeper breathing					
Short of breath					
Tight feelings in chest					
Bloated feeling in stomach					
Tingling fingers					
Unable to breathe deeply					
Stiff fingers or arms					
Tight feelings around mouth					
Cold hands or feet					
Palpitations					
Feeling of anxiety					

Reprinted from [27]. With permission from Elsevier

The HVPT has been long held to be the gold standard of tests designed to reproduce the symptoms of and therefore diagnose hyperventilation. However, its sensitivity and specificity to determine whether symptoms occur as a result of hypocapnic alkalosis or the stress of the procedure has been called into question. Hornsveld et al. [30] studied 115 patients with suspected hyperventilation in terms of their ability to recognize symptoms during a HVPT versus a placebo test consisting of isocapnic overbreathing. Thirty patients with a positive HVPT then underwent ambulatory $tcCO_2$ monitoring to determine hyperventilation during spontaneous symptom attacks at home. Of the 115 patients, 85 (74%) reported symptoms during the HVPT. However, 56 of those also reported symptoms during isocapnic overbreathing (false positive), while 29 did not report symptoms under this condition (true positive). Fifteen false-positive and 15 true-positive patients underwent the home $tcCO_2$ monitoring and experienced 22 symptom attacks. $tcCO_2$ decreased in only 7, was slight, and followed the onset of hyperventilation, suggesting that hyperventilation was a consequence rather than cause of the symptoms. In another study, patients with hyperventilation symptoms underwent a HVPT and a mental load task [20]. About the same number of patients recognized symptoms during the mental load (52%) versus the HVPT (61%). Both HVPT and a mental load (word-color conflict test) with measurement of $ETCO_2$ have been shown to have some usefulness in discriminating patients with asthma-like symptoms associated with negative tests for asthma and hyperventilation from true asthmatics [31]. Although the HVPT is theoretically a quick and easy test to do in the office, in our pediatric pulmonology clinic, we have often found it difficult for young patients to complete with accompanying emotional breakdown and tears.

Other provocation tests have been proposed including responses to exercise, as hyperventilation is often provoked by exercise (also see exertional dyspnea below). Kinnula and Sovijarvi [32] measured ventilatory parameters including ventilatory equivalents for oxygen (volume expired [VE]/volume oxygen consumed [VO_2] or VE/VO_2) and carbon dioxide (VE/volume carbon dioxide produced [VCO_2] or VE/VCO_2) in order to determine wasted ventilation during overbreathing (in excess of metabolic needs) while undergoing maximal bicycle exercise and collecting expired gases in adults with previously diagnosed hyperventilation and normal controls. They found that ventilatory equivalents for both O_2 and CO_2 were significantly higher in hyperventilation patients than in controls at most work levels. A significant negative correlation is also found between $PaCO_2$ and the ventilatory equivalents at both light and maximal exercises. However, ventilatory equivalents as a diagnostic tool for hyperventilation have not been systematically studied in children and adolescents.

Conditions Representing Variations of Hyperventilation

Sighing Dyspnea

Sighing is a normal physiological function that prevents alveolar collapse due to early airway closure at low lung volumes during normal tidal respirations. It is represented by periodic deeper than normal inspirations followed by prolonged expirations, not associated with increased respiratory rate, but sometimes with use of accessory respiratory muscles [26, 33, 34]. It is also a normal consequence of emotional states such as anxiety. It becomes a problem when it is distressing to the patient and/or his/her family and disruptive of normal social interaction. Frequent sighing respirations were described in the early literature of "effort syndrome" which was later termed the hyperventilation syndrome [35]. Less has been studied and written about this probable variation of hyperventilation, and therefore, the epidemiology is less clear. It is said to be more common in women between the second and fourth decade but has been also described in adolescents, and it is not uncommonly seen in a pediatric pulmonary clinic [36, 37].

Clinical

As with hyperventilation, a thorough history and physical examination is important to rule out other cardiopulmonary or metabolic conditions and eliminate "organic" causes of dyspnea including asthma. These can include pulmonary function testing, bronchial challenge with methacholine, chest X-ray, serum pH, glucose, electrolytes, and a thyroid screen.

A frequent complaint is that of a sense of suffocation accompanied by a feeling of chest restriction or heaviness [37]. The patient may undertake environmental manipulation such as running to an open window in an attempt to "get enough air" [34]. As with other functional respiratory disorders, a history of life stressors should be sought.

The typical patient presents with a series of deep, sighing respirations with normal respiratory frequency, often using accessory muscles. When distracted, the sighing may decrease spontaneously and when faced with a stressful situation becomes more frequent and pronounced. Although sighing dyspnea has been described most commonly associated with psychological stress, including anxiety, this has not been invariable. Wong et al. [33] showed similar personality profiles in children with sighing dyspnea as compared to normal children in terms of anxiety, somatic complaints, and internalizing behavior.

Testing for Sighing Dyspnea

There are no physiological tests that distinguish sighing dyspnea, and the laboratory workup is the same as for hyperventilation. Inconsistent pulmonary function abnormalities have been described including higher residual volume (RV) and residual volume to total lung capacity (TLC) ratio (RV/TLC%) but with normal TLC and functional residual capacity (FRC) measured with the body plethysmograph [38]. Aljadeff et al. [39] showed normal TLC and increased RV in adults with sighing dyspnea. In another study, office spirometry was normal in children with sighing dyspnea [33]. The significance of these pulmonary function findings is unknown. With treatment, including simple reassurance, the prognosis appears to be good for this condition.

Exertional Dyspnea

Dyspnea with exercise is often an early manifestation of cardiopulmonary disease including both restrictive and obstructive pulmonary disease. In healthy children and adolescents, exercise-induced dyspnea is most commonly thought to be associated with exercise-induced asthma [40]. It is also present when patients are poorly conditioned for the attempted activity and frequently accompanies obesity. When symptoms are out of proportion to the patient's level of conditioning and the history, physical examination, and appropriate testing do not suggest an underlying cardiopulmonary disorder, a functional respiratory diagnosis should be considered. These include VCD and exercise-induced hyperventilation. VCD is extensively discussed in Chap. 6.

Clinical

A typical presentation of exercise-induced hyperventilation (EIHV) as a functional cause of exertional dyspnea consists of often abrupt onset of shortness of breath associated with a sense of extreme air hunger occurring much earlier in exercise than one would expect based on the patient's level of conditioning. The patient appears anxious but can talk through the episode and may have associated symptoms such as paresthesias of the extremities, light-headedness or dizziness, a sensation of being hot or cold, diaphoresis, and chest discomfort, among others. If stridor or wheezing is heard, another functional or "organic" diagnosis needs to be considered. Typically, the episode resolves quickly with rest but reoccurs with new onset of activity. As performance anxiety may drive the symptoms, these may occur more commonly or severely with competition rather than practice. Upon careful history taking, other somatic complaints may be elicited and other psychological dysfunction or trauma uncovered. A family pattern of anxiety-associated symptoms may be present.

The physical examination is generally normal, although the patient may show signs of anxiety such as hyperreflexia, sinus tachycardia, or hyperhidrosis. Other causes of cardiopulmonary or metabolic diseases, as outlined in Table 4.2, should be considered based on the history and physical examination before making a functional diagnosis.

Testing for Exercise-Induced Functional Dyspnea

Exercise testing with or without measurement of expired gases is useful in trying to discriminate those with underlying physiologic abnormalities associated with dyspnea and normal physiologic limitation. Abu-Hassan et al. [40] reviewed the records of 142 children and adolescents (6–21 years) referred to a pediatric pulmonary clinic for exercise-induced dyspnea to determine the etiologies of the exercise-induced dyspnea with no signs and symptoms of asthma and no response to inhaled beta-adrenergic agents. Ninety-eight had had a primary diagnosis of exercise-induced asthma (EIA) made by their referring provider. During exercise testing, symptoms of dyspnea were reproduced in 117. However, only 11 (8%) had evidence of EIA defined by a decrease on forced expiratory volume over 1 s (FEV_1) of at least 15%. Seventy-four patients (52%) had normal physiological limitations, 15 (11%) had restrictive pulmonary function due to minor thoracic cage abnormalities, 13 (9%) had VCD, 2 (1%) had exercise-induced laryngomalacia, and one patient demonstrated exercise-induced primary hyperventilation (EIHV). Selecting patients for chest discomfort (frequently associated with hyperventilation/panic) and no evidence of exercise-induced decrease in FEV_1 appears to be more selective in diagnosing EIHV. Hammo [41] studied 32 patients (8–18 years) presenting to their pediatric pulmonary clinic with a history of EIA and chest discomfort with exercise. Patients underwent treadmill exercise with monitoring of $ETCO_2$, oxygen saturation

(SPO_2), and postexercise spirometry. Eleven patients experienced chest discomfort during the test with minimal decrease in SPO_2 and spirometry. However, this group showed an average decrease in $ETCO_2$ of 23% versus 9.8% for the rest of the group (17 with no reproducible symptoms and no significant drop in FEV_1 and 4 diagnosed with EIA).

The value of measuring $ETCO_2$ during exercise testing for cardiopulmonary disease has also been shown in adults with typical and atypical chest pain [42]. Among a group of 113 adults with exercise-induced chest pain, 92 did not show significant ST depression, i.e., evidence of coronary artery disease. These were divided in a group ($n=30$) with history compatible with hyperventilation and without ($n=62$). Hypocapnia was demonstrated in 21/30 of those with a positive history of hyperventilation, but also in 25/62 of the negative history group. Hypocapnia also occurred in 3 patients with ST depression and in one control. Fourteen of the 49 patients also had borderline or mild reductions in postexercise peak flow measurements. The authors felt that measurement of $ETCO_2$ as an adjunct to cardiopulmonary exercise testing was a useful tool to assess symptoms associated with hyperventilation. They also felt that mild lung disease may also be responsible for triggering overbreathing during exercise in some subjects.

Ventilatory equivalents during exercise testing have been used as a provocative test to differentiate those patients who hyperventilate versus normal controls (see specific testing for hyperventilation above) [32]. However, they have also been used to assess the relationship between mild lung disease and hyperventilation. Twenty-two mild asthmatics (11 males, 11 females), 11 patients with hyperventilation, and 22 (11 males, 11 females) controls underwent exercise testing with gas exchange measurement [43]. VE/VO_2 and VE/VCO_2 were no different between the controls and mild male asthmatics but were significantly elevated in those previously determined to hyperventilate and in female asthmatics. Although postexercise spirometry was positive in 50% of asthmatics (>15% decrease), it did not correlate with the ventilatory equivalents. From this study, exercise-induced hyperventilation in female mild asthmatics did not appear to be related to EIA, although there was no immediate explanation for this other than possible psychological factors. Of note is a similar female preponderance in hyperventilation without asthma.

Specific Treatment for Functional Dyspnea

Treatment for functional dyspnea is generally the same as for other functional respiratory disorders and is outlined in detail in several chapters of this text. Several specific treatments for functional dyspnea have been studied, and some are discussed below. Our general approach to psychological evaluation and treatment of patients with any functional disorder is outlined in Table 4.5. This approach including psychological testing has not infrequently uncovered psychological disturbance requiring further intervention as in case #1 presented below.

Table 4.5 Psychological evaluation and treatment of functional disorders

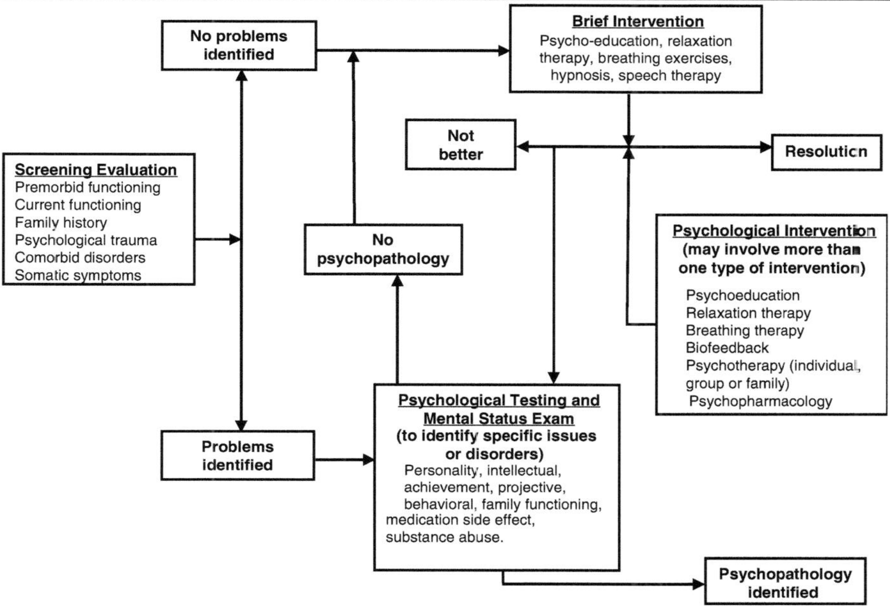

Reprinted from [28]. With permission from Elsevier

Although not well documented in the medical literature, patients have traditionally used a paper bag for rebreathing during an acute episode of hyperventilation. Although, in theory, this can reduce hypocapnia in association with the hyperventilation, it also offers the opportunity for the patient to observe the depth and frequency of their respirations in order to make a conscious effort to slow them. Suggestion and expectation of relief of symptoms also has been shown to be a factor in bag rebreathing under experimental conditions [44]. However, bag rebreathing also has some risks. Callaham [45] reported three cases where bag rebreathing erroneously applied to patients with myocardial ischemia resulted in death. A subsequent experiment in normal volunteers showed significant hypoxia associated with hypercapnia in some individuals depending on length of rebreathing therapy.

Simple reassurance has also been used successfully to relieve symptoms of hyperventilation. In the case study of Enzer and Walker [7], reassurance was stated as the primary treatment, although all patients employed bag rebreathing to abort acute attacks. Nine of the 44 subjects studied also receive sedative medications for varying period of times, and several underwent cognitive-behavioral therapy. Extensive discussions of cognitive-behavioral and pharmacologic therapies are found in Chaps. 9 and 14.

Acupuncture has also been shown to be an effective treatment for hyperventilation in one study. In a pilot, randomized, crossover trial of 4 weeks of acupuncture therapy versus breathing retraining, Gibson et al. [46] showed a statistically significant decrease in Nijmegen scores and in the Hospital Anxiety and Depression

Scale in subjects with hyperventilation. Use of acupressure may yield similar benefit (Chap. 15).

Self-hypnosis has also been shown to be effective in reducing chronic dyspnea in children and teens (Chap. 12). Anbar [47] studied 17 youths (ages 8–18) who were taught hypnotic self-induction techniques and imagery related to their dyspnea. Sixteen of the patients had resolution or improvement of their symptoms within one month of practicing the techniques and experienced no recurrences during follow-up of up to 15 months.

Others have used biofeedback, breathing techniques, and breathing retraining to reduce or eliminate functional dyspnea associated with panic attacks/disorder [48–50]. Biofeedback, breathing techniques, and speech therapy techniques are thoroughly reviewed in Chaps. 10, 11, and 13.

Case Studies

Case 1

YS is a 14-year-old girl seen in emergency department for severe respiratory distress. This included rapid and deep respirations with slight increase in respiratory rate, chest pressure, blurring of vision, headache, diaphoresis, rapid heart rate, and normal cardiopulmonary auscultation. She is able to verbally describe her symptoms during an episode. This is the third trip to the emergency department in 2 months. Workup in the ED has included an electrocardiogram, electroencephalogram, computerized tomography of her head, serum electrolytes, bicarbonate, calcium, magnesium, thyroid screen, sedimentation rate, arterial blood gas, and chest X-ray. The ED workup has been negative except for a slightly abnormal ABG showing pH 7.51, pCO_2 32, and pO_2 99 in room air.

Further history shows that these episodes have occurred spontaneously: once during Spanish class, twice while home alone in the afternoon after school, and never at night. YS was able to call a neighbor and subsequently her mother for the two episodes at home and was transported by paramedics all three times. She also complains of frequent headaches and stomach aches and has had other episodes of shortness of breath which she has been able to relieve by sitting in front of a fan. She has not responded to albuterol prescribed in the ED and, in fact, states that the inhaler makes her shaky and more short of breath. The exam in the office is normal except for mild tachycardia, mild diaphoresis, and slightly increased respiratory rate. She appears anxious and complains of shortness of breath during the examination, but her respiratory rate is normal and there is no clinical evidence of respiratory distress. Spirometry is normal.

You obtain further history that reveals she is missing school at least 1 day per week because of headache and stomach ache. The history and workup suggests a functional respiratory disorder and she is referred to psychology for evaluation. During the subsequent psychological testing and interview, it is revealed that she has been the victim of bullying at school that has been going on for about 6 months. The testing is suggestive of an ongoing anxiety disorder.

Questions:

1. Items from the medical history that would suggest a functional respiratory disorder include which of the following:
   (a) Symptoms are not occurring at night.
   (b) Urgent, repeated visits to the emergency department.
   (c) She is able to verbalize her symptoms during an episode of respiratory distress.
   (d) a and c.
   (e) a, b, and c.
2. The arterial blood gas done in the emergency department probably represents which of the following conditions:
   (a) Acidosis secondary to renal disease
   (b) Undiagnosed bulimia
   (c) Chronic hyperventilation
   (d) Acute airway obstruction
   (e) Acute hyperventilation
3. From the history, clinical presentation, and psychological evaluation, the most likely diagnosis is dyspnea secondary to:
   (a) Schizophrenia
   (b) Hypercarbia
   (c) Panic attack/disorder with hyperventilation
   (d) Hyperventilation syndrome
   (e) None of the above

Answers:

1. (d): The majority of patients with functional causes of dyspnea demonstrate disappearance of their symptoms during sleep and during the day when distracted. They are also able to talk through an episode where patients with "organic" causes of dyspnea such as acute asthma are not able to verbalize more than a word or two at a time. Repeated ED visits occur with acute "attacks" of anxiety-driven functional disorders as well as true cardiorespiratory disease.
2. (e): A mild, uncompensated respiratory alkalosis is not unusual in a recovering acute episode of hyperventilation. The workup in the ED is negative, and the patient's symptoms resolve spontaneously. Additionally, there has been no airway noise detected during the examination and no response to albuterol, suggesting the absence of acute airway obstruction. Normal electrolytes are against renal

disease or bulimia, and blood gases in chronic hyperventilation are usually normal or show a mild compensated respiratory alkalosis.
3. (c): Hyperventilation is a sign with symptoms most consistent with panic attack often as part of panic disorder or chronic anxiety; although controversial, it is now thought not to be a distinct syndrome. Bullying has likely led to the anxiety disorder with understandable school phobia as psychological testing has not shown evidence of psychosis. Hypercarbia is a result of *under*ventilation.

Case 2

AJ is a 15-year-old boy brought to your office for evaluation by his mother with the complaint that he feels that "he can't get enough air." This consists of intermittent deep sighing respirations occurring up to 20 per minute, lasting for several minutes and occurring up to ten times per day or more, and beginning about one month before his visit. He appears distressed during these episodes, uses accessory respiratory muscles, complains of chest heaviness, and often becomes light-headed. Turning a fan on and sitting in its stream or going outside house for a few minutes helps relieve the symptoms, which eventually resolve spontaneously. He makes no respiratory noises during the episodes, and intermittent use of an inhaled beta-adrenergic inhaler has only made him "shaky." His past medical history is generally unremarkable except for frequent "migraine" headaches and occasional stomach aches. His physical examination and spirometry are normal. He demonstrates occasional deep sighs during the examination. Of note in the social history is the death 1 year ago of his father, recent decrease in his academic performance, and frequent missed days of school due to his breathing problems.

Subsequent workup including a chest X-ray, metabolic screen, drug screen, and complete pulmonary functions is normal.

Questions:

1. AJ's symptoms are most consistent with which of the following condition:
   (a) Metabolic acidosis
   (b) Sighing dyspnea
   (c) Vocal cord dysfunction
   (d) Asthma
   (e) None of the above
2. True statements about this condition include all of the following EXCEPT:
   (a) Pulmonary functions can reliably diagnose this condition.
   (b) Most patients with this condition have underlying anxiety.
   (c) Manipulation of the environment is a typical finding.
   (d) With treatment, the prognosis is good.
   (e) Patients may have other somatic complaints.

Answers:

1. (b): Sighing dyspnea. A normal metabolic screen and intermittent increased respiratory distress are inconsistent with a metabolic acidosis such as might occur in diabetic ketoacidosis. Normal pulmonary functions and lack of noise during breathing and normal auscultation would be against VCD. Normal lung functions and lack of response to a short-acting beta-adrenergic inhaler make asthma unlikely.
2. (a): It is true that most patients with sighing dyspnea have underlying anxiety and they may also manipulate the environment by, for example, sitting in front of a fan or running to an open window to help relieve their symptoms. The prognosis appears to be good in this condition. There are no consistent pulmonary function abnormalities found.

Case 3

LW is a 16-year-old girl who comes to the office with mother complaining of shortness of breath associated with her extensive sports activities. LW, a straight A student, plays varsity soccer on the high school team and is also involved in club soccer with an extensive travel schedule. She has attained a high level of skill and is anticipating being recruited by colleges after high school.

However, during this season, she has periodically experienced acute shortness of breath occurring about 10 min into play and worse during games versus practices. Her primary physician suspects exercise-induced bronchospasm, but she has had no relief using a short-acting beta-adrenergic agent prior to exercise or with symptom onset, with daily use of an inhaled corticosteroid and a leukotriene modifier. Her episodes come on quickly; she complains of light-headedness, tingling in her hands and feet, and chest discomfort. These disappear within a few minutes after stopping her activity, although upon resumption of the activity, the symptoms often return. Both her coach and mother have observed these episodes, and other than deep, rapid breathing, no respiratory noise or other symptoms have been noticed. Her examination in the office is entirely normal except from some hyperhidrosis of the palms. Spirometry done in the office is normal.

Questions:

1. The clinical history and signs are compatible with?
   - (a) Vocal cord dysfunction
   - (b) Poorly controlled and undiagnosed exercise-induced asthma
   - (c) Exercise-induced tracheomalacia
   - (d) Hyperventilation
   - (e) All of the above

2. What additional history would be useful in helping differentiate a functional respiratory disorder from an "organic" disorder?
   (a) Do symptoms occur at times other than exercise?
   (b) Is there a history of stomach or headache complaints?
   (c) Have there been any family disruptions, i.e., divorces, new babies, family illnesses, deaths, etc.?
   (d) b and c
   (e) All of the above
3. What test(s) would be most useful to utilize first in distinguishing functional respiratory disorder from an "organic" disorder?
   (a) Flexible bronchoscopy
   (b) Flexible bronchoscopy while undergoing exercise testing on a treadmill
   (c) Cardiorespiratory metabolic testing on a bicycle ergometer
   (d) Simple exercise testing on a treadmill with cardiac monitoring and postexercise spirometry
   (e) Complete lung functions

Answers:

1. (d): Patients with acute upper airway obstruction due to VCD or lower airway obstruction due to tracheomalacia will often demonstrate noisy breathing, i.e., inspiratory stridor or expiratory, monophonic wheezing. Undiagnosed exercise-induced asthma is most often a feature of poorly controlled persistent asthma and, assuming good adherence to therapy, should get better. The fact that there is no noisy breathing and the symptoms resolve within minutes suggests a functional respiratory disorder other than VCD, most likely overbreathing due to performance anxiety. Complete lung functions without a challenge of exercise are often unrevealing unless significant "organic" disease is present.
2. (e): All of the above pieces of historical information can lead the examiner in the direction of a functional respiratory disorder as all are compatible with anxiety or other psychological disturbance. Similar symptoms occurring at times other than exercise as during test taking in school, etc., strongly point to a functional etiology.
3. (d): The simplest and most comprehensive way to screen for cardiorespiratory disease due to an "organic" etiology is exercise testing on a treadmill with cardiac monitoring and postexercise spirometry. The pattern of the flow volume loop and ratios of inspiratory to expiratory flows can distinguish between exercise-induced upper airway obstruction and lower airway bronchoconstriction (see Chap. 6). Also, when deep and frequent respirations out of proportion to level of conditioning and amount of work are observed during the test, this can be helpful in making a functional diagnosis.

Conclusions

Functional dyspnea is represented by VCD, acute and chronic hyperventilation, sighing dyspnea, and exertional dyspnea. The prognosis for these conditions remains guarded with variable success in attaining long-term remission or cure. In long-term follow-up of children and adolescents with hyperventilation, it was found that 40% still had symptoms of hyperventilation as adults. This often occurred with signs and symptoms of chronic anxiety [8, 51]. However, many techniques have been useful for at least short- to moderate-term improvement in symptoms. These combined with a thorough medical evaluation to rule out "organic" disease and psychological testing and intervention, when appropriate, have the best chance of providing for long-term benefit.

References

1. De Groot EP. Breathing abnormalities in children and breathlessness. Paediatr Resp Rev. 2011;12:83–7.
2. Goldman A. Clinical tetany by forced respiration. JAMA. 1922;78:1193–95.
3. Kerr WJ, Dalton JW, Gliebe PA. Some physical phenomena associated with the anxiety states and their relationship to hyperventilation. Ann Intern Med. 1937;11:961–92.
4. Lum LC. Hyperventilation: the tip and the ice berg. J Psychosom Res. 1975;19:375–83.
5. Rice RL. Symptom patterns of the hyperventilation syndrome. Am J Med. 1950;8:691–700.
6. Thomas M, McKinley RK, Freeman E, Foy C, Price D. The prevalence of dysfunctional breathing in adults in the community with and without asthma. Prim Care Respir J. 2005;14: 78–82.
7. Enzer NB, Walker PA. Hyperventilation syndrome in childhood. J Pediatr. 1967;70(4): 521–32.
8. Herman SP, Stickler GB, Lucas AR. Hyperventilation syndrome in children and adolescents: long-term follow-up. Pediatrics. 1981;67:678–80.
9. Gardner WN, Bass C, Moxham J. Recurrent hyperventilation tetany due to mild asthma. Respir Med. 1992;86:349–51.
10. Bass C, Gardner WN. Respiratory and psychiatric abnormalities in chronic symptomatic hyperventilation. BMJ. 1985;290:1387–90.
11. De Ruiter C, Garssen B, Rijken H, Kraaimaat F. The hyperventilation syndrome in panic disorder, agoraphobia, and generalized anxiety disorder. Behav Res Ther. 1989;27(4):447–52.
12. Bass C. Hyperventilation syndrome: a chimera. J Psychosom Res. 1997;42:421–26.
13. Fensterheim H, Wiegand B. Group treatment of the hyperventilation syndrome. Int J Group Psychother. 1991;4:399–403.
14. Garssen B, Buikhuisen MD, van Dyck R. Hyperventilation and panic attacks. Am J Psychiatry. 1996;153:513–18.
15. Hornsveld HK, Garssen B, Fiedeldij Dop M, et al. Double-blind, placebo-controlled study of the hyperventilation provocation test and the validity of the hyperventilation syndrome. Lancet. 1996;348:154–8.
16. Howell JB. The hyperventilation syndrome: a syndrome under threat? Thorax. 1997;52: S30–4.
17. Margarin GJ, Middaugh DA, Linz DH. Hyperventilation syndrome: a diagnosis begging for recognition. West J Med. 1983;138:733–36.

18. Marshall JR. Hyperventilation syndrome or panic disorder: what's in a name? Hosp Pract. 1987;15:105–18.
19. Diagnostic and Statistical Manual of Mental Disorders (DSM IV). American Psychiatric Association. Arlington, VA. 4th ed., July 2000.
20. Hornsveld HK, Garssen B, Fiedeldij Dop M, et al. Symptom reporting during voluntary hyperventilation and mental load: implications for diagnosing hyperventilation syndrome. J Psychosom Res. 1990;34:687–97.
21. Perkins GD, Joseph R. Neurological manifestations of the hyperventilation syndrome. J R Soc Med. 1986;79:448–50.
22. Haldane JS, Poulton EP. The effects of want of oxygen on respiration. J Physiol. 1908;37: 390–407.
23. Wood P. Da Costa's syndrome (or effort syndrome). BMJ. 1941;1:767–72.
24. Rasmussen K, Ravnsbaek J, Funch-Jensen P, et al. Oesophageal spasm in patients with coronary artery spasm. Lancet. 1986;1:174–76.
25. Niggemann B. How to diagnose psychogenic and functional breathing disorders in children and adolescents. Pediatr Allergy Immunol. 2010;21:895–99.
26. Homnick DN, Pratt HD. Respiratory diseases with a psychosomatic component in adolescents. Adol Med SARS. 2000;11(3):547–64.
27. Gardner WN, Meah MS, Bass C. Controlled study of respiratory responses during prolonged measurement in patients with chronic hyperventilation. Lancet. 1986;ii:826–30.
28. van Dixhoorn J, Dunvenvoorden HJ. Efficacy of the Nijmegen questionnaire in recognition of the hyperventilation syndrome. J Psychosom Res. 1985;29:199–206.
29. Hardonk HJ, Beumer HM. Hyperventilation syndrome. In: Vinken PJ, Bruyn GW, editors. Handbook of clinical neurology, vol. 38. Amsterdam: North Holland Biomedical Press; 1979. p. 309–60.
30. Hornsveld H, Garssen B. The low specificity of the hyperventilation provocation test. J Psychosom Res. 1996;41(5):435–49.
31. Ringsberg KC, Akerland I. Presence of hyperventilation in patients with asthma-like symptoms but negative asthma test responses: provocation with voluntary hyperventilation and mental stress. J Allergy Clin Immunol. 1999;103:601–8.
32. Kinnula VL, Sovijarvi ARA. Elevated ventilatory equivalents during exercise in patients with hyperventilation syndrome. Respiration. 1993;60:273–78.
33. Wong K, Huang Y, Huang Y, Chiu C. Personality profiles and pulmonary function of children with sighing dyspnea. J Paediatr Child Health. 2007;43:280–83.
34. Perin P, Perin R, Rooklin A. When a sigh is just a sigh…and not asthma. Ann Allergy. 1993;71:478–80.
35. Soley MH, Shock NW. The etiology of the effort syndrome. Am J Med Sci. 1938;196: 840–51.
36. Butani J, O'Connell EJ. Functional respiratory disorders. Ann Allergy Asthma Immunol. 1997;79:91–101.
37. Maytung CK. Sighing dyspnea: a clinical syndrome. J Allergy. 1938;10:50–5.
38. Wong K, Chiu C, Huang Y, Huang Y. Plethysmographic lung volumes in children with sighing dyspnea. Pediatr Int. 2009;51:405–8.
39. Aljadeff G, Molho M, Katz I, Shlomo B, Yemini Z, Shiner RJ. Pattern of lung volumes in patients with sighing dyspnea. Thorax. 1993;48:809–11.
40. Abu-Hassan M, Tannous B, Weinberger M. Exercise-induced dyspnea in children and adolescents: if not asthma then what? Ann Allergy Asthma Immunol. 2005;94:366–71.
41. Hammo A, Weinberger MM. Exercise-induced hyperventilation: a pseudoasthma syndrome. Ann Allergy Asthma Immunol. 1999;82:574–78.
42. Chambers JB, Kiff PJ, Gardner WN, Jackson G, Bass C. Value of measuring end tidal partial pressure of carbon dioxide as an adjunct to treadmill exercise testing. BMJ. 1988;296: 1281–85.
43. Kinnula VL, Sovijarvi ARA. Hyperventilation during exercise: independence on exercise-induced bronchoconstriction in mild asthma. Respir Med. 1996;90:145–51.

44. Van den Hout MA, Boek C, van der Molen GM, Jansen A, Griez E. Rebreathing to cope with hyperventilation: experimental tests of the paper bag method. J Behav Med. 1988;11(3): 303–10.
45. Callaham M. Hypoxic hazards of traditional paper bag rebreathing in hyperventilating patients. Ann Emerg Med 1989;18(6):622–628.
46. Gibson D, Bruton A, Lewith GT, Mullee M. Effects of acupuncture as a treatment for hyperventilation syndrome: a pilot, randomized crossover trial. J Altern Complement Med. 2007;13(1):39–46.
47. Anbar RD. Self-hypnosis for management of chronic dyspnea in pediatric patients. Pediatrics. 2001;107:e21.
48. Meuret AE, Wilhelm FH, Roth WT. Respiratory feedback for treating panic disorder. J Clin Psychol. 2004;60(2):197–207.
49. Meuret AE, Wilhelm FH, Roth WT. Respiratory feedback-assisted therapy in panic disorder. Behav Mod. 2001;25(4):584–605.
50. Grossman P, de Swart JC, Defares PB. A controlled study of a breathing therapy for treatment of hyperventilation syndrome. J Psychosom Res. 1985;29:49–58.
51. Hodgens JB, Fanurik D, Hanna DE, et al. Adolescent hyperventilation syndrome. Ala J Med Sci. 1988;25:423–26.

Chapter 5
The Habit Cough Syndrome and Its Variations

Miles M. Weinberger

Abstract Involuntary cough without an identified underlying organic reason has been given various names and recommended treatments. Current experience suggests that "habit cough" best describes this clinical entity and that various forms of suggestion therapy including hypnotic methods are the treatment of choice. Suggestion therapy is effective when it is directed at demonstrating to the patient that they have the ability to resist the urge to cough. Attempts at medical treatment or use of placebo therapy, even with the suggestion that the "medicine" will stop the cough, are generally not successful. In the absence of suggestion therapy, even when the diagnosis is correctly made, continued symptomatology for years is common. On the other hand, sustained relapse after suggestion therapy is uncommon.

Keywords Cough • Functional disorder • Habit • Habit cough

Background

Involuntary cough without an identified underlying organic reason has been repeatedly described. One of the earliest detailed case reports accompanied by 1 year of follow-up was published by Bernstein [1]. He described a 12-year-old girl with what he named "the barking cough of puberty." Two months later, Baker [2] placed "chronic cough from habit or psychosomatic disease" in the differential diagnosis for chronic cough in children. The actual term "habit cough" was first used by Berman in 1966 [3]. He reported six children (three in detail) in whom he "relied solely on the art of suggestion" to produce the cessation of cough. His 2-year follow-up supported the

M.M. Weinberger (✉)
Department of Pediatrics, University of Iowa Hospital, Iowa City, IA, USA
e-mail: miles-weinberger@uiowa.edu

R.D. Anbar (ed.), *Functional Respiratory Disorders: When Respiratory Symptoms Do Not Respond to Pulmonary Treatment*, Respiratory Medicine,
DOI 10.1007/978-1-61779-857-3_5,

success of his therapy. Since then, several descriptive terms have been used for this condition: "functional or psychogenic cough" [4], "psychogenic cough tic" [5], "operant cough" [6], "honking" [7], and "involuntary cough syndrome" [8].

Clinical Characteristics of the Classic Habit Cough

In 1991, we first reported our experience with the classic habit cough syndrome [9] describing the following 15-year-old girl:

Case 1

She had been coughing multiple times per minute during the clinic visit. The cough was the characteristic harsh tracheal cough sounding like a "barking dog" or "barking seal." She had experienced this intractable coughing for many months, had been subjected to extensive medical evaluation, and had experienced no consistent response even to several hospitalizations. Although interfering with getting to sleep, coughing did not awaken her once she was asleep, and parents observed no cough during sleep. She had been a good student with many friends and expressed regret about missing school because the cough made attending class unacceptably intrusive. The cough was stopped by me during a 15-min course of suggestion therapy in a manner used previously in similar cases.

That case stimulated a review of our experience with habit cough syndrome and examination of outcome. In that report [9], we identified nine patients with habit cough, all initially misdiagnosed as asthma. I or one of my colleagues had treated each of them during a period of sustained repetitive symptoms with a brief session of suggestion therapy. Symptoms had previously been present for up to 2 years (median of 2 months). Five had been hospitalized for the cough. Evaluation revealed no physiologic or radiologic abnormality. All patients became symptom-free during a 15-min session of suggestion therapy (described later in this chapter). During the subsequent week, one remained completely asymptomatic, and 8 had transient minor relapses that were readily self-controlled by our autosuggestion instructions. Seven of the 9 could be contacted for determination of long-term outcome at periods up to 9 years (median 2.2 years) after the session. Six were totally asymptomatic; one had occasional minor self-controlled symptoms.

A total of 153 patients from 17 publications were identified with sufficient descriptive detail for a previous review [10]. Of those, 149 were younger than 18 years, and four patients were adult women from 19 to 30 years of age. Several clinical characteristics of habit cough (Table 5.1) have been described with striking similarity by all of the authors despite some differences in diagnostic approach. Habit cough occurred only slightly more often in females than in males. Ages have ranged from 5 to 30 years, but the vast majority of patients were teenagers. The

Table 5.1 Clinical characteristics of habit cough

Very loud, repetitive, dry cough; may be accompanied by stereotypical "chin-on-chest" posture or "hands-to-mouth" gestures
Mostly teens (range: 5 to 30 years old)
Both sexes but with female preponderance
Duration of weeks to months
Weeks to months of school missed
No consistent response to bronchodilators, steroids, antibiotics, or antitussive medications
Multiple office or hospital "sick" visits
No other tics, normal physical exam except cough[a]
All the tests are normal
Initial respiratory insult is identified in 35% (viral, allergic reaction, trauma)
Misdiagnosis of "asthma" (at least 15% of 153 patients)[b]
Secondary gain, school phobias, psychological conflicts identified in 22%[c]

[a]Depressed or absent gag/corneal reflexes in some (From [15])
[b]All of our patients
[c]For all 4 adults, but only 19 of 149 children

duration of cough prior to diagnosis ranged from 1 week to 16 years, with the median for each report from weeks to months for children and 4 years for adults.

All the case reports noted a predominantly day-time cough that disappeared after patients actually fall asleep. The cough was characterized as dry, repetitive, generally nonproductive, "barking seal," loud cough that would increase whenever attention was being paid to it. In contrast to organic causes of cough, increase with exercise was not noted nor would the cough awaken the patient once asleep. Nineteen pediatric patients and all four adults carried the diagnosis of asthma that was disproved during the evaluation for habit cough. A recent respiratory insult such as viral infection, trauma to the airways, or severe allergic reaction with respiratory manifestations was identified in 35% (56 of 153 patients).

For most, multiple radiological, serological, clinical, pulmonary functions and endoscopic evaluations invariably showed negative results. The exceptions are the reports of localized tracheomalacia found by flexible bronchoscopy in seven patients [11]. Five of seven were treated with hypnosis with sustained improvement suggesting that a habit-like component had been acquired in these patients predisposed to irritate their tracheas due to the structural instability at the site of the malacia. However, the significant nocturnal cough in those patients with tracheomalacia distinguished them from other typical cases of habit cough. Lavigne also reported localized bronchomalacia due to vascular compression of the right main bronchus in one case [12].

"Chin-to-chest" posture or some stereotypical "hands-to-mouth" gestures accompanying the cough were described by some authors [1, 7, 13, 14]. The physical examination was generally normal. However, several authors did report some specific physical findings [4, 11, 12, 15, 16]. Cohlan checked the gag and corneal reflexes in 31 of his patients with habit cough and found abnormally decreased or absent gag reflex in all and depressed or absent corneal reflex in 21 [15]. Rabin brought attention to the "presence of edema of the lingual tonsils" that "impinge on the epiglottis, obliterating the vallecula space" [4]. In his view, this was the result of the severe cough itself. Cohlan [15] and then Wolff [14] reported patients' ability to reproduce the paroxysm of cough on command, but our own experience has been to the contrary.

The degree to which psychological abnormalities are responsible for or even present in habit cough is controversial. The extent of evaluation for possible psychological problems associated with habit cough reported in the literature varied from office interviews done by the allergist or pulmonologist (for most) to extended psychiatric evaluations done by psychologist or psychiatrist. Whether specific patients were referred for psychological evaluation appeared to depend on the authors' conception of the origin of this illness. Overall, school phobias, secondary gain, or significant psychological conflicts were reported in 34 of 153 patients. All four adults were reported to meet the criteria for conversion reactions or somatization with conversional symptoms [17, 18]. The contrast between those studies that found some sort of psychological problem to be present in (and responsible for) the habit cough phenomena in all or almost all of their patients [5, 7, 13, 19] and those that found no significant psychological problems among their patients suggests either marked differences in patient selection or biases of the observers [3, 15]. Only one of 33 patients of Cohlan was reported to need psychiatric treatment for a significant conversion disorder [15]. Berman suspected school phobia in only one of his 6 patients [3]. None of the nine patients we previously reported with habit cough had identifiable psychological or psychiatric problems. Moreover, follow-up with a standardized psychological questionnaire (SCL-90-R) did not reveal any apparent somatization or other psychopathology in any of our patients, although they did score somewhat higher than usual norms on an obsessive–compulsive scale [9]. It was also our clinical observations that they were brighter than average with generally excellent school performance.

Prevalence

The prevalence of habit cough is difficult to establish. Eighteen years of clinical experience from The Mayo Clinic revealed only 62 cases of habit cough diagnoses [8]. Cohlan reported 33 cases of habit cough from over 25 years of his clinical experience [15]. Later, Wolff, from the same clinic, described another two patients and mentioned a total of six over the next 4 years after the original report [14]. Houstek et al. reported 10 cases from 1971 to 1981 [19]. In our own retrospective study of close to 4,500 medical records covering over 12 years from a pediatric allergy and pulmonary referral service, we identified 23 patients with all categories of functional respiratory disorders, of whom nine had habit cough (Table 5.2) [9]. Although habit cough was the most frequent diagnosis in that report, this probably reflects more the severity and duration of symptoms of habit cough compared with some of the other diagnoses in Table 5.2 rather than the true relative incidence in the community; we suspect that hyperventilation attacks, for example, are much more common than

Table 5.2 Characteristics of patients diagnosed with functional respiratory disorders at the University of Iowa Pediatric Allergy and Pulmonary Clinic

Clinical pattern	Male/female	Age of diagnosis [median (range) in years]	Previous symptom duration: [median (range) in months]	Hospitalized
Coughing	3/6	11(6–17)	2(0.25–24)	5
Hyperventilating	2/3	15(12–16)	7(2–72)	1
Throat clearing	1/2	15(9–26)	48(0.5–120)	1
Laryngeal spasm	0/3	13(12–25)	36(4–84)	3
Sneezing	0/1	11	0.2	0
Sniffing	0/1	8	18	0
Nose blowing	1/0	12	5	0
Summary	*7/16*	*12(6–26)*	*7(0.25–120)*	*10*

Adapted from [10]. With permission from Mary Ann Liebert, Inc. publishers

indicated in Table 5.2 because of the greater recognition in the community and lesser likelihood of referral to our subspecialty service. From our personal observations and communications with our colleagues, it seems that most busy allergists would encounter about one to two cases of habit cough a year. It is probably underreported and underestimated due to the lack of clear definition and specific diagnostic tests as well as due to low awareness of it in the general medical community.

Variations of the Habit Cough Syndrome

A Common Variation of the Habit Cough Syndrome—Habit Throat Clearing

Case 2

A 6-year-old boy has been having a repeated throat clearing cough for several weeks following initial symptoms consistent with a viral upper respiratory infection. Unlike the barking cough described in case 1, this was characterized by a much softer sound appearing to be somewhere between a cough and throat clearing. Similar to case 1, the sound was repetitive occurring up to several times per minute during waking hours but was absent once asleep. A 15-min session of suggestion therapy was successful in stopping the repetitive activity.

This variation of the habit cough, perhaps better termed habit throat clearing (although parents frequently refer to this as coughing), tends to generate less concern because of its milder nature. It is nonetheless annoying to those around the patient, especially the parents, though less bothersome to the individual manifesting this disorder.

Less common variations I have seen include habit sniffing, habit nose blowing, and habit sneezing. All of these are characterized by the repetitive nature of the behaviors that are completely absent once asleep. All responded to suggestion therapy by the faculty of the Pediatric Allergy and Pulmonary Division.

Diagnostic Considerations

Asthma

Cough is certainly a prominent symptom of asthma, occurring as frequently as the wheezing that characterizes asthma. However, the cough of asthma is characteristically made worse with activity and, in contradistinction to the habit cough, occurs during sleep, and the individual with a cough from asthma is frequently awakened by cough.

Airway Malacia

Both tracheomalacia and bronchomalacia have previously been described as being misdiagnosed as asthma [20]. Inadequate rigidity of the tracheal or main stem bronchial cartilage results in collapse which causes cough by at least two mechanisms. Collapse of the trachea or main stem bronchi during increased intrathoracic pressure as in vigorous exhalation or coughing can cause the anterior and posterior walls to come into contact, resulting in an irritable focus that stimulates further cough. Additionally, when secretions are present in the airway, the airway collapse during expiration prevents normal airway clearance of mucus. The secretions then act as a further stimulus for cough. While tracheomalacia and bronchomalacia can be troublesome in the infant, some cases do not cause problems until later in childhood [11].

Protracted Bacterial Bronchitis

This is an entity not well appreciated and only infrequently described with variable terminology [21–24]. While chronic bacterial bronchitis is certainly a characteristic of cystic fibrosis, protracted bacterial bronchitis occurs predominantly in young children with no identifiable abnormalities of immunity or other underlying disease. They have prolonged periods of cough with neutrophilia and high colony counts of bacteria in their lower airways demonstrable by bronchoalveolar lavage. Some, but not all, have bronchomalacia that may be contributing both to cough and to retaining secretions in the lower airway which predisposes the child to secondary infection [25]. These patients are readily distinguished from the habit cough by the young age and troublesome cough at night that frequently disturbs sleep.

Pertussis (Whooping Cough)

Infection from *Bordetella pertussis*, known in the past as the 100-day cough, causes a prolonged period of cough, and we have seen several cases where the primary care physician prescribed antiasthmatic medication because pertussis was not adequately considered. While the cough is characteristically spasmodic and associated with post-tussive gagging or emesis, the classical clinical symptom of a whoop is often not present in an immunized population. In fact, evidence for *B. pertussis* infection has been identified in 10% to 30% of immunized children and adults with persistent cough for 2 or more weeks in the absence of a prior history consistent with an underlying disorder [26–30]. Establishing the diagnosis is important to prevent spread to contacts, especially to young infants who are at the greatest risk for hospitalization and fatality from this infection. Diagnosis is most readily made by polymerase chain reaction (PCR) identification of pertussis antigen from a properly collected nasal swab. As with other causes of organic cough, cough generally disturbs sleep, in contrast to the functional habit cough that is characteristically absent once the individual is asleep. However, pertussis, like other organic causes of cough, may result in undue persistence as a habit cough even after the initial cause of cough is gone.

Pseudo-considerations

Prolonged cough has also been frequently attributed to gastroesophageal reflux (GER). However, data have not been supportive of GER as an etiology of respiratory symptoms [31, 32]. When children with GER and cough have been examined for inflammation in the lower airway, it was protracted bacterial bronchitis and not reflux that was associated with the cough [33, 34]. When studied, GER itself has not been associated with increased airway inflammation [33]. Similarly, sinusitis and postnasal drainage cannot be argued as a cause of prolonged cough without having evidence for the absence of protracted bacterial bronchitis as the etiology for simultaneous inflammation of the upper and lower airway [35]. These two popular pseudo-diagnoses should not be confused with habit cough with its repetitive pattern and absence once asleep.

Treatment

Even when habit cough is diagnosed correctly, absence of a specific treatment plan can result in prolonged symptomatology. In a report of 60 patients from Mayo Clinic, 44 of 60 patients required an average of 6 months beyond the diagnosis for resolution and 16 continued to be symptomatic (mean duration of 5.9 years) later [8]. The therapeutic approaches reported in the literature can be divided into two major groups: (1) vigorous psychological intervention with behavioral techniques or psychotherapy with or without psychotropic drugs and (2) suggestion therapy using a variety of techniques.

Reports of adults with habit cough suggested that intense psychotherapy, counseling, and speech therapy (see Chaps. 9 and 13) resulted in decrease of symptom severity in a small number of patients who accepted it [17, 18]. The same authors treated other patients successfully with speech therapy alone but with no follow-up data or details of the cases involved. "Response suppression shaping" utilizing painful electric shocks was used successfully in two teenage boys with no relapses after 1.5–2.5 years of follow-up [36, 37]. Prior to this therapy, one coughed so severely that he lost consciousness. One of these patients required more than 100 sessions, when the other patient discontinued his cough immediately after one shock. An "elevated level of anxiety, neuroticism, affective lability, hyperactivity, and low tolerance to frustration" were found in all 10 patients from one report [19] with a good response to mild tranquilizers and prolonged psychotherapy.

One of the earliest references to a successful use of suggestion therapy for treatment of habit cough came from Bernstein in 1963 [1]. He described a dramatic and lasting resolution of a severe habit cough in a 12-year-old girl after one session of suggestion therapy. Follow-up of over 1 year showed no significant relapses. A few mild, self-controlled episodes of habit cough were noted during the first 3 days after the suggestion therapy session. Hypnosis (the specific technique was not described) had been used on the same child for habit cough two times prior to suggestion therapy with no success. In 1966, Berman reported 6 patients with habit cough successfully treated with therapy that "relied solely on the art of suggestion" [3]. The children were told that the cough was a habit, that there was no evidence of disease causing symptoms, and therefore, the cough was unnecessary and must stop. Within a few days, the habit cough gradually subsided and did not recur during a 2-year follow-up period. Special attention was paid in that report to the possibility of psychological or emotional disturbances as a cause of cough, but only in one case was there a suggestion to school phobia.

In a review of functional respiratory disorders, Rabin stated that "symptoms could be alleviated by reassurance from an understanding family physician" in most cases, but he also warned: "If the symptoms do not respond rather promptly to reassurance and suggestive measures, expert psychiatric help should be sought" [4]. Rabin's report, however, gave no indication of his success rate. Kravitz et al. [5] and later Weinberg [7] reported treatment of a total of 12 cases of habit cough using suggestion and reassurance for all, with addition of mild tranquilizers and psychotherapy in some cases. They felt that school phobia was a factor in all but one of their patients. Lorin et al. reported a striking case of an 11-year-old girl with habit cough coughing so severe that she had suffered rib fractures [16]. She was diagnosed with an "adjustment reaction with obsessive, hysterical, and phobic features." Her parents refused the psychotherapy. A single session of suggestion therapy utilizing a lollipop as a "distractor" was then tried with prompt cessation of symptoms; she remained asymptomatic 7 years later.

The largest group of habit cough patients treated with suggestion therapy utilized a bed sheet tightly wrapped around the patient's chest with strong verbal reinforcement that this would stop the cough [15]. Thirty-one of 33 patients treated in this manner then became cough-free in 24–48 h after suggestion therapy. The long-term outcome, which ranged from 10 months to 21 years (median of 14 months), reported success in 17 of 18 patients with follow-up data. There has been a subsequent report of success with the same technique on six patients with no further symptoms reported 1 week after the treatment [14]

Hypnosis has been successfully used in children by Anbar using a technique he terms use of self-hypnosis (see Chap. 12) [38, 39]. One patient was reported as successfully treated with self-hypnosis taught by telephone [40]. Biofeedback and cognitive coping were described in treating one 11-year-old girl with classical habit cough (see Chaps. 9 and 10) [41]. She was described as cough-free after 6 1 h sessions. Vocal fold injection with botulinum toxin was used in 3 children, ages 11–13, with transient improvement (Chap. 14) [42]. Subsequent control was reported attained with 4 to 8 sessions of behavioral therapy.

In our own study [9], all nine patients with habit cough were treated with suggestion therapy without psychotherapy or psychotropic medications. Eight responded well with no more than minor self-controlled symptoms reported during the long-term follow-up (8 days to 9.4 yrs; 2.2 yrs median). One patient required a second session of suggestion therapy 9 days after the original one and remained symptom-free since.

Approach to Successful Suggestion Therapy

We regard suggestion therapy as a means to empower the patient with the ability to resist the urge to cough. In the process of suggestion therapy, various "distracters" such as lollipops [16], sips of warm water [4, 9], tight chest rapping with a bed sheet [14, 15], hypnosis or medications [4, 5, 7, 11], and even electric shock [29, 30] have been used. The specific distracters, which essentially provide an alternative behavior to the cough, should match the physician's version of the origin of the habit cough as explained to the patient. An explanation of habit cough and the way the distracter will help should be given to the patient clearly and without any ambiguity. The distracter cannot be regarded as a placebo treatment in itself; our experience suggests that attempts at therapy where medication is prescribed to stop the cough result in failure.

Our success with suggestion therapy has been predominantly with those who were acutely symptomatic at the time. This treatment has generally consisted of a single short session of suggestion therapy by a staff physician that utilized a distractor, most commonly 0.5 ml of 1% lidocaine diluted to 3 to 5 ml with normal saline for most of our patients. A glass of warm water sipped slowly when the urge to cough was perceived has also been used as an alternative behavior. The cough was explained as a response to a perceived irritation in the airway that results in a vicious cycle of cough in response to irritation which causes more irritation and thereby more cough. The patient was instructed to focus on the distractor (slow deep breaths of the aerosol or sips of the body temperature water when the urge to cough was perceived) while listening to a constant patter by the physician telling the patient that the distractor would help soothe the irritation inducing the cough and that this would help the patient resist the urge to cough. Primary emphasis was placed on the fact that it was the patient who actually was resisting the urge to cough and that the distractor was only soothing the irritation which enable the patient to break the vicious cycle "cough–irritation–cough."

The major elements of the suggestion therapy sessions were as follows:

1. *Expressing confidence, communicated verbally and behaviorally, that the therapist will be able to show the patient how to stop the cough.*
2. *Explaining the cough as a vicious cycle of an initial irritant, now gone, that had set up a pattern of coughing which caused irritation and further symptoms.*
3. *Encouraging the suppression of cough in order to break the cycle. The therapist closely observes for the initiation of the muscular movement preceding coughing and immediately exhorts the patient to hold the cough back, emphasizing that each second the cough is delayed makes further inhibition of cough easier. Utilizing the distractor as an alternative behavior to coughing is emphasized.*
4. *Repeating expressions of confidence that the patient was developing the ability to resist the urge to cough.*
5. *When some ability to suppress cough is observed (usually after about 10 min), asking in a rhetorical manner if they are beginning to feel that they can resist the urge to cough, for example, "You're beginning to feel that you can resist the urge to cough, aren't you?"*
6. *Discontinuing the session when the patient can repeatedly answer positively to the question "Do you feel that you can now resist the urge to cough on your own?" This question is only asked after the patient has gone 5 min without coughing.*

A cough-free period was generally reached within the first 10 min. The complete session was then over in about 15 min. Patients are advised that, now that they have learned they can suppress the cough, they need to continue concentrating on suppressing the cough for the remainder of the day. They are further advised to treat minor recurrences promptly by isolating themselves, using sips of tepid (body temperature) water to "sooth the irritation" and concentrate on suppressing the urge to cough. It has been common for the patients to readily do this at home with generally prompt success.

Complications encountered

While success is usual in the treatment of habit cough with suggestion therapy, I have had experience with three cases of unusual, undesirable, and perplexing outcomes.

The first one was an 8-year-old girl with classical habit cough that was stopped with usual suggestion therapy. She returned the following week with excessive drinking and urinating consistent with polydipsia and polyuria that was behavioral in nature. Once that was managed by restricting intake of water, she developed polyphagia. Psychiatric consultation was obtained.

The second was a 10-year-old boy referred from Northwestern Iowa 300 miles from us with an initial history consistent with classical habit cough syndrome who had been seen initially by a local psychiatrist and eventually institutionalized. The nature of the treatment was unclear but appeared to have been somewhat verbally accusatory regarding the nature of the cough. Apparently, the coughing increased in severity to the extent that food ingestion was limited and considerable weight loss occurred. Upon arrival at our clinic, he exhibited a somewhat soft cough rather than the barking cough described at initiation of the problem several months earlier, but the cough occurred with each exhalation during all waking hours. Our usual suggestion therapy was ineffective. He was admitted to our extended care facility for attempted rehabilitation and only very gradually improved.

The third case was a 14-year-old boy, a very bright, straight A student, who had been diagnosed with depression the previous year according to the referring pediatrician. The boy himself stated that his problem had been chronic fatigue syndrome. His cough, present for about 2 months, was consistent with classical habit cough syndrome. The referring pediatrician had diagnosed this patient as having habit cough syndrome and had utilized local specialists to provide suggestion therapy and hypnosis without benefit prior to the referral. The boy and his parents were skeptical about further behavioral attempts at stopping the coughing, which had kept him out of school for the previous 2 months. There was no history to support school avoidance. To the contrary, he reported liking school, had friends, and excelled academically. An attempt at suggestion therapy by me was unsuccessful. A bronchoscopy found no airway malacia, but a large lingual tonsil impinging on his epiglottis was suspected to perhaps be a nidus of irritation acting as a stimulus for the cough. A lingual tonsil debulking by pediatric otolaryngology was associated with cessation of the cough, but 2 days later, he began having pharyngeal spasms associated with a gulping sound occurring several times per minute during waking hours. This was associated with decreased oral intake, weight loss, and continued inability to attend school. A further complaint was persistent headache. Sleep was impaired, but parents described cessation of the "gulping" once he was asleep. An attempt at habit cessations by one of our psychologists skilled in that technique and at teaching pharyngeal muscular control by our most experienced speech pathologist was not successful. He was subsequently referred to a psychologist experienced at biofeedback closer to home, but he and his parents remained skeptical of such efforts.

These 3 cases are notable as outliers during 35 years of seeing at least 2 cases of habit cough annually cured with suggestion therapy. They stand as exceptions to the general experience that habit cough is responsive to suggestion therapy and is not associated with evidence for underlying psychopathology or additional somatization.

Discussion

The origin of the habit cough remains unclear. However, it is associated with considerable morbidity, disruption of life, and can result in considerable iatrogenic problems due to misdiagnosis. Conflicting views are presented by those who approach it as a manifestation of severe psychological problems and those who concentrate on the respiratory symptoms alone. If the rationale for an approach can be judged by the results of the therapy, then the therapy with the fastest symptom resolution and the lowest relapse rate may be accepted as the answer to this clinical problem until more in-depth prospective studies are available.

The use of hypnosis, psychotropic medications, or psychiatric hospitalizations that did not incorporate some form of suggestion toward cough suppression has not resulted in cough cessation. The consequence of simply diagnosing and counseling the patient can result in a prolonged symptomatic course for many patients [8]. On the other hand, suggestion therapy aimed at empowering the patient with the ability to resist the urge to cough results in rapid and sustained resolution of symptoms in almost all the patients for whom it had been used.

Questions:

1. A 12-year-old boy has been coughing for 3 months. It is characterized by a loud barking sound. It occurs up to several times per minute for many days on end. It has interfered with ability to be in a classroom at school. It interferes with him getting to sleep. What would be the most valuable information?

   (a) Spirometry
   (b) Chest X-ray
   (c) Chest CT
   (d) Observation for the presence of cough during sleep
   (e) Bronchoscopy

2. If observation documents the complete absence of cough once asleep, the most appropriate initial treatment would be:

   (a) A course of prednisone
   (b) A collar that provides a safe electric shock when coughing occurs as used for barking dogs
   (c) A behavioral approach utilizing suggestion, autosuggestion, or autohypnosis
   (d) Psychotherapy
   (e) A codeine cough suppressant

3. If observation in that patient documented the presence of disturbing cough once asleep, the most appropriate measure would be:

   (a) A behavioral approach utilizing suggestion, autosuggestion, or autohypnosis
   (b) Bronchoscopy

(c) A codeine cough suppressant
(d) Psychotherapy
(e) A mucolytic

Answers:

1. (d): The presence of a cough of the nature described in the first question with complete absence once asleep is the *sine qua non* for the habit cough syndrome. Other diagnostic tests are then generally superfluous.
2. (c): Since the absence of cough provides evidence for the patient having the habit cough syndrome, medication is highly unlikely to be of value, which excludes a and e. b might be appropriate for annoying barking dogs but does not appear appropriate for a child. There is no data supporting psychotherapy but various forms of suggestion have been effective.
3. (b): Since the presence of night cough is inconsistent with a diagnosis of the habit cough syndrome, further evaluation is needed, and a bronchoscopy would allow determination if the cough was from airway malacia, other airway anomalies, or inflammatory processes. While pulmonary function testing and a chest X-ray might also be justified, the best answer of the choices provided is b.

Conclusions

From the point of view of therapeutic simplicity and immediate and long-term success, suggestion therapy appears to be an effective, rapid, and cost-effective means of treatment. Making the diagnosis requires that the clinician be alert to the clinical characteristics of the habit cough syndrome and have an index of suspicion based on the clinical characteristics. Organic disease needs to be effectively ruled out. For the majority of patients, a careful history, a chest roentgenogram, and pulmonary function tests should be sufficient to assure a physician as well as a patient's family that nothing has been missed. Early recognition of habit cough is essential to prevent overtreatment and unnecessary morbidity.

References

1. Bernstein L. A respiratory tic: "the barking cough of puberty." Report of a case treated successfully. Laryngoscope. 1963;73:315–9.
2. Baker Jr DC. Chronic cough in children. N Y State J Med. 1963;63:1535–9.
3. Berman BA. Habit cough in adolescent children. Ann Allergy. 1966;24:43–6.
4. Rabin CB. Disturbances of respiration of functional origin. J Asthma Res. 1968;5:295–308.

5. Kravitz H, Gomberg RM, Burnstine RC, Hagler S, Korach A. Psychogenic cough tic in children and adolescents. Nine case histories illustrate the need for re-evaluation of this common but frequently unrecognized problem. Clin Pediatr (Phila). 1969;8:580–3.
6. Munford PR, Liberman RP. Differential attention in the treatment of operant cough. J Behav Med. 1978;1:289–95.
7. Weinberg EG. 'Honking': Psychogenic cough tic in children. S Afr Med J. 1980;57:198–200.
8. Rojas AR, Sachs MI, Yunginger JW, O'Connell EJ. Childhood involuntary cough syndrome: a long-term follow-up study. Ann Allergy. 1991;66:106.
9. Lokshin B, Lindgren S, Weinberger M, Koviach J. Outcome of habit cough in children treated with a brief session of suggestion therapy. Ann Allergy. 1991;67:579–82.
10. Weinberger M. The habit cough syndrome. Pediatr Allergy Immunol Pulmonol. 2010;23: 125–9.
11. Wood RE. Localized tracheomalacia or bronchomalacia in children with intractable cough. J Pediatr. 1990;116:404–6.
12. Lavigne JV, Davis AT, Fauber R. Behavioral management of psychogenic cough: alternative to the "bedsheet" and other aversive techniques. Pediatrics. 1991;87:532–7.
13. Shuper A, Mukamel M, Mimouni M, Lerman M, Varsano I. Psychogenic cough. Arch Dis Child. 1983;58:745–7.
14. Wolff PS. An ingenious way to treat psychogenic cough. MCN Am J Matern Child Nurs. 1988;13:118–20.
15. Cohlan SQ, Stone SM. The cough and the bedsheet. Pediatrics. 1984;74:11–5.
16. Lorin MI, Slovis TL, Haller JO. Fracture of ribs in psychogenic cough. N Y State J Med. 1978;78:2078–9.
17. Gay M, Blager F, Bartsch K, Emery CF, Rosenstiel-Gross AK, Spears J. Psychogenic habit cough: review and case reports. J Clin Psychiatry. 1987;48:483–6.
18. Blager FB, Gay ML, Wood RP. Voice therapy techniques adapted to treatment of habit cough: a pilot study. J Commun Disord. 1988;21:393–400.
19. Houstek J, Vyhnalek M, Sukova B, Copova M. Psychogenic cough. Cesk Pediatr. 1983;38:405–10.
20. Weinberger M, Abu-Hasan M. Pseudo-asthma: when cough, wheezing, and dyspnea are not asthma. Pediatrics. 2007;120:855–64.
21. Saito J, Harris WT, Gelfond J, Noah TL, Leigh MW, Johnson R, Davis SD. Physiologic, bronchoscopic, and bronchoalveolar lavage fluid findings in young children with recurrent wheeze and cough. Pediatr Pulmonol 2006;41:709–19.
22. Marchant JM, Masters IB, Taylor SM, Cox NC, Seymour GJ, Chang AB. Evaluation and outcome of young children with chronic cough. Chest 2006;129:1132–41.
23. Chang AB, Redding GJ, Everard ML. Chronic wet cough: protracted bronchitis, chronic suppurative lung disease and bronchiectasis. Pediatr Pulmonol 2008;43:519–31.
24. Donnelly D, Critchlow A, Everard ML. Outcomes in children treated for persistent bacterial bronchitis. Thorax. 2007;62:80–4.
25. Kompare M, Weinberger M. Protracted bacterial bronchitis in young children: association with airway malacia. J Pediatr 2012;160:88–92.
26. Mink CM, Cherry JD, Christenson P, Lewis K, Pnedea E, Shlian D, Dawson JA, Blumberg DA. A search for Bordetella pertussis infection in university students. Clin Infect Dis 1992;14:464–71.
27. Wright SW, Edwards KM, Decker MD, Zeldin, MH. Pertussis infection in adults with persistent cough. JAMA 1995;273:1044–46.
28. Nennig ME, Shinefield HR, Edwards KM, Black SB, Fireman BH. Prevalence and incidence of adult pertussis in an urban population. JAMA 1996;275:1672–74.
29. Craig AS, Wright SW, Edwards KM, Greene JW, Haynes M, Dake AD, Schaffner W. Outbreak of pertussis on a college campus. Am J Med 2007;120:364–68.
30. Harnden A, Grant C, Harrison T, et al. Whooping cough in school age children with persistent cough: prospective cohort study in primary care. BMJ. 2006;333:174–77.

31. Størdal K, Johannesdottir GB, Bentsen BS, et al. Acid suppression does not change respiratory symptoms in children with asthma and gastro-oesophageal reflux disease. Arch Dis Child. 2005;90:956–60.
32. Chang AB, Connor FL, Petsky HL, et al. An objective study of acid reflux and cough in children using an ambulatory pHmetry-cough logger. Arch Dis Child. 2011;96:468–72.
33. Chang AB, Cox NC, Purcell J, et al. Airway cellularity, lipid laden macrophages and microbiology of gastric juice and airways in children with reflux oesophagitis. Respir Res. 2005;6:72.
34. Chang AB, Cox NC, Faoagali J, et al. Cough and reflux esophagitis in children: their co-existence and airway cellularity. BMC Pediatr. 2006;6:4.
35. Campanella SG, Asher MI. Current controversies: sinus disease and the lower airways. Pediatr Pulmonol. 2001;31:165–72.
36. Alexander AB, Chai H, Creer TL, et al. The elimination of chronic cough by response suppression shaping. J Behav Ther Exp Psychiat. 1973;4:75–80.
37. Creer TL, Chai H, Hoffman A. A single application of an aversive stimulus to eliminate chronic cough. J Behav Ther Exp Psychiat. 1977;8:107–9.
38. Anbar RD, Hall HR. Childhood habit cough treated with self-hypnosis. J Pediatr. 2004;144: 213–7.
39. Anbar RD. User friendly hypnosis as an adjunct for treatment of habit cough: a case report. Am J Clin Hypn. 2007;50:171–5.
40. Anbar RD. Childhood habit cough treated with consultation by telephone: a case report. Cough. 2009;5:2.
41. Labbe EE. Biofeedback and cognitive coping in the treatment of pediatric habit cough. Appl Psychophysiol Biofeedback. 2006;31:167–72.
42. Sipp JA, Haver KE, Masek BJ, Hartnick CJ. Botulinum toxin A: a novel adjunct treatment for debilitating habit cough in children. Ear Nose Throat J. 2007;86:570–2.

Chapter 6
Vocal Cord Dysfunction

Miles M. Weinberger and Devang R. Doshi

This chapter contains videos, please download from
http://www.springerimages.com/videos/10.1007/978-1-61779-857-3_6

Abstract Initially described as hysteria and then Munchausen's stridor, we now recognize vocal cord dysfunction as a functional group of disorders. Exercise and spontaneously occurring phenotypes exist that benefit from different treatments. The former appears to respond to pharmacological pretreatment with an anticholinergic aerosol and the latter may require vocal cord training to learn to relieve the symptoms. The differential diagnosis includes consideration of neurological and anatomical abnormalities. Recognition and effective treatment is important to permit the individual to be involved in activities important to them and to avoid unnecessary and ineffective medical care.

Keywords Functional disorder • Stridor • Vocal cord dysfunction • Vocal cords

Background

A medical textbook in 1842 by Robley Dunglison described a disorder of the laryngeal muscles brought on by "hysteria." This episodic upper airway obstruction was subsequently termed "Munchausen's stridor" [1]. The physiology of this disorder was characterized as paradoxical vocal cord movement [2], and the diagnostic terminology generally used has become the vocal cord dysfunction syndrome (VCD) [3]. VCD has been frequently misdiagnosed as asthma despite the difference between inspiratory stridor, the sound typical of upper airway obstruction, and the typical expiratory wheeze of asthma [3–6].

M.M. Weinberger (✉)
Department of Pediatrics, University of Iowa Hospital, Iowa City, IA, USA
e-mail: miles-weinberger@uiowa.edu

D.R. Doshi
William Beaumont School of Medicine, Oakland University, Bloomfield, MI, USA

R.D. Anbar (ed.), *Functional Respiratory Disorders: When Respiratory Symptoms Do Not Respond to Pulmonary Treatment*, Respiratory Medicine,
DOI 10.1007/978-1-61779-857-3_6,

Clinical Phenotypes

In reviewing various descriptions of VCD, it is apparent that several phenotypes can be identified [7]. A common pattern has been the observation of symptoms being limited to vigorous exertion [5]. Most of those patients demonstrate paradoxical vocal cord movement whereby inspiratory flow is obstructed when the vocal cords adduct rather than abducting on inspiration as they should. Normal flow generally occurs during expiration for those patients. More disruptive has been those characterized by spontaneous acute onset of severe symptoms. Two variations of the spontaneous form have been seen. Paradoxical movement appears to be the most common. A more serious phenotype has been those where severe adduction occurs during both phases of respiration.

Our own reported experience involved a review of 49 sequential patients diagnosed with VCD in the Pediatric Allergy and Pulmonary Clinic at the University of Iowa. Forty-one had been previously diagnosed as asthma that was confirmed by us in only 12. The diagnosis of vocal cord dysfunction was based on direct laryngoscopy while symptomatic in 24. Reversible flattening of the inspiratory portion of the flow-volume loop during observed symptoms was observed in 8 whose symptoms were insufficiently sustained to permit laryngoscopy. The other 17 had a sufficiently convincing history of episodic inspiratory stridor that was rapid in onset and rapidly reversible in the absence of any other findings.

Of the 49 patients, 29 had only exercise-induced VCD. Twenty patients had spontaneously occurring VCD, only 4 of whom had symptoms also brought on by exercise. The median age at the time of diagnosis for those with exclusively exercise-induced VCD was 14.9 years (range 9–20 years); those with spontaneously occurring VCD averaged 13.5 years (range 8–25 years). The female to male ratio demonstrated a higher number of female patients affected in each group (1.6:1 in exercise-induced vocal cord dysfunction group; 2.2:1 in the spontaneous vocal cord dysfunction group).

Clinical Presentation

The common exercise-induced phenotype is typically triggered by vigorous athletic activity and presents as dyspnea on exertion associated with inspiratory stridor. Physiologically, this causes upper airway obstruction on inspiration with normal expiratory physiology. The patient may complain of tightness in the throat and difficulty getting air in. However, those symptoms themselves are not diagnostic of VCD since similar symptoms can occur even with dyspnea related to normal physiologic limitation [8].

Less common but associated with the more severe pattern of upper airway obstruction are those patients who experience adduction of the vocal cords on both inspiration and expiration, often associated with adduction also of the false vocal cords [9, 10]. This produces an inspiratory and expiratory wheezing-like sound, chest tightness, and shortness of breath. The acute onset and severity of symptoms in some patients with this pattern of VCD has resulted in emergency intervention with endotracheal intubation or tracheotomy for severe upper airway obstruction [11, 12].

Another phenotypical variation is expiratory VCD. In one series of VCD, 11% were reported to have only the expiratory closure, 31% had the combined inspiratory and expiratory closure, while the remainder had the more typical paradoxical movement with closure only on inspiration [4].

Examples of the most common phenotypes are illustrated with the two following cases:

Case 1

A 15-year-old girl takes a typical teenage summer time job in Iowa called detasseling.[1] She developed severe dyspnea with respiratory sounds that were described as wheezing and was taken to the local emergency room where an injection of epinephrine relieved her symptoms. The next day, she again attempted detasseling with the same result. She then abandoned her goal of detasseling but continued for the next 3 weeks to have similar episodes of dyspnea described by the patient, emergency room caregivers, and her primary care pediatrician as wheezing. These episodes would occur both spontaneously and with exertion and would not respond to epinephrine as they did on the first 2 days. Trials by her primary care pediatrician of antiasthmatic medications, including inhaled albuterol, oral corticosteroids, and inhaled corticosteroids, failed to either prevent or relieve acute symptoms when they occurred. Symptoms would last up to several hours, considerably limiting activity of this normally very active adolescent.

After 3 weeks of these daily symptoms, she was referred to our pediatric allergy and pulmonary clinic. She was initially asymptomatic. However, a treadmill exercise test reproduced her dyspnea and the respiratory sound previously described as wheezing. The sound precipitated during exercise testing was high-pitched and limited to inspiration. Spirometry before and after the onset of dyspnea demonstrated inspiratory airway obstruction (Fig. 6.1). Flexible laryngoscopy during the episode demonstrated paradoxical vocal cord movement (Video 6.1).

This demonstrated that her dyspnea was from the vocal cord dysfunction syndrome. The evaluation included a large positive skin prick test to corn pollen, which explained the initial episodes as being consistent with allergen-specific IgE-mediated laryngeal edema from intense exposure to the corn pollen during the detasseling

[1] Detasseling is done to crossbreed or hybridize two different varieties of corn. Fields of corn that will be detasseled are planted with two varieties of corn. By removing the tassels from all plants of one variety, all the grain growing on those plants will be fertilized by the other variety's tassels. Detasseling work is typically performed by teens; as such, it serves as a typical rite of passage (for many, it is their first job) in rural areas of the Corn Belt.

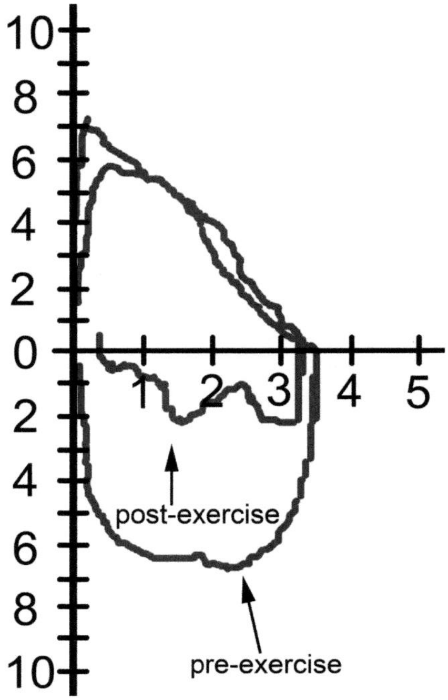

Fig. 6.1 Spirometry before and after exercise in the girl described in Case 2 showing the marked decrease in the inspiratory portion of the flow-volume loop in association with dyspnea and an inspiratory wheeze-like sound (technically a high-pitched stridor). (Reprinted from [13]. With permission from American Academy of Pediatrics)

procedure. The clinically indicated epinephrine was consequently effective. The subsequent episodes were from the functional disorder of vocal cord dysfunction with paradoxical motion whereby the vocal cords paradoxically closed on inspiration with relaxation and consequent opening on expiration. Epinephrine then was ineffective as were all of the other pharmacologic measures.

Instructions by a speech pathologist provided this girl with the ability to stop the paradoxical movement when it would start, but it continued to occur during vigorous activity, interfering with her activities as a cheer leader. Suspecting a vagal mechanism for this, a trial of pre-exercise treatment with an anticholinergic inhaler, ipratropium *(Atrovent oral inhaler)*, reliably prevented the exercise-induced vocal cord dysfunction [7]. This allowed her to resume her usual athletic activities, including cheer leading.

Case 2

This 15-year-old girl had a 1½-year history of recurrent extremely severe dyspnea. Episodes were sufficiently impressive to observers that paramedics were repeatedly called for urgent transportation to a local hospital emergency room. Symptoms would last for variable periods of time and occurred with sporadic frequency without apparent inciting factors. She had been treated with various antiasthmatic medications including inhaled and oral corticosteroids with no benefit. She had

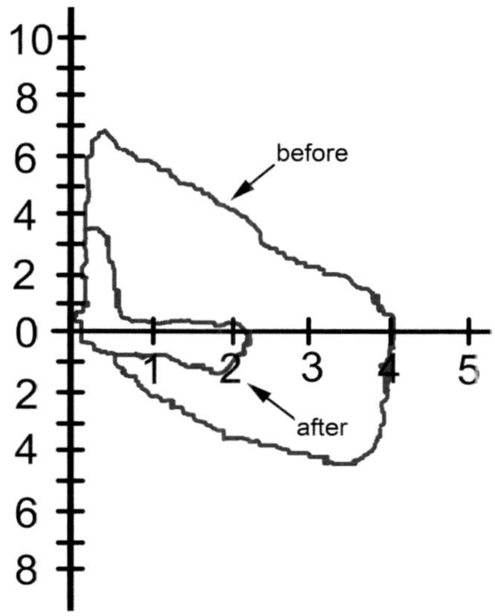

Fig. 6.2 Spirometry before and after the onset of dyspnea in the girl described in Case 2 showing the marked decrease in the inspiratory and expiratory portion of the flow-volume loop in association with an inspiratory wheeze-like sound (technically a high-pitched stridor on inspiration and a monophonic wheeze on expiration). (Reprinted from [13]. With permission from American Academy of Pediatrics)

been hospitalized several times where she received intravenous corticosteroids and vigorous use of inhaled bronchodilators, also without benefit.

When first seen at our pediatric allergy and pulmonary clinic, she was free of any symptoms of dyspnea, and her physical exam was normal. Initial spirometry was completely normal. Since the nature of her recurrent dyspnea was not apparent from the history but sounded atypical for asthma, a bronchoprovocation with histamine was planned in order to assess if asthma was the cause of her recurrent dyspnea. While preparing the vials of the various concentrations of histamine needed for the progressive inhalational provocation and before any had been administered, she began having severe respiratory distress with both inspiratory and expiratory wheezing-like sounds. Her spirometry changed from showing normal inspiratory and expiratory flow to severe obstruction in both phases of respiration (Fig. 6.2). Flexible laryngoscopy during the episode demonstrated virtually complete closure of the vocal cords leaving only a small aperture for air movement with no abduction except briefly during speech (Video 6.2).

Treatment focused on speech pathology to teach the patient control over her vocal cords when symptoms occurred. Response to treatment was only partially effective. She was able to control some episodes but not others. Lack of continuity for her care hampered progress. She and her single mother subsequently moved to Texas, and she was lost to follow-up.

A special category of vocal cord dysfunction has been described in elite athletes. Rundell and Spiering evaluated 370 developing or elite athletes for symptoms consistent with inspiratory stridor and exercise-induced bronchospasm. Their findings showed 5% or 19 patients (18 female) with symptoms consistent with vocal cord dysfunction occurring only during exercise [14]. They also observed that an observation of inspiratory stridor was significantly more common among outdoor rather than indoor athletes. A concern regarding these data among elite athletes, however, is the absence of direct observation to confirm vocal cord dysfunction, a deficiency they acknowledge in their publication. These authors also describe flattened or truncated inspiratory flow-volume loops to be insensitive in identifying VCD. They identified VCD purely by eliciting stridor during exercise and listening over the larynx and chest to confirm their impression that the inspiratory sound they identified as stridor was heard in the laryngeal area.

Contrary to the conclusions of Rundell and Spiering, we have repeatedly heard substantial inspiratory noise at maximal effort in well-conditioned and highly motivated athletes without evidence for upper airway obstruction, either by the flow-volume loop or direct visualization with a flexible laryngoscope. The explanation appears to be simply very high air movement through the narrowest portion of the normal upper airway. Moreover, we have never visualized vocal cord dysfunction without having seen truncation of the inspiratory portion of the flow-volume loop where the FIF_{50}/FEF_{50} was very low when symptomatic rather than the usual ratio of about 1 that was present when the same patient was asymptomatic. Therefore, the assumption that increased inspiratory laryngeal noise itself is sufficient to confirm the diagnosis of VCD appears fallacious to us.

Differential Diagnosis

There are other causes of upper airway obstruction that may be confused with VCD. They include virtually any cause of acquired stridor. A particularly relevant consideration for exercise-induced stridor is exercise-induced laryngomalacia. Vocal cord dysfunction and exercise-induced laryngomalacia both can cause exercise-induced dyspnea due to upper airway obstruction. The flow-volume loop will result in virtually identical flattening of the inspiratory portion of the flow-volume loop. However, the effect for VCD occurs from paradoxical vocal cord movement, while collapse of the laryngeal structures is the cause of the upper airway obstruction with laryngomalacia [15–19].

Vocal cord dysfunction has also been seen with Chiari 1 malformations. In a review of 31 young children with Chiari 1 malformations, vocal cord dysfunction was seen in 26%, all under the age of 3 [20]. The following case illustrates such a patient seen by us:

Case 3

A 17-month-old child had harsh nocturnal coughing and occasional stridor. She was initially treated as asthma without response. Intermittent paradoxical vocal cord moment was seen during flexible bronchoscopy. The age was so atypical for classical functional VCD that a head MRI was performed to examine for a Chiari 1 malformation. When that was confirmed (Fig. 6.3), decompressive neurosurgery eventually eliminated the respiratory symptoms.

Other disorders that can be confused with vocal cord dysfunction included vocal cord paresis or paralysis [21]. Subglottic stenosis may also present in a manner that can initially be suggestive for vocal cord dysfunction as illustrated by the following case:

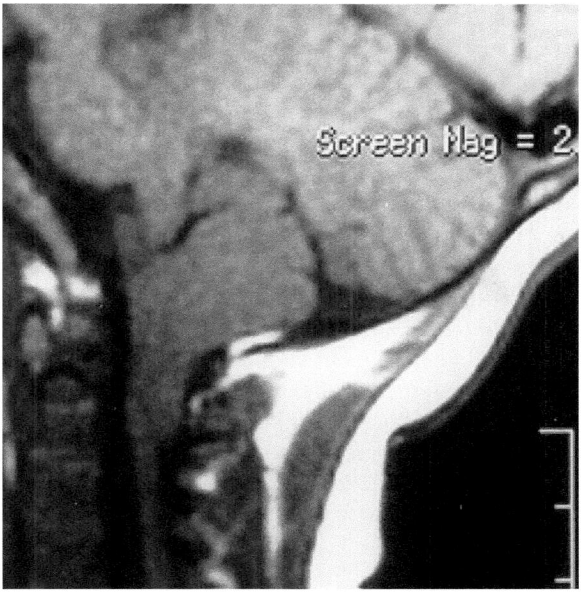

Fig. 6.3 Chiari 1 malformation with herniation of the cerebellar tonsil below the foramen magnum

Case 4

A 14-year-old girl was seen for recurrent respiratory distress associated with stridor. Since she was asymptomatic when first seen and had normal appearing spirometry other than a mild decrease in the inspiratory flow rate, she was advised to return the next time she had similar symptoms. When seen several weeks later with an acute episode of dyspnea and stridor, there was marked flattening of the inspiratory portion of her flow-volume loop. A flexible fiber-optic laryngoscopy visualized completely normal vocal cord movement. Flexible bronchoscopy then demonstrated profound subglottic stenosis when the 3.5-mm-diameter bronchoscope completely obstructed her airway just below the vocal cords. She was subsequently diagnosed with relapsing polychondritis similar to a previous report of dyspnea and stridor with normal vocal cord movement [22].

Pathophysiology of Functional Vocal Cord Dysfunction

Support for the rationale of vagal mediation in exercise-induced VCD is found in two recent case reports that described prolonged stimulation of the vagal nerve by vagal nerve stimulators, used in patients for intractable seizures, causing vocal cord dysfunction as a complication [23, 24]. Laryngopharyngeal dysfunction, coughing, and voice changes were also reported in these patients. Ayres and Gabbot suggested an altered autonomic balance as a cause of vocal cord dysfunction since true and false vocal cords derive motor innervation from the vagus nerve [25].

Several studies have suggested that a spontaneous onset of vocal cord dysfunction is often associated with underlying psychiatric disorders. Psychiatric consultation for further therapy and consideration of underlying somatoform disorders has also been recommended [26]. In a report by Selner et al. [27], three patients were described with spontaneous onset of VCD symptoms attributed to psychological factors, and a psychological assessment was recommended for patients with vocal cord dysfunction. Another study by Gavin et al. [28] described 12 patients with vocal cord dysfunction occurring only at times of anxiety with no relationship to activity or exercise. There is a report suggesting an association of VCD with sexual abuse [12]. Newman et al. [4] reported a previous psychiatric diagnosis in 73% of patients with vocal cord dysfunction. This observation has also been noted in other studies suggesting a higher incidence of vocal cord dysfunction in female patients with an underlying psychological condition [12]. Stress and emotions as well as times of increased panic or anxiety have been suggested as triggers for vocal cord dysfunction [29]. Social stressors were also described in 12 of 22 pediatric patients with vocal cord dysfunction, particularly in those involved with organized sports [30].

Treatment of Vocal Cord Dysfunction

The use of an anticholinergic inhaler was considered by us for patients with exercise-induced VCD based on the suggestion that a vagally mediated reflex was the mechanism (see Chap. 14) [23–25]. Six of our initially described patients with exercise-induced VCD for whom ipratropium bromide aerosol (Atrovent MDI) was prescribed and used reported prevention of symptoms associated with exercise. Use of an albuterol MDI prior to exercise in 4 of those 6 previously diagnosed with asthma had been ineffective. We have utilized the anticholinergic aerosol for many more patients subsequent to our initial report and have continued to see effectiveness as prophylaxis when used prior to exercise but not as a means of reversing symptoms after they occur.

A study by Sullivan et al. [31] described teaching 20 female athletes "coordinated thoracic–abdominal breathing exercises" when symptoms of VCD occurred during exercise with 19 of the 20 indicated as being able to control their symptoms after 6 months. However, it was not clear whether complete resolution of the problem had occurred in any. In our patients with exercise-induced VCD, symptoms generally subsided with a decrease or cessation of exercise. Breathing exercises such as those described by Sullivan et al. [31] appeared to us to be difficult to apply during the athletic activity affected. While there is a need for a controlled clinical trial of the anticholinergic agent, ipratropium (Atrovent MDI), our continued series of successful responses with no failures for those with confirmed VCD from exercise is efficient, benign, and encouragingly successful.

Speech therapy (see Chap. 13), relaxation and hypnosis (Chap. 12), biofeedback (Chap. 10), and breathing techniques (Chap. 11) have been interventions described previously for vocal cord dysfunction [29, 32–35]. Christopher et al. [3] described improvement in symptoms 3–21 months after speech therapy in five patients. In our published report, 8 of 11 contacted patients with spontaneously occurring VCD followed our recommendations for speech therapy [7]. Although the patients reported that the techniques taught by our speech therapist enabled them to control symptoms when they occurred, the subsequent duration for recurrences varied from a week to 12 months among them. Of 3 who did not follow our recommendation for speech therapy, recurrent symptoms persisted for 4, 12, and 60 months, respectively [7].

Anbar used hypnosis to assist in confirming the diagnosis by inducing spontaneously occurring severe VCD, which was then observed with flexible laryngoscopy. He then utilized hypnosis to have the patient "relax his neck" with conversion of the vocal cord movement from previous adduction to normal abduction during inspiration [35].

Natural History of VCD

In 28 of 49 patients in our report who we were able to contact, the median onset of exercise-induced VCD was 12 months prior to our diagnosis with a range of 3 weeks to 7 years [7]. For spontaneously occurring VCD, the median onset was 6 months prior to our assessment (range 1 week to 4 years). Seventeen of the 28 patients (10 female, 7 male) had only exercise-induced VCD. Eleven of the 28 patients (8 female, 3 male) had spontaneously occurring VCD with two of them (both female) additionally experiencing exercise-induced VCD. The median time until resolution of symptoms was 5 and 4 months for exercise-induced VCD and spontaneously occurring VCD, respectively, although with a great deal of variability ranging from 1 week to 5 years, irrespective of intervention. Once symptoms were reported as stopped, there were no descriptions of recurrences. However, six patients with exercise-induced VCD for whom the ipratropium MDI was not prescribed indicated when contacted that they had quit the competitive athletic activity that had been associated with their symptoms.

Only one previous report described the long-term outcome of patients following the diagnosis of vocal cord dysfunction. In that report, resolution of symptoms within 8.2 months was described in five patients by Murry et al. [36].

Questions:

1. A 14-year-old girl is diagnosed with severe chronic asthma based on multiple observations of wheezing described by the girl and previous observers but not responding to inhaled or oral corticosteroids, even in high doses. What would be most appropriate for evaluation?

   (a) Recommend a laryngoscopy
   (b) Chest X-ray

   (c) Ask the girl to reproduce the wheezing she makes
   (d) Request a psychiatric evaluation immediately
   (e) Consider addition of Xolair

2. What would be found from a laryngoscopy?

   (a) No abnormalities if she is asymptomatic at the time of the exam
   (b) The reason for resistant asthma could be determined
   (c) Observation of anxiety from the procedure would provide useful information regarding the diagnosis
   (d) Laryngoscopy would fail to help distinguish VCD from laryngomalacia, even when the patient is symptomatic
   (e) Laryngoscopy could distinguish VCD from laryngomalacia, even when not symptomatic

3. Requesting that the girl reproduce the wheezing made when symptomatic

   (a) Would provide evidence to support the diagnosis of asthma
   (b) Provide the examiner with information regarding whether the reported wheezing was an inspiratory or expiratory sound
   (c) Would assist in determining if a psychiatric consultation was indicated
   (d) Would help in determining if sexual abuse were an issue
   (e) Would not be any diagnostic value

Answers:

1. (c): A diagnosis of asthma should be considered as likely incorrect if symptoms do not respond to an adequate dose of a systemic corticosteroid. Since VCD is known to be frequently misdiagnosed as asthma, ask the patient to reproduce the sound they make that has previously been called wheezing. If the "wheeze" is inspiratory, that would be consistent with upper airway obstruction and warrant consideration for vocal cord dysfunction syndrome.
2. (a): Laryngoscopy is likely to be of value in distinguishing VCD from laryngomalacia only when the patient is symptomatic. It would be of no value in providing evidence for or against asthma.
3. (b): Reproducing the sound described as wheezing would be of value in identifying if symptoms were from upper or lower airway obstruction. That would not aid in diagnosing asthma or the specific therapy that might be needed.

Conclusions

Vocal cord dysfunction has several clinical and physiologic phenotypes which should be individually identified. Treatment should relate to those variations. Exercise-induced VCD appears to be readily prevented by pretreatment with an anticholinergic aerosol. Spontaneously occurring VCD may require training by a speech pathologist to learn effective voluntary control over the vocal cords or other techniques such as biofeedback, breathing techniques, or hypnosis. It is critical to consider the differential diagnosis of vocal cord disorders which can include neurological abnormalities such as the Chiari I malformation and abnormalities of the larynx causing exercise-induced laryngomalacia.

References

1. Patterson R, Schatz M, Horton M. Munchausen's stridor: non-organic laryngeal obstruction. Clin Allergy. 1974;4:307–10.
2. Rogers JH, Stell PM. Paradoxical movement of the vocal cords as a cause of stridor. J Laryngol Otol. 1978;92:157–8.
3. Christopher KL, Wood 2nd RP, Eckert RC, Blager FB, Raney RA, Souhrada JF. Vocal-cord dysfunction presenting as asthma. N Engl J Med. 1983;308:1566–70.
4. Newman KB, Mason 3rd UG, Schmaling KB. Clinical features of vocal cord dysfunction. Am J Respir Crit Care Med. 1995;152:1382–6.
5. McFadden Jr ER, Zawadski DK. Vocal cord dysfunction masquerading as exercise-induced asthma. A physiologic cause for "choking" during athletic activities. Am J Respir Crit Care Med. 1996;153:942–7.
6. Thomas PS, Geddes DM, Barnes PJ. Pseudo-steroid resistant asthma. Thorax. 1999;54: 352–6.
7. Doshi D, Weinberger M. Long-term outcome of vocal cord dysfunction. Ann Allergy Asthma Immunol. 2006;96:794–9.
8. Abu-Hasan M, Tannous B, Weinberger M. Exercise-induced dyspnea in children and adolescents: if not asthma then what? Ann Allergy Asthma Immunol. 2005;94:366–71.
9. Wood RP, Milgrom H. Vocal cord dysfunction. J Allergy Clin Immunol. 1996;98:481–5.
10. Goldstein R, Bright J, Jones SM, Niven RM. Severe vocal cord dysfunction resistant to all current therapeutic interventions. Respir Med. 2007;1–1:857–8.
11. Hayes JP, Nolan MT, Brennan N, FitzGerald MX. Three cases of paradoxical vocal cord adduction followed up over a 10-year period. Chest. 1993;104:678–80.
12. Freedman MR, Rosenberg SJ, Schmaling KB. Childhood sexual abuse in patients with paradoxical vocal cord dysfunction. J Nerv Ment Dis. 1991;179:295–8.
13. Weinberger M, Abu-Hasan M. Pseudo-asthma: when cough, wheezing, and dyspnea are not asthma. Pediatrics. 2007;120(4):855–64.
14. Rundell KW, Spiering BA. Inspiratory stridor in elite athletes. Chest. 2003;123:468–74.
15. Smith RJ, Bauman NM, Bent JP, Kramer M, Smits WL, Ahrens RC. Exercise-induced laryngomalacia. Ann Oto Rhinol Laryngol. 1995;104:537–41.
16. Bent JP, Miller DA, Kim JW, Bauman NM, Wilson JS, Smith RJ. Pediatric exercise-induced laryngomalacia. Ann Oto Rhinol Laryngol. 1996;105:169–1675.
17. Björnsdóttir US, Gudmundsson K, Hjartarson H, Bröndbo K, Magnússon B, Juliusson S. Exercise-induced laryngochalasia: an imitator of exercise-induced bronchospasm. Ann Allergy Asthma Immunol. 2000;85:387–91.
18. Manell DL, Arjmand EM. Laryngomalacia induced by exercise in a pediatric patient. Int J Ped Otorhinolaryngol. 2003;67:999–1003.
19. Christensen P, Thomsen SF, Rasmussen N, Backer V. Exercise-induced laryngeal obstructions objectively assessed using EILOMEA. Eur Arch Otorhinolaryngol. 2010;267:401–7.
20. Greenlee JDW, Donovan KA, Hasan DM, Menezes AH. Chiari I malformation in the very young child: the spectrum of presentations and experience in 31 children under age 6 years. Pediatrics. 2002;110:1212–9.
21. Morris MJ, Christopher KL. Diagnostic criteria for the classification of vocal cord dysfunction. Chest. 2010;138:1213–23.

22. Kim C-M, Kim B-S, Cho K-J, Hong S-J. Laryngotracheal involvement of relapsing polychondritis in a Korean girl. Pediatr Pulmonol. 2003;35:314–7.
23. Vassilyadi M, Strawsburg RH. Delayed onset of vocal cord paralysis after explantation of a vagus nerve stimulator in a child. Childs Nerv Syst. 2003;19:261–3.
24. Zalvan C, Sulica L, Wolf S, Cohen J, Gonzalez-Yanes O, Blitzer A. Laryngopharyngeal dysfunction from the implant vagal nerve stimulator. Laryngoscope. 2003;113:221–5.
25. Ayres JG, Gabbott PLA. Vocal cord dysfunction and laryngeal hyperresponsiveness: a function of altered autonomic balance? Thorax. 2002;57:284–5.
26. Fritz GK, Fritsch S, Hagino O. Somatoform disorders in children and adolescents: a review of the past 10 years. J Am Acad Child Adolesc Psychiatry. 1997;36:1329–38.
27. Selner JC, Staudenmayer H, Koepke JW, Harvey R, Christopher K. Vocal cord dysfunction: the importance of psychologic factors and provocation challenge testing. J Allergy Clin Immunol. 1987;79:726–33.
28. Gavin LA, Wamboldt M, Brugman S, Roesler TA, Wamboldt F. Psychological and family characteristics of adolescents with vocal cord dysfunction. J Asthma. 1998;35:409–17.
29. Leo RJ, Konakanchi R. Psychogenic respiratory distress: a case of paradoxical vocal cord dysfunction and literature review. Prim Care Companion J Clin Psychiatry. 1999;1:39–46.
30. Powell DM, Karanfilov BI, Beechler KB, Treole K, Trudeau MD, Forrest LA. Paradoxical vocal cord dysfunction in juveniles. Arch Otolaryngol Head Neck Surg. 2000;126:29–34.
31. Sullivan MD, Heywood BM, Beukelman DR. A treatment for vocal cord dysfunction in female athletes: an outcome study. Laryngoscope. 2001;111:1751–5.
32. Earles J, Kerr B, Kellar M. Psychophysiologic treatment of vocal cord dysfunction. Ann Allergy Asthma Immunol. 2003;90:669–71.
33. Miller S. Voice therapy for vocal fold paralysis. Otolaryngol Clin North Am. 2004;37:105–19.
34. Sandage M, Zelazny S. Paradoxical vocal fold motion in children and adolescents. Lang Speech Hear Serv Sch. 2004;35:353–62.
35. Anbar RD, Hehir DA. Hypnosis as a diagnostic modality for vocal cord dysfunction. Pediatrics. 2000;106:e81.
36. Murry T, Tabaee A, Aviv JE. Respiratory retraining of refractory cough and laryngopharyngeal reflux in patients with paradoxical vocal fold movement disorder. Laryngoscope. 2004;114:1341–5.

Chapter 7
Functional Sleep Disorders

Zafer N. Soultan and Ran D. Anbar

Abstract Sleep-related disorders are common, and when left untreated, they can negatively impact health, cognitive development and learning, behavior, and emotional regulation. This chapter will focus on sleep disorders with no known primary organic trigger, which thus can be defined as falling within the spectrum of functional disorders. Fortunately, these disorders are amenable to adjustment of patients' behavior and/or cognition. Patients with sleep disorders are often treated by specialists who deal with pulmonary disease, and many of the therapies employed in the treatment of such sleep disorders are the same as those for functional respiratory disorders. Sleep-related disorders that are treated primarily by medical or surgical therapies such as sleep-disordered breathing (SDB), narcolepsy, idiopathic hypersomnolence, and restless legs syndrome will not be discussed. However, application of positive airway pressure (PAP) therapy for SDB is demanding, and many patients have difficulties with its application. Thus, management of the functional issues associated with application of this therapy is discussed.

Keywords Apnea • Enuresis • Insomnia • Parasomnia • Positive airway pressure • Sleep

Sleep-related disorders are common, and when left untreated, they can negatively impact health, cognitive development and learning, behavior, and emotional regulation [1, 2]. This chapter will focus on sleep disorders with no known primary organic

Z.N. Soultan (✉)
Department of Pediatrics, SUNY Upstate Medical University,
Syracuse, NY, USA
e-mail: soultanz@upstate.edu

R.D. Anbar
Department of Pediatrics, SUNY Upstate Medical University, 750 East Adams St.,
13210-1834, Syracuse, NY, USA

R.D. Anbar (ed.), *Functional Respiratory Disorders: When Respiratory Symptoms Do Not Respond to Pulmonary Treatment*, Respiratory Medicine,
DOI 10.1007/978-1-61779-857-3_7,

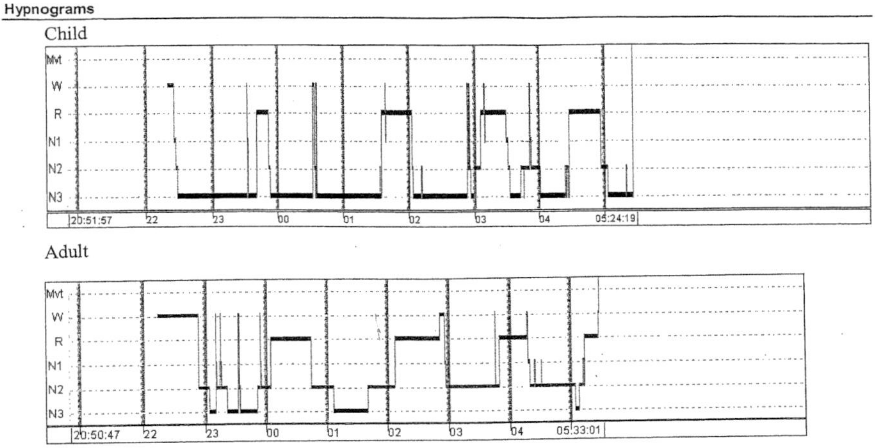

Fig. 7.1 Note the ultradian cycles of REM and NREM sleep stages and the predominance of SWS (stage N3) in childhood, which decreases through the lifespan

trigger, which thus can be defined as falling within the spectrum of functional disorders. Fortunately, these disorders are amenable to adjustment of patients' behavior and/or cognition. Patients with sleep disorders are often treated by specialists who deal with pulmonary disease, and many of the therapies employed in the treatment of such sleep disorders are the same as those for functional respiratory disorders. Sleep-related disorders that are treated primarily by medical or surgical therapies such as sleep-disordered breathing (SDB), narcolepsy, idiopathic hypersomnolence, and restless legs syndrome will not be discussed. However, application of positive airway pressure (PAP) therapy for SDB is demanding, and many patients have difficulties with its application. Thus, management of the functional issues associated with application of this therapy is discussed.

Sleep is divided into two stages according to the polysomnographic features of electroencephalographic (EEG) patterns, eye movements, and muscle tone. These are non-rapid eye movement (NREM) sleep and REM sleep (or dream sleep). NREM sleep is further divided into stage 1 (N1), stage 2 (N2), and stage 3 (N3), which also is known as "deep" sleep or slow wave sleep (SWS) [3].

NREM and REM sleep rotate throughout the night in what is called "ultradian cycles." Each of these "sub-cycles" lasts about 90–110 min (Fig. 7.1). The parts of NREM and REM per cycle change throughout the night. NREM sleep predominates in the first third of the night and REM sleep in the last third [3].

Sleep architecture changes with age. The average duration of sleep during a 24-h period declines from infancy through adolescence (Table 7.1). The proportion of REM sleep decreases from birth through early childhood and adulthood (from 50% to 25–30%). Further, an initial predominance of SWS drops off after puberty and continues to decrease over the life span (Fig. 7.1) [3].

Table 7.1 Average duration of sleep during a 24-h period

	Recommended sleep time (hours)	
	Nighttime	Naps
Infants	9–10	3–4
Toddlers (2–3 years)	9–10	2–3
Preschool (3–5 years)	9–10	0–1
Elementary school (6–12 years)	9–10	0
Adolescents (12–20 years)	9	0
Adults	7–8	0

Adequate sleep is essential for normal cognitive function and development. SWS restores cognitive function, while REM sleep is involved in enhancement of cognition, such as consolidation of memory, and in the growth and development of the central nervous system of children. Insufficient sleep results daytime sleepiness, neurocognitive dysfunction, and mood disturbances [1, 2].

The following sleep-related disorders, without a known physical trigger will be discussed:

- Parasomnias
  - Disorders of arousal from NREM sleep: sleepwalking, sleep terrors, and confusional arousals
  - Parasomnia associated with REM sleep: nightmares
  - Other parasomnias: sleep enuresis
- Sleep-related movement disorders
  - Sleep-related bruxism
- Insomnia
  - Behavioral insomnia of childhood: sleep-onset association and limit-setting types
  - Psychophysiological insomnia

Parasomnias are events of unwanted behaviors and experiences that accompany sleep.

Disorders of arousal from NREM sleep are initiated almost exclusively from SWS and are more common in children than adults. They occur in the first few hours of sleep when NREM sleep is predominant. They involve skeletal muscle disturbances, autonomic behaviors, agitation, and disorientation. There is usually amnesia for the events [4].

Anything that causes an increase in the SWS would trigger these episodes in susceptible individuals. For example, sleep deprivation causes rebound of SWS and subsequent increase in the occurrence of these parasomnias. In addition, arousals by a noise, a light, or a sleep apnea event trigger the episodes [4].

Sleepwalking can begin as soon as the child is able to walk and occur at any age. Most of the time, it resolves on its own by adolescence. The prevalence is as high as 17% in childhood, with a peak incidence between ages 8 and 12 years.

The incidence is 4% in adults including *de novo* cases. In adults, it is more common in males, but there is no gender difference in childhood [4].

During a typical sleepwalking episode, the patient sits up in bed and appears confused before walking. Sometimes, patients walk or bolt out of bed and run immediately. During an episode, the sleepwalker appears awake and confused. The eyes are open with a confused look. The event may terminate spontaneously at inappropriate places. If forced to respond, agitation and shouting may occur. There are safety concerns when sleepwalking is associated with wandering outside, jumping out of windows, or engaging in behavior that could be potentially injurious to a patient's bed partner [4].

Sleep terrors consist of sudden arousals from SWS with intense fear as manifested by a cry or blood-curdling scream and autonomic nervous system manifestations related to the intense fear of hyperventilation, tachycardia, and diaphoresis. The person sits up in bed, is unresponsive to stimuli, and when awakened is confused and disoriented. Bolting out of bed and running is not uncommon in adults and can be associated with harm to self and others. Amnesia of the event occurs, but sometimes there are reports of dream fragments involving imminent danger, particularly in adults. The incidence is up to 6.5% in children and 2.2% in adults. A substantial number of adults with sleep terrors have a history of bipolar disorder, depressive disorders, or anxiety disorders [4].

Confusional arousals are manifest by confusion and grogginess upon awakening from SWS early in the night or in the morning. Sometimes, there may be thrashing and movement in bed. The usual episode lasts 15–30 min. Stress and anxiety exacerbate these episodes [4].

These parasomnias can have significant impact on children and their parents. Children may limit their social interactions, such as sleepovers, because of fear of the embarrassment from occurrence of the episodes. Parents' sleep may be disturbed as a result of their children's parasomnias, and they frequently worry about the possibility that their children may have underlying health problems and about the risk of physical harm to their children [5].

Treatments include assuring the children and parents regarding the self-limited and benign nature of the events. In addition, ensuring adherence to adequate sleep hygiene and avoidance of sleep deprivation should lead to a decrease in the frequency of these episodes. Good sleep habits include:

- Ensuring adequate total sleep time for age.
- Consistent sleep schedule on weekdays and weekends.
- Avoiding napping or restricting them to early afternoon.
- Avoiding caffeine entirely or at least after 12 noon.
- Beginning wind-down activities an hour before bedtime.
- Avoiding television, radio, cell phones, and computer game playing at bedtime.
- Avoiding strenuous exercise in the evening.
- Avoiding a big meal an hour before bedtime.
- The bedroom should be used for sleep only and not for play.
- The television and computers should be removed from the bedroom.
- The room should be cool and quiet.

With sleepwalking, care should be taken to ensure the children's safety. Additional treatments are indicated when the episodes recur frequently or cause physical harm or significant anxiety to parents and the children. In partial arousal parasomnias, benzodiazepines or tricyclic antidepressants have been used for their effect on shortening SWS [5]. Scheduled awakenings prior the time of the events are sometimes helpful in preventing the episodes from occurring. Teaching children self-hypnosis in one or two visits has been used successfully to eliminate sleepwalking in children and adults and alleviating the associated daytime anxiety (see Chap. 12) [6–10].

Nightmares occur in the second half of the night, when the REM stage is prominent. The patients experience coherent dreams. They are frightening as they unfold and may sometimes cause awakening. Nightmares disorder occurs when nightmares recur frequently. As compared to partial arousal insomnia, the patient is usually frightened but coherent and remembers the events. Sometimes, children are too frightened to go back to sleep and often request parental reassurance. Nightmares usually start between the ages 3 and 6 years, and it is estimated that 10–50% of children aged three to 5 years have nightmares severe enough to disturb their parents. Approximately 2–8% of general population has a current problem with nightmares. Nightmares occur consistently in patients with posttraumatic stress disorder (PTSD). Stress and traumatic events, anxiety, sleep deprivation, and insomnia are associated with an increased incidence of nightmares. Frequent nightmares are associated with certain personality traits. Antidepressants, antihypertensive drugs, and dopamine-receptor agonists are associated with nightmares. Associated features of nightmares include nighttime fears, bedtime resistance, and sometimes daytime anxiety [4, 5].

Treatment is offered for severe and persistent nightmares that are associated with sleep avoidance and subsequent sleep deprivation or daytime sleepiness and anxiety. For younger children, active reassurance by the parents usually is sufficient [5]. For older children, teaching and positive reinforcement for independent coping skills is helpful. Avoiding frightening movies, books, and computer games; reducing stressors; and ensuring adequate sleep are useful measures to prevent nightmares. Safety objects, such as blankets or stuffed animals, and providing of dim nighttime lighting can be helpful [4]. Hypnotherapy has been used successfully in eliminating frequent nightmares. The same strategies of hypnotherapy have been used successfully for eliminating night terrors. Given the amenability of young children to hypnotic suggestions, the parents can stay with the child as he or she shows evidence of beginning to sleep (hypnagogic state) and start making positive suggestions such as that they will keep the child safe and secure. The children can construct a dream catcher above their bed. According to Native American tradition, the net will catch the bad dreams and allow good dreams to go through. In addition, using self-hypnosis-induced relaxation at bedtime allows the children to be more comfortable in going to bed [6–9].

Nighttime fears manifest by resisting falling asleep because of fears that occur independently from any intra-sleep disorder such as nightmares. Most children develop fear of potential harm as part of normal cognitive development. Such fears typically start in preschool. Risk factors include anxiety, stress, traumatic events, parental anxiety, and family conflicts. Nighttime fears usually are benign and self-limited although can extend to adolescence. In one study, 79% of children reported nighttime fear, including 49% of adolescents, and a severe form associated with significant insomnia is seen in 20–30% of children. Sometimes, nighttime fears are masked by bedtime resistance and curtain calls that manifest by the patient leaving his or her bedroom and returning to the family room for different excuses such as saying goodnight or for one more goodnight kiss. The fears can be so intense such that the patient cries and leaves the bedroom seeking parental assurance at bedtime or in the middle of the night. Typically, children alleviate their fears by sharing the bedroom with parents or household members. They are sometimes associated by daytime fears and somatic complaints at bedtime such as headaches and stomachaches [4, 5, 11].

Most children develop coping mechanisms on their own or with help of parents with no need for referral for therapy. Using security objects such as blankets and stuffed animals and having a nightlight can be comforting and decrease the fear of the child and they are encouraged. Treatment is needed in severe cases that disrupt the sleep of the child and the family. The therapist assures the parents about the benign nature of nighttime fears and instructs them to avoid reinforcing the fears, to teach children coping skills, and helps develop solutions (see Chap. 9 for discussion of cognitive behavior therapy in this context). Creating a reward system for appropriate bedtime behavior can be useful. At the same time, limits should be set to disallow the child's behavior that could reinforce the child's fears, such as reading and watching scary movies and books that reinforce the belief of the presence of predators. The child should be told that screaming in the middle of the night for the purpose of reporting the fears is unhelpful, and in this case, the parents may say, "Remember: Stay calm and quiet." Hypnotherapy can alleviate nighttime fears by teaching children relaxation techniques (e.g., involving imagery of a favorite place or focusing on slow deep breathing) and by suggesting that they can practice self-hypnosis to help them relax at bedtime that allows them to fall sleep easily [6–9].

Sleep-Related Movement Disorders

Bruxism is abnormal clinching or grinding of teeth during sleep. The incidence increases in early childhood, and it becomes relatively uncommon in older individuals following eruption of the secondary teeth. The risk of bruxism tends to increase in association with anxiety, depression, attention deficit hyperactivity disorder, medications such as selective serotonin reuptake inhibitors (SSRI) and amphetamines, obstructive sleep apnea, occlusal misalignment, mental retardation, autism, and cerebral palsy [4, 5, 12].

Bruxism is self-limited, and treatment usually is unnecessary. In managing these patients, the source of stress should be explored. Therapy should be directed at eliminating the anxiety associated with stress. Self-hypnosis as a relaxation technique has been reported to be useful. Mouth guards are used in severe cases to protect teeth from erosion [4, 5, 12].

Insomnia is a subjective experience of difficulty in initiating and/or maintaining sleep with subsequent effects on daytime function and mood [4]. In early childhood, *parents* usually complain that their children experience difficulties with falling asleep and/or frequent awakenings. The issue is often due to parents' difficulty in limit setting (behavioral insomnia limit-setting type) or to children's association of sleep onset with parents' presence (behavioral insomnia sleep-onset association type).

Treatment is directed toward the parents by teaching skills in setting limits and encouraging adequate sleep hygiene and weaning their children gradually from requiring and depending on their presence while falling asleep [13].

Psychophysiologic or primary insomnia occurs in adolescents. The incidence is estimated to be 9–13%. This diagnosis is rare in prepubertal children. Psychophysiologic insomnia develops in adolescents with certain personality traits that probably are genetically determined [4, 5]. These traits include heightened physiologic arousals (hyperarousal state) and cognitive hypervigilance. The usual course is that a *precipitating* event such as an acute stress triggers the insomnia in the *predisposed* patient. When developed, the insomnia is maintained by the *perpetuating* factors including poor sleep habits, such as irregular sleep–wake schedule and excessive consumption of caffeine. Anxiety can develop about the lack of sleep and potential consequences of missing school and social functions. Associations can develop that are incompatible with sleep, such as learning to associate the bedroom with being awake rather than asleep with increased somatic and muscle tension at bedtime. As the cycle develops in which the more one strives to sleep, the more agitated one becomes and less able to fall asleep, the more the bedroom becomes associated with lack of sleep. Further, conditioned environmental cues can cause insomnia to develop. For example, playing violent videogames, watching television, or socializing (including through social media) at bedtime conditions the patient to associate being in their bedroom with behaviors that are not conducive to sleep. Thus, the bedroom can become a conditioned stimulus that prevents sleep, and some patients report that they sleep better when away from their bedroom.

The recommended first line of treatment for psychophysiologic insomnia is cognitive-behavioral treatment (Chap. 9) and hypnotherapy (Chap. 12). Hypnotherapy may also be used in combination with cognitive-behavioral therapy. The principles of these therapies are observation of adequate sleep hygiene. Cognitive-behavioral treatment targets learned sleep-preventing associations and combines sleep restriction with stimulus control. Stimulus control involves asking the patient to get out of bed when awake more than 20 min; to engage in quiet, nonstimulating activity; and to return to bed only when sleepy. Sleep restriction is part of stimulus control, and the principle is to shorten time in bed to the amount usually spent sleeping and to gradually increase the length of time in bed after sleep efficiency improves. Self-hypnosis often is successful in facilitating falling asleep and diminishing preoccupation with anxious thoughts [14]. Mindfulness meditation also may be helpful in the treatment of insomnia (Chap. 16) [15].

Nocturnal enuresis is characterized by recurrent involuntary voiding during sleep. It is defined as occurring at least twice a week after 5 years of age. *Primary enuresis* is diagnosed when a patient has never had a dry period for 6 consecutive months. *Secondary enuresis* occurs in children who have recently suffered a psychosocial stress, such as parental divorce, physical or sexual abuse, or neglect. Chronic constipation and encopresis are frequent comorbidities in children with secondary sleep enuresis [5, 16].

Enuresis has significant impact on children and their families. Children feel embarrassed, limit their social functioning, and may develop low self-esteem, shame, or emotional, behavioral, and conduct problems. The parents are worried and may punish the children for their behavior.

The spontaneous cure rate is 15% per year. Treatments include behavioral adjustments by improving bladder health via regular voiding, avoiding drinking at night, and avoiding caffeine. An enuresis alarm can be helpful. Since the enuresis occurs usually early in the night, awakening the child at the anticipated time of enuresis sometimes is useful. Pharmacological treatment has been used successfully, including imipramine, and DDAVP is useful in the short term, but recurrence is common when medication is discontinued [5, 15]. Hypnotherapy has been reported as useful in the treatment of children with primary nocturnal enuresis. Hypnosis was shown to be more effective than imipramine for children with enuresis older than 5–7 years of age, and the results usually are evident after few sessions [6, 7].

Positive Airway Pressure Therapy for Obstructive Sleep Apnea

It is estimated that OSA occurs in 2–10% of children and adolescents and 28% of adults. Tonsillectomy and adenoidectomy (T&A) is the treatment of choice for children. PAP therapy is the treatment of choice for adults and in children not responsive to T&A [17, 18]. PAP therapy involves forcing air with high pressure through a tightly fit mask with a headgear. Although it was found to be effective, it has been reported that only 53% of adults and 33% of children adhere to this therapy [17, 18]. Please see case 4 below for a discussion regarding possible reasons for lack of adherence to PAP and how this might be addressed.

Case Studies

Case 1

Sarah is a 6-year-old girl who was brought by her parents for abnormal behavior during sleep. She has a 2-year history of sleepwalking. She arises after 1.5 h of falling asleep and walks to her parents' room. During the episode, her eyes appear to be open, but she seems to be looking through the parents and not at them and does not respond to them typically. Sarah becomes agitated and screams when her parents try to awaken her from an episode. She does not remember the event in the morning.

Sarah otherwise is healthy. Her sleep history indicates that she goes to bed at 9 pm and falls sleeps within 15–20 min. The parents report that she snores loudly enough that they can hear her in their room across the hall. The snoring sometimes is interrupted by pauses that are followed by gasping. Her breathing is labored when snoring.

Despite sleeping for 10 h overnight, she naps for 1½ h after returning from school.

Her physical examination is remarkable for the presence of grade 3 tonsils and adenoid facies.

Questions:

1. What is the likely diagnosis?
   (a) Seizures
   (b) Sleepwalking
   (c) Sleepwalking and possible sleep-disordered breathing
   (d) Night terrors
   (e) None of the above
2. How do you confirm the diagnosis?
   (a) Sleep study (overnight polysomnography)
   (b) Sleep EEG
   (c) Lateral neck film to evaluate the size of the adenoids
   (d) Chest X-ray
   (e) All the above
3. How do you manage the patient?
   (a) Assure her parents that sleepwalking is benign and review the safety measures that should be undertaken.
   (b) Tonsillectomy and adenoidectomy.
   (c) Clonazepam half an hour before sleep.
   (d) Teach the child self-hypnosis.
   (e) a and b.

Answers:

1. (c): Sarah's history is consistent with sleepwalking. The history of continuous loud snoring and the findings on her physical examination suggest sleep-disordered breathing. In this case, the sleep deprivation and frequent arousals that are typically associated with obstructive sleep apnea likely trigger the sleepwalking [10]. The history of daytime napping indicates the possibility of poor sleep quality associated with obstructive sleep apnea because the patient's history indicates

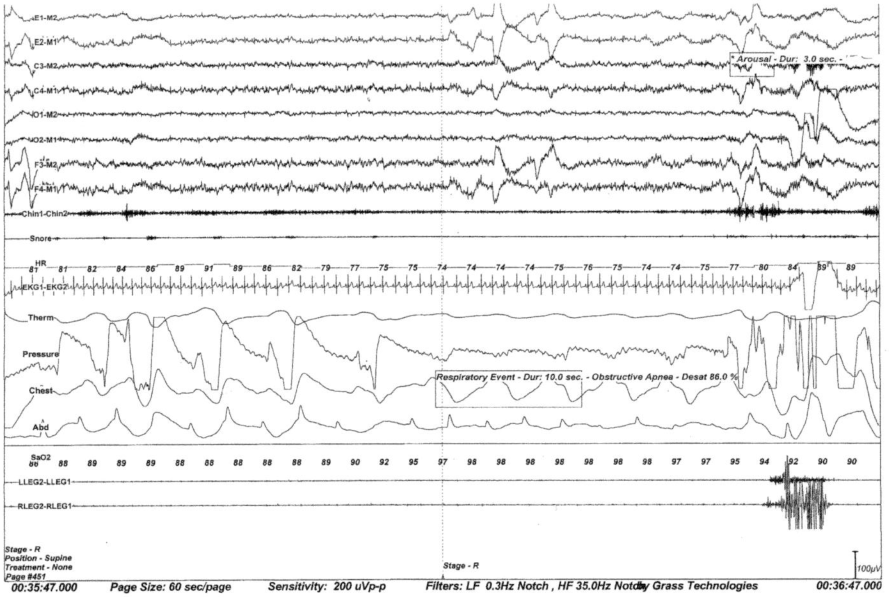

Fig. 7.2 These 2 epochs (60 s) are from R stage of Sarah's sleep. The obstructive episode is evident by the flattening of the nasal flow waveform as transmitted by the thermistor and the pressure cannulas and is associated by continuing abdominal and chest wall movements and followed by arousal and oxygen desaturation

adequate 10-h nighttime sleep. Children at 6 years of age do not usually nap, unless they are sleep deprived. It is unlikely that she has seizures since she does not demonstrate stereotypical movements and sleep-related enuresis that are typical of sleep-related seizures.

2. (a): Although the history and physical examination are suggestive, polysomnography is indicated in order to confirm the presence of sleep-disordered breathing and determine its severity. A sleep study is not indicated to confirm sleepwalking per se because the diagnosis of sleepwalking can be made on the basis of the history. Sleep study with extensive EEG montage is indicated sometimes when the history is not clear and there is suspicion of seizures causing the nighttime activities. Sarah's sleep study revealed 11 obstructive episodes per hour of sleep and some that were associated with arousals (Fig. 7.2). This is consistent with moderately severe obstructive sleep apnea. The arousals and sleep deprivation associated with sleep-disordered breathing are potent triggers of sleepwalking. We did not observe sleepwalking during the study, but that does not rule out sleepwalking.
3. (e): In this case, it is to be expected that treating the sleep-disordered breathing will eliminate arousals, improve sleep quality, and thus eliminate the triggers for sleepwalking. Therefore, referral for tonsillectomy and adenoidectomy (T&A) was made. The parents were educated about taking safety measures to

ensure the child safety. Clonazepam is a benzodiazepine that has been used for its effect on shortening SWS with a resultant decrease in the frequency of sleepwalking. It is recommended in difficult to treat cases that have led to injuries. Hypnotherapy also has been utilized successfully in treating sleepwalking, but we decided in this case to treat the sleep apnea first in order to eliminate the trigger and then follow for the need for further therapies. Sarah underwent T&A, and following the treatment, the parents reported resolution of the snoring and disturbed sleep, and the frequency of sleepwalking diminished substantially.

Case 2

Joe is a 7-year-old boy brought by his parents for difficulty falling asleep. Despite following adequate sleep hygiene and bedtime routine, Joe resists sleep and comes out of his bedroom for different excuses such as asking for water, more kisses, or to use the bathroom. He will not fall sleep unless the light is kept on in his bedroom and one of his parents stays with him. Eventually, he falls asleep at around 11 PM. In 1 or 2 h, he wakes up and goes to the parents' bedroom to complain of fears of intruders. He ends up falling back to sleep in his parents' bedroom and remains there for the rest of the night. The parents allow him to sleep in their bed so they can sleep.

During the daytime, Joe takes 2 h naps on most weekdays. He is doing well in school and does not experience problematic daytime anxiety or fears. When asleep, he does not exhibit symptoms suggestive of disordered breathing. Otherwise, the medical history is insignificant.

Questions:

1. What is the diagnosis?
   (a) Nighttime fears
   (b) Night terrors
   (c) Nightmares
   (d) Sleepwalking
   (e) None of the above
2. How should this be managed?
   (a) No need to treat.
   (b) Encourage the parents to invite the child to sleep with them to make him feel safe and protected.
   (c) Educate the parents regarding helping the child to develop coping skills.
   (d) Allow the child to fall asleep in the living room while the parents are available, and then the child can be transferred to his room.
   (e) None of the above.

Answers:

1. (a): Joe appears to resist sleep in his room because of his fears. The fact that he sleeps well as long as he is with his parents supports this impression. Nightmares and night terrors occur during sleep and not while the patient is trying to fall asleep. Severe forms of nightmares (associated with awakening from fearful dreams) and terrors (associated with screaming) can lead to bedtime resistance similar to Joe's manifestations, but he does not have symptoms while asleep, as long as he sleeps with the parents. Joe's arousals and going to his parents' room are inconsistent with sleepwalking since he appears to be fully awake when he goes to his parents and complains about fear of intruders.
2. (c): Treatment is indicated because the fears are severe and affecting the child's and the family's sleep. The sleep disruption is evident by the history of daily napping, which is indicative that Joe is sleep deprived, because 7-year-olds do not usually sleep in the daytime. The following strategies can be used: The parents are taught to assure the child of their presence nearby to ensure his safety. It is important that the parents maintain a balance between reassuring the child and avoiding reinforcement of the fears. For example, effective parental assurance of safety includes saying, "Mommy and daddy are next-door and we'll always make sure that you are safe." Joe can be taught appropriate coping skills and ways to respond to nighttime fears, such as "being brave" and making positive self-statements such as, "I can take care of myself." The parents can assure the child by checking on the child in a mutual agreed schedule (e.g., every 15 min) of personal assurance. Reading stories that provide examples of coping role models who conquer their fears can be helpful. The family can encourage the child to develop creative solutions such as monster spray.

Case 3

Samantha is a 16-year-old with a 2-year history of "poor sleep." She believes that she sleeps for 2–3 h in the night. It takes her 2–3 h to fall asleep, and on many nights, she awakens in early morning and has difficulty falling back to sleep or may not be able to fall back to sleep. While in bed, she is anxious about her inability to fall asleep and the consequences of sleep deprivation. Despite of being tired in the daytime, it is difficult for her to take naps even when she has the opportunity. She consumes up to 5 cups of coffee a day and still is unable to concentrate in classes, and her grades subsequently have declined. This year, she decided to drop out of school. She has not been able to participate in her favorite sport, lacrosse, because of her daytime fatigue. Samantha's parents say she always has been a poor sleeper, and she becomes anxious easily. Her insomnia started after she broke her arm while playing lacrosse 2 years ago and was unable to participate in the sport for 3 months. She could not sleep well at first because of the pain, but even after the pain resolved, her sleep did not improve. Her parents stated that Samantha's sleep issues were not associated with such severe daytime consequences in the past. She is depressed about her inability to meet friends, participate in social activities, the decline in her grades, and her decreased chances of receiving a college lacrosse scholarship as a result of insufficient playing time. Otherwise, the history indicates that she had been healthy. Her physical examination is remarkable for an anxious and tired-appearing adolescent but otherwise is unremarkable.

Questions:

1. In the development of Samantha's insomnia, which of the following are either predisposing, precipitating, or perpetuating factors?
   (a) History of being "poor sleeper and becoming anxious easily"
   (b) Breaking the arm 2 years ago
   (c) Poor sleep hygiene and anxiety about lack of sleep
   (d) All the above
2. The recommended therapy for Samantha is:
   (a) Hypnotic medication
   (b) Replacement of her bedroom furniture so that she can develop new sleep-time associations
   (c) Cognitive-behavioral therapy and hypnotherapy
   (d) Combination of the above
   (e) None of the above

Answers:

1. (d): The history that Samantha has always been poor sleeper and becomes anxious easily demonstrates a *predisposition* to develop insomnia. The sport injury *precipitated* the insomnia 2 years ago perhaps because of her associated decreased physical activity, withdrawal from playing on the team, and withdrawal from social activities. The insomnia has been *perpetuated* because of maladaptive behavior such as spending prolonged time in bed ruminating about the consequences of lack of sleep, the changes in her life, her lost friends, and the fact that her chance of receiving a scholarship for college was decreased as she was unable to play lacrosse with the varsity team.
2. (c): CBT is the standard of care. For Samantha, the bedtime was delayed to 2:00 a.m. (consistent with her reported sleep-onset time) to minimize sleep-onset latency. The rise time was set at 6:30 a.m., which was consistent with her school schedule. Once asleep within 20 min on a consistent basis, her bedtime was gradually moved earlier by 30 min to the goal of an 11:00 pm bedtime. She was instructed not to nap during the day. Samantha was offered hypnotherapy and used it successfully to relax at bedtime and to alleviate her anxieties. Within 3 weeks of therapy, Samantha's sleep-onset latency was shortened. She continued

to have some nocturnal awakenings, but decreased in frequency and duration. In the daytime, her mood improved, and she decided to return to school.

Case 4

Kevin is a 16-year-old male who came for ongoing continuous positive airway pressure (CPAP) management. He had been diagnosed previously with severe obstructive sleep apnea. His apnea–hypopnea index (AHI) was 46/hour, indicating severe obstructive sleep apnea. He underwent T&A. The surgery did not resolve the snoring, and he continued to experience daytime tiredness and sleepiness, and his post-surgery AHI was 22/h. Therefore, CPAP therapy was recommended. His medical history was significant for morbid obesity, hypertension (his blood pressure was 158/95), and dyslipidemia. His physical examination was notable for obesity (body mass index 38, with a normal range of 20–25).

Kevin was given a CPAP with nasal mask with auto-titration, which automatically increases the pressure of forced air to treat and prevent apnea. The auto-titration equipment was given in order for Kevin to acclimate with the equipment, in anticipation of the need for overnight therapy titration study at the sleep lab. The visit was scheduled 1 week after he was given the PAP equipment. Kevin reported using the PAP sporadically for less than a minute at a time. He explained that he found it impossible to breathe with the air forced on his nose with high pressure. He said he felt as if he was going to "suffocate." He developed anxiety that he would feel palpitations from seeing or hearing the CPAP.

Questions:

1. How would you change Kevin's attitude toward the CPAP?
   (a) Just give him more time and ask him to keep trying since he has the equipment for 1 week only.
   (b) Refer him for cognitive-behavioral and desensitization therapy.
   (c) Teach him self-hypnosis to cope with the anxieties.
   (d) Offer him a bribe, such as a car, in exchange for using the CPAP.
   (e) b and c.

Answers:

1. (e): CBT has been found to substantially increase the rate of adherence to CPAP in adults and in children, in particular when used early. In fact, this follow-up visit in 1 week is very important because studies have shown that skipping CPAP for one or more nights in the first weeks is a marker of a group of patients who likely will go on to use CPAP poorly [17, 18]. Giving patients more time or

offering a bribe would not be sufficient to help overcome significant anxiety. For Kevin, we educated him about obstructive sleep apnea and the benefits of the treatments. We reviewed his symptoms such as excessive daytime sleepiness and discussed the positive consequences of his potential improvement. We reviewed the results of the sleep study to highlight how the therapy addresses the problems. We discussed the advantages and disadvantages of treatment and developed goals for his therapy. Given his anxieties, we recommended gradual desensitization. He was instructed to practice breathing with the mask only in the daytime. Gradually, the headgear was placed and, when comfortable, a low positive airway pressure was introduced. The pressure was increased gradually according to his tolerance. Self-hypnosis was offered and accepted by the patient in order to relax and relieve his anxieties associated with using the CPAP. After he became comfortable and able to breathe in the daytime with the prescribed pressure, the therapy was applied while he was sleep.

Conclusions

Functional sleep-related disorders are common. They have negative effects on the sleep efficiency and architecture and thus substantially impact the cognitive function of patients. Simple measures to adjust the behaviors of the patients and their parents can resolve these disorders and improve the quality of life and function of the patients.

References

1. Banks S, Dinges D. Chronic sleep deprivation. In: Kryger M, Roth T, Dement W, editors. Principle and practice of sleep medicine. 5th ed. St. Louis Missori: Elsevier; 2011.
2. Sadeh A, Gruber R, Raviv A. Sleep, neurobehavioral functioning, and behavior problems in school age children. Child Develop. 2002;73(2):405–17.
3. Kryger MH. Atlas of clinical sleep medicine. Philadelphia: Elsevier; 2010.
4. American Academy of Sleep Medicine. The international classification of sleep disorders; diagnostic and coding manual. 2nd ed. Westchester: American Academy of Sleep Medicine; 2005.
5. Mindell JA, Owens JA, editors. A clinical guide to pediatric sleep: diagnosis and management of sleep problems. 2nd ed. Philadelphia: Lippincott Williams & Wilkins; 2010.
6. By N, Lee TS. Hypnotherapy for sleep disorders. Ann Acad Med Singap. 2008;37(8):683–8.
7. Graci GM, Hardie JC. Evidenced-based hypnotherapy for the management of sleep disorders. Intl J of Clin Exp Hypn. 2007;55(3):288–302.
8. Hurwitz TD, Mahowald MW, Schenck CH, Schluter JL, Bundlie SR. A retrospective outcome study and review of hypnosis as treatment of adults with sleepwalking and sleep terror. J Nerv Ment Dis. 1991;179(4):228–33.
9. Kramer RL. The treatment of childhood night terrors through the use of hypnosis—a case study: a brief communication. Int J Clin Exp Hypn. 1999;37(4):283–4.
10. Guilleminault C, Palombini L, Pelayo R, Chervin RD. Sleepwalking and sleep terrors in prepubertal children: what triggers them? Pediatrics. 2003;111(1):e17–25.

11. Gordon J, King NJ, Gullone E, Muris P, Ollendick TH. Treatment of children's nighttime fears: the need for a modern randomized controlled trial. Clin Psychol Rev. 2007;27(1): 98–113.
12. Nissani M. A bibliographical survey of bruxism with special emphasis on non-traditional treatments modalities. J Oral Sci. 2001;43(2):73–83.
13. Morgenthaler TI, Owens J, Alessi C, et al. American academy of sleep medicine. Practice parameters for behavioral treatment of bedtime problems and night wakings in infants and young children. Sleep. 2006;29(10):1277–80.
14. Morgenthaler T, Kramer M, Alessi C, et al. American academy of sleep medicine. Practice parameters for the psychological and behavioral treatment of insomnia: an update. Sleep. 2006;29(11):1415–9.
15. Gross CR, Kreitzer MJ, Reilly-Spong M, et al. Mindfulness-based stress reduction versus pharmacotherapy for chronic primary insomnia: a randomized controlled clinical trial. Explore (NY). 2011;7(2):76–87.
16. Robson WL. Evaluation and management of enuresis. N Engl J Med. 2009;360(14):1429–36.
17. Koontz KL, Slifer KJ, Cataldo MD, Marcus CL. Improving pediatric compliance with positive airway pressure therapy: the impact of behavioral intervention. Sleep. 2003;26(8):1010–5.
18. Aloia MS, Di Dio L, Ilniczky N, Perlis ML, Greenblatt DW, Giles DE. Improving compliance with nasal CPAP and vigilance in older adults with OAHS. Sleep Breath. 2001;5(1):13–21.

Part III
Treatment of Functional Respiratory Disorders

Chapter 8
When Should a Patient Be Referred to a Mental Health Provider?

Brett G. Toelle, Juliet M. Foster, and Christine R. Jenkins

Abstract Psychological comorbidity in functional respiratory disorders is common and, if not fully appreciated, may lead to inaccurate investigations, treatments, and diagnosis. For this reason, it is important to recognize that comorbid psychological conditions may interact with functional respiratory symptoms for a prolonged period of time without identification by patient or clinician. We propose a model of care that uses screening questions and assessment tools early on in the investigation of the respiratory presentation that uses both patient and clinician time efficiently. A range of simple tools are available for use in primary care to help inform the decision about whether referral to a mental health professional is appropriate. In addition, the severity, age of patient, and/or complexity of the presentation of symptoms are other factors to consider when deciding whether to refer to a mental health professional. Many focused psychological strategies can be delivered successfully in primary care, and the ultimate decision about referral will depend on a range of factors including the ability, competence, remuneration, and willingness of primary care staff to deliver these approaches. Because patients with functional respiratory disorders often have a psychological component to their presentation, it is important to address psychological issues in primary care early through treatment strategies or mental health-care referral.

B.G. Toelle (✉)
Respiratory & Environmental Epidemiology Group, Woolcock Institute of Medical Research, Box M77, Missenden Road Post Office, Camperdown, NSW 2050, Australia
e-mail: brett.toelle@woolcock.org.au

J.M. Foster
Respiratory & Environmental Epidemiology Group, Woolcock Institute of Medical Research, Box M77, Missenden Road Post Office, Camperdown, NSW 2050, Australia

C.R. Jenkins
Clinical Professor, University of Sydney, Co-operative Research Centre for Asthma Woolcock Institute of Medical Research, Thoracic Physician, Concord Hospital, Australia

Department of Thoracic Medicine, Concord Hospital, Hospital Road, Concord, NSW 2137, Australia
e-mail: christine.jenkins@sydney.edu.au

R.D. Anbar (ed.), *Functional Respiratory Disorders: When Respiratory Symptoms Do Not Respond to Pulmonary Treatment*, Respiratory Medicine,
DOI 10.1007/978-1-61779-857-3_8, © Springer Science+Business Media, LLC 2012

Keywords Anxiety • Depression • Mental health • Psychological • Referral • Screening

The most common approach to the management of symptoms of breathlessness, habit cough, vocal cord dysfunction, or chest pain is to run the standard battery of respiratory and cardiac investigations to search for a cause or physiological explanation for the symptoms. Often, psychological or psychogenic explanations are kept as a consideration of last resort once all other causes or disorders have been ruled out. However, there is a good argument for concurrent investigation of both physiological and psychological aspects of respiratory symptoms. The concurrent investigation of both is an efficient way to proceed and may result in time and cost savings to the patient and health-care system as well as avoid unnecessary investigations and treatments that may bring about a range of side effects and potential adverse effects. Investigation of psychological and psychosocial factors may help to identify them as a cause for the symptoms, but even when these factors are not causal, an appreciation of them is important because they so frequently interact with symptoms to influence response to treatment and ultimately health outcomes.

Background

Psychological disorders of mood and affect are commonly seen in primary care. An Australian review estimated that their prevalence in primary care patients was 25% [1]. In addition, a number of reviews and studies have identified the high prevalence of psychological comorbidity among patients with respiratory symptoms and diseases. In a review of anxiety and depression in chronic obstructive pulmonary disease (COPD), the authors report an overall estimate of approximately 50% of COPD patients having clinically significant symptoms of anxiety and/or depression [2]. In an audit of 406 Canadian adult outpatients attending an asthma clinic, a total of 34% of patients had one or more psychiatric diagnoses, including major depression (15%), minor depression (5%), dysthymia (4%), panic disorder (12%), generalized anxiety disorder (5%), and social phobia (4%) [3].

Many psychosocial issues impact on the well-being of patients with chronic respiratory disease, from the moment of receiving a diagnosis and adjusting to the disease through coping with worsening symptoms and quality of life in progressive diseases such as COPD or managing highly variable symptoms in uncontrolled asthma. In patients with chronic disease, low socioeconomic status, poverty, and poor education are associated with more stressful life events and fewer social resources to buffer them, which result in poorer mental health [4, 5]. Smoking, poor housing, and financial barriers to quality health care and medication may also contribute to poorer health and suboptimal self-management in patients with asthma [6, 7].

There may be a downward shift in the socioeconomic status of patients with chronic disease [8]. Physical or functional limitation may lead to changes in income and social networks and may threaten the life goals of patients and their families. This can lead to feelings of uncertainty about the future [5].

Individual patients cope with their disease in different ways, but most fall somewhere on the active-avoidant coping continuum. Active copers will seek information and social and medical support and find outlets for emotional expression, whereas avoidant copers may deny or disengage with their medical condition, ignore symptoms, and avoid treatment. In asthma, for example, avoidant coping is associated with a greater frequency of emergency room visits and hospital admissions in the next 12 months [9, 10].

Social support appears to be somewhat protective against psychological comorbidity in asthma [11] and may promote appropriate health behaviors [12], but inappropriate or negative social support (e.g., resentment from the support provider or feelings of guilt from the patient) is associated with greater depression and anxiety in COPD [13]. When a spouse or partner is the main support provider, both patient and partner (spouse) may suffer from loneliness and depression. This is often due to functional limitation, particularly in severe chronic respiratory illness, where the opportunity to socially interact is restricted or impossible for both parties because of poor mobility and dependence on oxygen therapy. The additional burden that spouses carry in order to assume the partner's responsibilities as well as maintaining their own [14] leaves them less time and opportunity to remain socially engaged beyond their immediate domestic setting. In children, the family is the primary source of support, and family dysfunction may act directly as a barrier to optimal asthma management through inadequate supervision of disease management [15] or psychological distress and poor coping strategies [11, 16].

Poor adherence to prescribed medication regimens is associated with poor quality of life, increased health-care use, and fatal and near-fatal asthma exacerbations [17–19]. There is a strong, consistent relationship between poor adherence and depression across many different chronic diseases (e.g., asthma, end-stage renal disease, angina, and rheumatoid arthritis) with the odds being three times greater that depressed patients, versus the nondepressed, will be poorly adherent with medical treatment recommendations [20].

Poor perception of dyspnea is strongly associated with treatment delay, near-fatal events, and death during acute severe asthma [21, 22]. In asthma, alexithymia—i.e., difficulty in perceiving or expressing feelings—is associated with higher rates of exacerbation and hospitalization, poorer quality of life, and near-fatal asthma [23, 24]. Patients with COPD may have poorer perception of dyspnea than patients with asthma perhaps due to habituation to the more prolonged dyspnea experienced in COPD and the very gradual development of impairment that occurs over 20 or more years. Age-related loss of perceptual ability [25] almost certainly plays a role as well, although for a given level of energy expenditure, as would be expected, COPD patients do experience greater levels of dyspnea than healthy individuals [26].

Table 8.1 Characteristics of an open empathic communication style

1.	Encourage patient dialogue through asking open questions, not interrupting, maintaining eye contact, and tolerating silence
2.	Active listening: respond to nonverbal cues and summarize what the patient has said to clarify your understanding and to establish rapport
3.	Use empathic statements to show you understand the patient's perspective
4.	Ask direct psychologically oriented questions early in the interview

In paradoxical vocal cord dysfunction, psychological comorbidity is estimated at an extremely high rate of up to 75% [27]. Comorbidities may include mood, anxiety, somatoform, or personality disorders, as well as psychosocial distress [28]. Such high rates suggest the need for early psychological screening when assessing vocal cord dysfunction, and treatment may need to be initiated for both vocal cord dysfunction and psychological comorbidity. Particularly where patients have somatoform conversion disorders, the early identification of psychological disorders may assist the physician in ruling out a physiological cause/diagnosis and prevent the reinforcement of inappropriate medical ideation and unnecessary treatments [29].

Dyspnea can be an important and frightening feature of asthma and COPD that may have a profound impact on the patient's experience of their condition. Limitations to quality of life, functional status, and increased socioeconomic burden may all be associated with dyspnea, and the accurate assessment of the experience of dyspnea is important so that the symptom is not over- or under-interpreted. Poor perception has been associated with treatment delay that increases the risk of adverse outcomes, whereas high or overperception of dyspnea has been linked to unnecessary treatments and investigations. A number of studies have demonstrated the interaction between affect and perception, showing that participants who had a blunted affect were more likely to overperceive their breathlessness. Thus, there has been an increased focus on combining physical and psychological techniques to successfully manage the symptoms of breathlessness [30].

Identifying Psychological Comorbidity

Psychological comorbidity is often difficult to identify; it is estimated that up to half of all patients who present with psychological disorders in primary care, such as anxiety and depression, may not be diagnosed and others may not be treated [1]. To optimize detection of these disorders, general practitioners need at least a basic knowledge of the common presenting symptoms and syndromes. But patients with depression or anxiety often present with physical symptoms which mask psychological issues and delay or prevent diagnosis, so the use of an open, empathic communication style in consultations is key to diagnosis of psychological comorbidity (see Table 8.1). Physicians are more likely to recognize or diagnose depression when they ask questions about feelings or psychosocial issues [31].

Screening and Assessment Tools

Because psychological problems are so common in primary care and also commonly observed as a comorbidity in respiratory patients, we are strongly of the view that, at the very least, simple screening tools should be used in the assessment of all respiratory patients.

In a New Zealand study of 476 primary care patients, two simple verbal screening questions were used to identify depression (see Table 8.2) [32]. The sensitivity and specificity of both questions for detecting depression were 97% and 67%, respectively, when validated against depression identified by the mood module of the Composite International Diagnostic Interview (CIDI) [36].

A study conducted in 15 U.S. primary care clinics among 965 patients investigated the utility of simple screening questions for the identification of generalized anxiety disorder, panic disorder, social anxiety disorder, and posttraumatic stress disorder [33]. The study showed that the use of the generalized anxiety disorder 7 item (GAD-7) and the shorter two-item GAD-2 (score $\geq$3) provided good sensitivity and specificity for identification of anxiety when compared to structured psychiatric interview by a trained mental health professional blinded to results of the screening questions.

Table 8.2 presents both the short screening questions useful in primary care but also some of the more detailed assessment tools that are available for use. Some of these tools are subject to copyright and therefore require a license to use in clinical practice. Others are available free of charge, and there are now several websites that allow you to download pen and paper copies or to complete the questionnaire online. Of course, as with any instrument, it is important to use one that is appropriate for the population. There is a range of instruments available and some may be more appropriate for the cultural background, age (younger or older), and cognitive ability of your patients.

Psychosocial issues may play a meaningful role in the expression of symptoms, the maintenance of symptoms, or the inability to satisfactorily diagnose symptoms. The taking of a good psychosocial history may help to uncover otherwise unrecognized associations between the expression of symptoms and dimensions of the patient's life (see Table 8.3). Historically, some have argued that the expression of symptoms has been due to an internal intrapsychic conflict and that the partial expression of this conflict is through the expression of physical symptoms [37]. A consultation between practitioner and patient with good rapport and a genuine interest in a holistic understanding of the patient, their symptoms, and their life experience can assist to understand the direction in which to refer the patient.

When to Refer to a Mental Health Professional?

The clinical decision about when to refer a patient with a functional respiratory disorder needs to be made after carefully weighing up a range of factors. Firstly, what indicators from among the clinical investigations are inconsistent with a physiological

Table 8.2 Screening questions and assessment tools

Disorder	Questions	Response options	Reference
Screening questions			
Depression	– During the past month, have you often been bothered by feeling down, depressed, or hopeless?	Yes or no	Arroll et al. [32]
	– During the past month, have you often been bothered by little interest or pleasure in doing things?	Yes or no	
Anxiety	– Over the last 2 weeks, how often have you been bothered by the following problems?	Not at all = 0	Kroenke et al. [33]
	– Feeling nervous, anxious, or on edge?	Several days = 1	
	– Not being able to stop or control worry?	More than half the days = 2 Nearly every day = 3	
Assessment tools			
Anxiety depression	Hospital anxiety and depression scale (HADS)	14 items 7 items per scale Each item scores 0–3 Each scale ranges 0–21 Requires purchase	Zigmond et al. [34]
Depression anxiety stress	Depression anxiety stress scales (DASS)	42 or 21 (short version) items 14 or 7 items per scale Each item scores 0–3 Each scale ranges 0–42 or 21 No charge (available on web) http://www2.psy.unsw.edu.au/groups/dass/	Lovibond et al. [35]
Depression	Patient health questionnaire 9 (PHQ-9)	9 items Each item scores 0–3 No charge (available on web) http://www.phqscreeners.com/	
Anxiety	General anxiety disorder 7 (GAD-7)	7 items Each item scores 0–3 No charge (available on web) http://www.phqscreeners.com/	

Table 8.3 Important areas to cover in psychosocial assessment

Psychosocial assessment areas	How does the symptomatology, management, or ongoing care relate to these particular areas?
Relationships	Significant personal relationships Family relationships
Employment	Pattern and hours of work Satisfaction with work and work relationships
Housing	Nature of housing, own/rent Connection with neighbors/local community
Finances	Ability to meet rent, bills, expenses of daily living Ability to withstand job loss, significant impact to earning ability
Coping strategies	What coping strategies does the patient use to deal with stressors and illness Alcohol, cigarettes, gambling, withdrawal, isolation, self-destructive actions/behaviors
Cultural issues	Aspects of culture that may be important such as practices, rituals, expectations
Social, leisure, hobby activities	Activities that are of interest
Health and well-being	Overall assessment in relation to construct of health and well-being

explanation for the symptoms/disorder? If there are questions around the cause of symptoms, clinical investigations might be combined with information gleaned from psychological screening tools and a more detailed psychological/psychosocial patient history. Where the primary care physician has a strong suspicion, supported by evidence from screening or assessment tools, that there may be a mental health component to the functional respiratory disorder, then the decision about when to refer to a mental health professional becomes much more straightforward.

Both patient and doctor may find it difficult to discuss referral due to the stigma associated with mental illness and the role of a mental health professional in their ongoing care. Potential referral needs to be discussed sensitively with the patient and their agreement must be secured. Explaining that it is very common for patients with respiratory illness to have anxiety or depression is important so that the patient does not feel that their respiratory symptoms are being dismissed as purely psychological. Informing the patient that multidisciplinary care can reduce the prescription of unnecessary and unhelpful medications may assist in helping the patient see the advantages of such a referral. It may be helpful to engage in a discussion with the patient about their perceptions of psychologist or psychiatric services to address patients' concerns or misconceptions.

When deciding whether to refer to a mental health professional, the primary care physician may need to consider a range of factors. Firstly, what is my capacity to provide therapy in this context to the patient? To what extent do I or others in my office have the time available to commit to the delivery of therapeutic approaches outlined in other chapters of this book—interventions such as biofeedback (Chap. 10), hypnosis (Chap. 12), or breathing techniques (Chap. 11)?

Table 8.4 When to refer to a mental health-care professional in the primary care setting

Referral should be considered in the following cases:
1. Significant depression or anxiety (especially in adolescent patients)
2. High suicide risk
3. Failure to respond to treatment
4. Uncertainty about the diagnosis
5. Possible organic brain disease or dementia
6. The need for greater resources
7. Comorbidity with drugs or alcohol
8. Patients not accepting recommended advice or treatment
9. Symptoms or impact that are out of keeping with objective assessment of severity

See [38]. © Copyright 1997. *The Medical Journal of Australia*—reproduced with permission

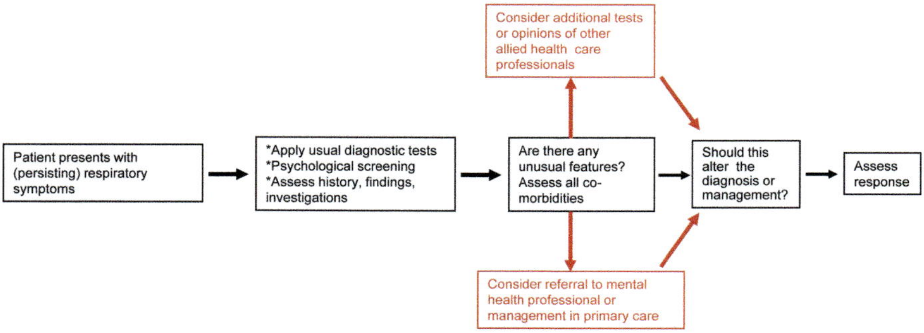

Fig. 8.1 Approach to managing a patient with respiratory symptoms and psychological comorbidity

All professionals need to be confident of their competence in delivering therapeutic approaches to their patients. In some settings, there may be adequate remuneration for this approach, where a range of management approaches can be delivered in primary care, while in others, the system may be designed such that referral is the most efficient for patient care.

Additionally, the decision of when to refer will be largely influenced by the severity of the symptoms and and/or the underlying psychological state which determine the impact on and the risk to the patient (see Table 8.4).

Screening tools that provide a positive indication or a psychosocial interview and history that is strongly suggestive of underlying psychological distress and disorder in and of itself may be worthy of referral to a mental health professional. The fostering of a multidisciplinary approach where primary care and mental health professionals work in tandem to help the patient address their disorder will facilitate a smooth referral process and effective collaboration when both physical and psychological aspects of airways disease need to be addressed (see Fig. 8.1). In the Australian context in which we work, the Australian Government has recognized the importance of collaborative mental health care and has provided significant funding for an initiative called the Mental Health Professionals Network (MHPN). The funding of this network was recently rolled out throughout Australia to bring together geographically colocated general practitioners (primary care physicians), psychiatrists, psychologists, pediatricians, mental health nurses, and other allied mental health professionals. The aim is to ensure that these professionals are aware of each other and the role that each can play in the management of mental health issues. We are unaware of other similar models of care around the world, but the evaluation of this new multidisciplinary network approach will be helpful to inform whether it may be considered in other health systems.

Case Studies

Case 1

A male aged 36 years presented with breathing difficulties associated particularly with singing. He felt his symptoms were related to diaphragmatic weakness or incoordination. He had been a successful performer in musicals, sustaining full-time employment in major roles in high-profile productions. His teacher said he had great note holding capacity, and he had no problems with his singing or breathing until 5 years earlier when he was given five new notes to sing in a tenor range, which were particularly challenging as he is a baritone.

He had kept a diary over the last few years and felt that he had to "think" about when to breathe. He described feeling his diaphragm not doing what it should, and feeling like "cement." Lying down aggravated this. He mentioned he did not feel confident about his breathing when he first lay down to go to sleep. His partner commented that his breathing seemed normal at night and he does not snore, have erratic breathing, or apneas.

He had been exercising to try and overcome this problem, particularly doing diaphragmatic breathing exercises and vocal exercises that require diaphragmatic and intercostal breathing and which encourage better breath management through lower abdominal support. He found these very challenging even though he made some progress. He had recently stopped professional singing but was committed to sing in a children's drama soon and was apprehensive about this.

The patient recalled wheezing episodes from the age of 5 although he had never been given a diagnosis of asthma and never had a regular controller medication. He wheezed and developed chest tightness on exposure to nonspecific irritants such as cold air, fumes, and smoke and after walking in the cold air. He was a lifelong nonsmoker.

On examination, the patient looked well. There was no chest wall asymmetry on deep expiration and chest expansion and air entry were normal bilaterally. Breath sounds were normal and there were no added sounds on auscultation. Spirometry revealed airflow limitation and a bronchodilator response, FEV1/FVC being 3.08/4.46 L (FEV1/FVC ratio 69%) with an improvement to 3.36/4.57 L (76% and 83% of predicted, respectively). Laryngoscopy showed secretions on the cords and no narrowing on inspiration. Chest X-ray was normal. Diaphragmatic screening indicated a normal sniff test (a test that uses fluoroscopy to evaluate the function of the diaphragm during "sniffing maneuvers" that exaggerate diaphragmatic movement) with no evidence of paradoxical movement to suggest phrenic nerve palsy. Functional diaphragmatic tests and measurement of maximum inspiratory and expiratory pressures showed values over 100% predicted, thus indicating no diaphragmatic weakness.

Questions:

1. What do you consider is the cause of the patient's difficulty in breathing?
2. Are there additional causes of his singing difficulty?
3. Should further investigations be undertaken?
4. Should the patient be assessed by a psychologist?
5. Would questionnaires to assess presence of anxiety or depression be helpful?
6. What interventions might assist the patient?

Answers and Clinician's Comments:

1. Despite having mild airflow limitation, this is unlikely to be the cause of the patient's singing and breathing problem, which has features of dysfunctional breathing.

   From the Nijmegen questionnaire [39] (see Table 4.4), it can be seen that dysfunctional breathing is characterized by a broad range of symptoms some of which are nonspecific and do not particularly apply to either the sensation of breathlessness or a patient's response to it. Specific symptoms in the questionnaire include chest pain, fast or deep breathing, shortness of breath, chest tightness, and difficulty breathing in or taking a deep breath. Nonspecific symptoms may be a manifestation of hyperventilation or of the somatic manifestations of anxiety, and these include feeling tense, having blurred vision, dizziness, a sense of loss of touch with reality, or anxiety. Symptoms that clearly would be related to hyperventilation include dizziness, tingling in fingers and hands, stiffness or cramps in fingers and hands, tightness around the mouth, cold hands or feet, and palpitations. This questionnaire has been validated, and a total score over 23 has been shown to be characteristic of patients with hyperventilation, having a sensitivity of 91% and a specificity of 95% as a screening instrument in patients diagnosed with hyperventilation syndrome [40, 41]. Hyperventilation is but one form of dysfunctional breathing.

   The patient described in the case history described a range of symptoms that would fit well with dysfunctional breathing, including being unable to breathe deeply, having a feeling of tightness in his chest, feeling tense, and feeling anxious. His Nijmegen score was 25, perhaps not as high as would be expected in somebody whose symptoms were simply due to apprehension and performance anxiety. It was therefore crucial to investigate his respiratory and diaphragmatic function, as he was convinced that this was the reason for his

difficulty in singing. In fact, his diaphragmatic pressures, lung volumes, sniff test for paradoxical diaphragmatic movement, and chest expansion were all completely normal.
2. The cause of the patient's dyspnea is multifactorial. Although he had no chest wall or diaphragmatic muscle weakness, he described feeling he could not fully exhale and commented that he might be breath-holding. His description of difficulty coordinating his breathing in a normal tidal breathing pattern suggested a degree of respiratory dyspraxia (breathing incoordination), possibly due to tension and increased tone in his lower chest wall and upper abdominal wall.
3. Most patients need to be reassured that there is no underlying disease contributing to their breathing difficulty, and most physicians feel far more confident discussing the possibility that symptoms are driven by anxiety when they have excluded significant alternative diagnoses. In some instances, especially in patients who have previously already been thoroughly investigated, it should be possible to progress to discussing the role of anxiety and to reinforcing the appropriate nature of the previous investigations. Exploring patients' health beliefs and their own view of the previous investigations and reassurance offered to them often will give clinicians an opening to discuss key psychological issues that may underlie dyspnea.
4. Patients who describe at least some of their symptoms as relating to situations of tension or anxiety may be more receptive to an early referral for psychological assessment. Even panic attacks, however, can occur without a clear temporal relationship to an anxiety-provoking context, and many patients will have difficulty believing that panic disorder underlies their breathlessness, particularly believing that the reasons for such a response should be very evident to them. Some patients are convinced that their symptoms have an organic physiologic basis and an early referral to a psychologist will not instill confidence but will rather lead them to the view that they are not being taken seriously. Judgements about the timing for psychological assessment therefore are often difficult to make and should be tailored to a clinician's perceptions of the patients' needs and the weight of evidence in favor of a psychological contributor to their symptoms.
5. Clinicians have some very useful "desktop" tools at their disposal for the diagnosis of dysfunctional breathing, such as the Nijmegen questionnaire (Table 4.4) and the Hospital Anxiety and Depression scale [34]. These are easy to use, self-completed questionnaires which can very quickly help clinicians to appraise accompanying symptoms and the psychological issues that may contribute to the respiratory presentation. Abnormal scores using these validated questionnaires should help point clinicians in the direction of an early consultation with a mental health professional rather than repeating investigations which are expensive and time-consuming and have previously been shown to be normal.
6. With the demonstration of normal lung function and diaphragmatic strength, the patient was able to appreciate that there was no structural limitation to his performance, and he was much more responsive to the idea that a significant proportion of his sensation of dyspnea was due to anxiety, specifically in his case, performance

anxiety. His hospital anxiety and depression score indicated that anxiety was a significant component in his mood, his score being 15 for anxiety, indicating moderately high level clinical anxiety but only 6 for depression, which is normal. His loss of confidence had led to a sense of feeling overwhelmed by the demands of the stage performance. This loss of confidence had resulted in his having to abandon his singing career and he had come to believe that he could no longer sing. We were able to show him that functionally, there is no reason why this would be the case. With the help of a physiotherapist with pulmonary rehabilitation experience, a clinical psychologist and a speech pathologist, he has made excellent progress. He has continued to see a clinical psychologist and speech pathologist and is gradually returning to his full singing range with the assistance of his voice trainer. He is currently auditioning for a major new role.

Case 2

A 42-year-old woman presented for investigation of dyspnea and cough. She had a prior diagnosis of asthma, made by another respiratory physician, without spirometric evidence of airflow limitation, so presumed to be on the basis of her history that was complex. She recalled that this physician had commented to her that she would "always have trouble with her lung function being extraordinary" perhaps suggesting that other physicians may have difficulty feeling confident about an asthma diagnosis. She also was concerned that she was prone to frequent respiratory infections and that these may be secondary to immune compromise as a result of her intense training schedule. Specific questioning about these infections did not suggest increased frequency, but protracted symptoms, especially cough and fatigue for weeks afterward.

The patient presented as a somewhat tense person with significant anger that previous investigations had not uncovered an organic reason for her fatigue and dyspnea.

Full pulmonary function tests on this occasion were normal, including the flow volume curve, lung volumes, and diffusing capacity. Her history was particularly of exercise limitation, but she was a regular recreational exerciser, running around 10–15 km comfortably several days a week. She therefore had excellent exercise capacity, but toward the end of exercise would feel extremely fatigued and, at these times, experienced a limitation to deep breathing, more intense breathlessness, and mild cough. She expressed significant frustration about having to deal with these symptoms. She had no associated wheezing, although she commented that she had wheezed on other occasions spontaneously particularly in association with viral respiratory tract infections. Although she related the presence of wheeze during respiratory tract infections, it was unclear if this symptom was actually noisy breathing possibly due to secretions, rather than a typical high-pitched expiratory sound suggestive of asthma.

The patient's cough generally was irritating and productive of very small amounts of mucoid sputum, occurring in the mornings and after exercise. She had not recently had any sputum purulence or had acute infective symptoms. She had no wheeze associated with the cough or breathlessness. Generally, fatigue rather than chest tightness caused her to stop exercising, but she experienced persistent dyspnea for 5–10 min after stopping exercise, suggesting the possibility of exercise-induced bronchoconstriction.

In view of this history, she underwent a eucapnic hyperventilation challenge. This test identifies the presence of exercise-induced bronchoconstriction (EIB) by a stepped up series of ventilatory challenges while breathing on a closed circuit in a laboratory, a fall in lung function (FEV1) of 15% indicating EIB. This showed a 5% fall in FEV1 to the maximum voluntary ventilation rate, thus *excluding* exercise-induced bronchoconstriction. Inspiratory flow volume curves performed during this test did not reveal any evidence of reduced inspiratory flow to suggest the possibility of exercise-related vocal cord dysfunction. Comparisons of her lung function in 2002 and 2010 showed identical values, indicating that despite the fact she had not received asthma medication, there was no evidence of variability in lung function nor deterioration over this time. A thoracic high-resolution computed tomography (HRCT) scan was performed to exclude bronchiectasis given the history of a productive cough, which showed no focal or diffuse abnormality in the lung fields.

Questions:

1. Are there any features in this patient's history to suggest a psychological component to her breathlessness?
2. How should this possibility be explored—before commencing investigations of lung function or once the results have been shown to be normal?
3. In view of a patient's resistance to a psychological examination largely contributing to her breathlessness and fatigue, how would you approach this?

Answers and Clinician's Comments:

1. The patient had a generally negative view of the health professionals who had indicated they thought there was no significant lung problem and a more positive view of others who had suggested explanations that had no psychological component. She had a high level of expectation about her physical performance and a low tolerance of the current frustrations imposed by her fatigue and the failure of the health system generally to sort out the problem for her. While no single feature pointed to a psychological problem, and the patient herself was intensely resistant to such a suggestion, the combination of these features certainly raised the possibility.
2. Exploration of the psychological issues involved in this patient's breathlessness would need to take place after establishing trust and the patient's confidence in the clinician's capacity to be sympathetic with her concerns and to thoroughly investigate the problem. Early introduction of a psychological explanation would probably not be well received by such a patient. As it is not possible for the

clinician to know definitely that investigations will reveal completely normal results, in this situation it is probably better to wait and then be justified in presenting possible alternative explanations. Patients such as this one, with high expectations of their own physical performance, may feel very strongly that a psychological explanation represents a dismissal and implies a personal weakness about which they may be quite defensive.

3. It is often helpful to prompt the patient to explore explanations themselves once investigations have been unhelpful in uncovering significant underlying pathology, instead of presenting a psychological diagnosis as a last resort alternative possibility. Even at this stage, many patients will find this a formulaic approach and will see the fault lying with the clinician who has failed to fully tease out the physical problem. For this reason, a dialogue that prompts the patient to explore possible reasons themselves can be harnessed by the clinician to endorse a particular interpretation offered by the patient rather than to force on them a perspective they are reluctant to take.

Case 3

The patient is a 66-year-old man who presented to the emergency department with an acute exacerbation of COPD associated with a lower respiratory tract infection. He had a history of slowly deteriorating exercise tolerance over the previous 12 months and increasing difficulty with activities of daily living in the last 2 months, but had not been assessed fully. On presentation, he was acutely dyspneic and moderately hypoxemic but was not in hypercapnic respiratory failure. He responded to bronchodilators acutely, but as his hypoxemia persisted, he was admitted to a hospital. He improved on bronchodilators, antibiotics, and corticosteroids, and the nature of his respiratory disease was explained to him following investigations confirming moderately severe airway obstruction consistent with COPD. He was discharged with an action plan for identifying and managing exacerbations, a booking for the pulmonary rehabilitation program, and a planned review for full assessment when stable.

After returning home, he began to experience episodes of acute breathlessness, some of which resulted in unscheduled out of hours visits to his GP and others in a return to the emergency department but without evidence of clinical worsening nor more marked hypoxemia. The attending medical officers noted the patient appeared very anxious but was responsive to oxygen and reassurance in the emergency department. Additionally, the arterial blood gases suggested a respiratory alkalosis, consistent with hyperventilation. The patient subsequently completed an 8-week course of pulmonary rehabilitation, and his exercise capacity improved, as demonstrated by his six-minute walk distance. He was able to return to his previous level of independence and to social activities, which he had had to abandon. Despite this, he continued to experience acute episodes of dyspnea sometimes resulting in presentation to the emergency department. During most of these episodes, it was not possible to demonstrate any change in his clinical status.

Questions:

1. This patient has a history of recurrent emergency department attendances which after the first moderately severe COPD exacerbation, do not appear to be associated with worsening clinical status nor more marked hypoxemia. How would you consider investigating the cause of this problem?
2. What are the risks associated with pharmacological management of anxiety in patients with COPD?
3. Should this patient be referred for psychological assessment?
4. What strategies could be developed to help this patient manage his acute breathlessness and to distinguish anxiety and episodes of panic from worsening dyspnea due to an acute exacerbation of COPD?

Answers:

1. Because an acute exacerbation of COPD is frequently manifested by worsening dyspnea, the first priority in this situation is to be certain that the acute breathlessness experienced by the patient is not due to an evolving exacerbation. Features consistent with an exacerbation would include infective symptoms particularly sputum purulence or fever, subacute onset in the context of a recent cold, easy fatigability, loss of appetite, sleep disturbance ,or worsening manifestations of comorbid illnesses such as heart failure or diabetes. Features suggesting a panic attack or acute anxiety would include sudden onset, associated apprehension and fear, recent stability of the underlying lung disease, no associated infection, improvement with reassurance, and lack of benefit from interventions that usually are helpful, such as bronchodilators. Although there may be distinguishing features, it can sometimes be exceptionally difficult to determine whether anxiety is overlaid on an episode of worsening disease that must be treated in its own right. Deteriorating breathlessness in patients with COPD may be a trigger for anxiety, amplifying the dyspnea through psychological and physiological mechanisms. Hyperventilation in patients who are already hyperinflated may result in shortened expiratory time, increased gas trapping, and hyperinflation, thus contributing to worsening dyspnea and putting the patient at greater disadvantage in relation to increased work of breathing and optimal ventilation.
2. Pharmacological management of anxiety in patients with COPD is likely to involve classes of medications such as benzodiazepines or antipsychotic drugs which can suppress respiratory drive and aggravate hypercapnia. Patients with CO_2 retention should only be given sedating agents, including narcotic analgesics, under supervision and with great care. There are very few studies investigating the potential of anxiolytic and antidepressant medications to assist COPD patients who have a significant component of anxiety; however, a recent review suggests that small doses of benzodiazepines may be helpful [42].

   This patient experienced recurrent episodes of acute breathlessness, out of keeping with the severity of his background COPD, which appeared to be stable at the time. These initially occurred following an acute presentation, when he had, for the first time, experienced much more intense dyspnea and the feelings of helplessness and foreboding that naturally accompany a life-threatening event. He is likely to benefit from a psychological assessment addressing his underlying fears and concerns that have probably been significantly amplified by his recent acute exacerbation and diagnosis of COPD, which he now knows may be associated with progressively worsening breathlessness and greater physical limitation. A psychologist's assessment to confirm the presence of anxiety and panic attacks is likely to be helpful in identifying this as a problem which can be managed effectively [42, 43].

3. Cognitive behavior therapy (Chap. 9) has been shown to be an effective strategy for COPD patients with panic attacks. COPD patients can be taught many techniques to reduce their dyspnea and to give them a sense of control over their breathlessness [44–47].
4. This patient may well benefit from a structured pulmonary rehabilitation program which has been shown to have benefits for comorbid anxiety and depression in the breathless patient. A structured program will provide opportunity for exercise, reduce social isolation through regular participation in program activities, and promote independence. All of these factors are often viewed as perpetuating factors in relation to anxiety and depression, and managing them in the context of breathlessness will have concurrent benefits for the patient's psychological health. Components of the program will also operate through a psychoeducation pathway whereby the patient gains a greater more accurate understanding of the characteristics, causes, and management of their symptoms.

Interoceptive exposure may also be employed in a safe environment where the patient can induce panic symptoms then when experiencing the symptoms, they can desensitize themselves to the anxiety. Primary care practitioners who feel competent and mental health professionals are skilled in the use of these techniques [48]. It is also important to discuss with the patient the potential physiological effects of medication on feelings of breathlessness but also upon feelings of anxiety such as palpitations, agitation, and hyperarousal.

Conclusions

Many focused psychological strategies can be delivered successfully in primary care, and the ultimate decision about referral will depend on a range of factors including the ability, competence, remuneration, and willingness of primary care staff to deliver these approaches. Because patients with functional respiratory disorders often have a psychological component to their presentation, it is important to address psychological issues in primary care early through treatment strategies or mental health-care referral.

References

1. Ellen SR, Norman TR, Burrows GD. MJA practice essentials. 3. Assessment of anxiety and depression in primary care. Med J Aust. 1997;167(6):328–33.
2. Mikkelsen RL, Middelboe T, Pisinger C, Stage KB. Anxiety and depression in patients with chronic obstructive pulmonary disease (COPD). A review. Nord J Psychiatry. 2004;58(1): 65–70.
3. Lavoie KL, Cartier A, Labrecque M, et al. Are psychiatric disorders associated with worse asthma control and quality of life in asthma patients? Respir Med. 2005;99(10):1249–57.
4. Mitchell EA, Stewart AW, Pattemore PK, Asher MI, Harrison AC, Rea HH. Socioeconomic status in childhood asthma. Int J Epidemiol. 1989;18(4):888–90.
5. Stanton AL, Revenson TA, Tennen H. Health psychology: psychological adjustment to chronic disease. Annu Rev Psychol. 2007;58:565–92.
6. Thai AL. The effects of health literacy on asthma self-management. J Asthma Allergy Educators. 2010;1:50–5.
7. Fattahi F, Hylkema MN, Melgert BN, Timens W, Postma DS, ten Hacken NH. Smoking and nonsmoking asthma: differences in clinical outcome and pathogenesis. Expert Rev Respir Med. 2011;5(1):93–105.
8. Stommel M, Kurtz ME, Kurtz JC, Given CW, Given BA. A longitudinal analysis of the course of depressive symptomatology in geriatric patients with cancer of the breast, colon, lung, or prostate. Health Psychol. 2004;23(6):564–73.
9. Gonzalez-Freire B, Vazquez-Rodriguez I, Marcos-Velazquez P, de la Cuesta CG. Repression and coping styles in asthmatic patients. J Clin Psychol Med Settings. 2010;17(3):220–9.
10. Adams RJ, Smith BJ, Ruffin RE. Factors associated with hospital admissions and repeat emergency department visits for adults with asthma. Thorax. 2000;55(7):566–73.
11. Wright RJ, Rodriguez M, Cohen S. Review of psychosocial stress and asthma: An integrated biopsychosocial approach. Thorax. 1998;53(12):1066–74.
12. Barton C, Clarke D, Sulaiman N, Abramson M. Coping as a mediator of psychosocial impediments to optimal management and control of asthma. Respir Med. 2003;97(7):747–61.
13. McCathie HC, Spence SH, Tate RL. Adjustment to chronic obstructive pulmonary disease: the importance of psychological factors. Eur Respir J. 2002;19(1):47–53.
14. Keele-Card G, Foxall MJ, Barron CR. Loneliness, depression, and social support of patients with COPD and their spouses. Public Health Nurs. 1993;10(4):245–51.
15. Fritz GK, Rubinstein S, Lewiston NJ. Psychological factors in fatal childhood asthma. Am J Orthopsychiatry. 1987;57(2):253–7.
16. Miller BD, Wood BL, Lim J, Ballow M, Hsu C. Depressed children with asthma evidence increased airway resistance: "vagal bias" as a mechanism? J Allergy Clin Immunol. 009; 124(1):66–73 e61-10.
17. Romagnoli M, Caramori G, Braccioni F, et al. Near-fatal asthma phenotype in the ENFUMOSA Cohort. Clin Exp Allergy. 2007;37(4):552–7.
18. Rea HH, Scragg R, Jackson R, Beaglehole R, Fenwick J, Sutherland DC. A case-control study of deaths from asthma. Thorax. 1986;41(11):833–9.
19. Popa V. Emergency department visits in asthma: Should all be prevented? Chest. 2001;120(4): 1058–61.
20. DiMatteo MR, Lepper HS, Croghan TW. Depression is a risk factor for noncompliance with medical treatment: Meta-analysis of the effects of anxiety and depression on patient adherence. Arch Intern Med. 2000;160(14):2101–7.
21. Restrepo RD, Peters J. Near-fatal asthma: Recognition and management. Curr Opin Pulm Med. 2008;14(1):13–23.
22. Magadle R, Berar-Yanay N, Weiner P. The risk of hospitalization and near-fatal and fatal asthma in relation to the perception of dyspnea. Chest. 2002;121(2):329–33.
23. Vazquez I, Sandez E, Gonzalez-Freire B, Romero-Frais E, Blanco-Aparicio M, Verea-Hernando H. The role of alexithymia in quality of life and health care use in asthma. J Asthma. 2010;47(7):797–804.
24. Serrano J, Plaza V, Sureda B, et al. Alexithymia: A relevant psychological variable in near-fatal asthma. Eur Respir J. 2006;28(2):296–302.

25. Rutgers SR, ten Hacken NH, Koeter GH, Postma DS. Borg scores before and after challenge with adenosine 5′-monophosphate and methacholine in subjects with COPD and asthma. Eur Respir J. 2000;16(3):486–90.
26. Ofir D, Laveneziana P, Webb KA, Lam YM, O'Donnell DE. Mechanisms of dyspnea during cycle exercise in symptomatic patients with GOLD stage I chronic obstructive pulmonary disease. Am J Resp Crit Care Med. 2008;177(6):622–9.
27. Newman KB, Mason 3rd UG, Schmaling KB. Clinical features of vocal cord dysfunction. Am J Respir Crit Care Med. 1995;152(4 Pt 1):1382–6.
28. Thurston NL, Fiedorowicz JG. Improvement of paradoxical vocal cord dysfunction with integrated psychiatric care. Psychosomatics. 2009;50(3):282–4.
29. Selner JC, Staudenmayer H, Koepke JW, Harvey R, Christopher K. Vocal cord dysfunction: The importance of psychologic factors and provocation challenge testing. J Allergy Clin Immunol. 1987;79(5):726–33.
30. von Leupoldt A, Dahme B. Psychological aspects in the perception of dyspnea in obstructive pulmonary diseases. Respir Med. 2007;101(3):411–22.
31. Williams Jr JW, Noel PH, Cordes JA, Ramirez G, Pignone M. Is this patient clinically depressed? JAMA. 2002;287(9):1160–70.
32. Arroll B, Khin N, Kerse N. Screening for depression in primary care with two verbally asked questions: Cross sectional study. BMJ. 2003;327(7424):1144–6.
33. Kroenke K, Spitzer RL, Williams JB, Monahan PO, Lowe B. Anxiety disorders in primary care: prevalence, impairment, comorbidity, and detection. Ann Intern Med. 2007;146(5):317–25.
34. Zigmond AS, Snaith RP. The hospital anxiety and depression scale. Acta Psychiatr Scand. 1983;67(6):361–70.
35. Lovibond PF, Lovibond SH. The structure of negative emotional states: comparison of the depression anxiety stress scales (dass) with the beck depression and anxiety inventories. Behav Res Ther. 1995;33(3):335–34.
36. Kessler RC, Ustun TB. The world mental health (WMH) survey initiative version of the world health organization (WHO) composite international diagnostic interview (CIDI). Int J Meth Psychiatr Res. 2004;13(2):93–121.
37. Butani L, O'Connell EJ. Functional respiratory disorders. Ann Allergy Asthma Immunol. 1997;79(2):91–9; quiz 99–101.
38. Ellen SR, et al. Assessing anxiety and depression in primary care. MJA. 1997;167:14–9.
39. van Dixhoorn J, Duivenvoorden HJ. Efficacy of Nijmegen Questionnaire in recognition of the hyperventilation syndrome. J Psychosom Res. 1985;29(2):199–206.
40. Ringsberg KC, Akerlind I. Presence of hyperventilation in patients with asthma-like symptoms but negative asthma test responses: provocation with voluntary hyperventilation and mental stress. J Allergy Clin Immunol. 1999;103(4):601–8.
41. Thomas M, McKinley RK, Freeman E, Foy C. Prevalence of dysfunctional breathing in patients treated for asthma in primary care: cross sectional survey. BMJ. 2001;322(7294):1098–100.
42. Hill K, Geist R, Goldstein RS, Lacasse Y. Anxiety and depression in end-stage COPD. Eur Respir J. 2008;31(3):667–77.
43. Eisner MD, Blanc PD, Yelin EH, et al. Influence of anxiety on health outcomes in COPD. Thorax. 2010;65(3):229–34.
44. Brenes GA. Anxiety and chronic obstructive pulmonary disease: prevalence, impact, and treatment. Psychosom Med. 2003;65(6):963–70.
45. Livermore N, Sharpe L, McKenzie D. Panic attacks and panic disorder in chronic obstructive pulmonary disease: a cognitive behavioral perspective. Resp Med. 2010;104(9):1246–53.
46. Livermore N, Sharpe L, McKenzie D. Prevention of panic attacks and panic disorder in COPD. Eur Respir J. 2010;35(3):557–63.
47. Raupach T, Bahr F, Herrmann P, et al. Slow breathing reduces sympathoexcitation in COPD. Eur Respir J. 2008;32(2):387–92.
48. Cantor L, Jacobson R. COPD: how to manage comorbid depression and anxiety. J Family Pract. 2003;2 www.jfponline.com/Pages.asp?AID=691.

Chapter 9
Basic Cognitive Behavioral Therapy: Applications for Functional Respiratory Disorders and Other Medically Unexplained Symptoms

Courtney E. Du Mond and David A. Johnson

Abstract Cognitive behavioral therapy encompasses a variety of therapeutic approaches involving the interaction of cognition, emotion, and behavior. It is widely considered the gold standard therapy for most psychologically based disorders and is currently considered the technique of choice for the treatment of medically unexplained symptoms and behaviorally based sleep disorders. The following chapter explores its application to the treatment of functional respiratory disorders in the primary care and consultative setting.

Keywords Cognitive behavioral therapy • Dyspnea • Functional respiratory disorders • Habit cough • Insomnia • Medically unexplained symptoms • Noncardiac chest pain

Background

Cognitive behavioral therapy (CBT) is a broad term used to refer to a variety of therapeutic approaches that emphasize interactions among cognition (thought), behavior, and emotion (feeling) with a goal of affecting favorable and practical change in a patient's chronic illness. CBT is an evidence-based technique that has been extensively studied in a variety of disorders. It is widely considered the gold standard of treatment for the majority of psychologically based disorders [1–4]. While some models emphasize cognitive over behavioral factors and vice versa, the

C.E. Du Mond (✉)
Department of Pediatrics, SUNY Upstate Medical University, Syracuse, NY, USA
e-mail: dumondc@upstate.edu

D.A. Johnson
Adirondack Internal Medicine and Pediatrics, 2249 State Route 86,
Suite 3, Saranac Lake, NY, USA

R.D. Anbar (ed.), *Functional Respiratory Disorders: When Respiratory Symptoms Do Not Respond to Pulmonary Treatment*, Respiratory Medicine,
DOI 10.1007/978-1-61779-857-3_9, © Springer Science+Business Media, LLC 2012

basic tenets are the same; there is interplay among what patients think, what they feel, and what they do. CBT seeks to interrupt this cycle by modifying a patient's thoughts and beliefs and by changing their behavioral habits. Since these elements are interdependent, change in one domain by necessity results in change in the others.

Functional respiratory disorders (FRD) and functional sleep disorders (e.g., insomnia, hypersomnia, and fatigue) are common and sometimes misdiagnosed. Despite their common occurrence, little research has examined effective treatments for most functional respiratory disorders. These disorders fall under a rather large umbrella, which includes more generalized diagnoses such as somatoform disorder, conversion disorder, and the broad category "medically unexplained symptoms" (MUS). While important differences exist among these diagnostic categories, the underlying mechanisms are similar: the existence of one or more physical symptoms that are distressing to the patient and/or family but lack a medical explanation. By their very nature, these disorders are often complex and difficult to treat. For the purposes of this chapter, we will use MUS to refer to the broad categories of functional respiratory, somatoform, and conversion disorders. Medically unexplained symptoms naturally lend themselves to a cognitive behavioral understanding and approach to treatment.

A useful cognitive behavioral conceptualization for MUS suggests that these patients selectively attend to one or more basic bodily functions and lack the ability to normalize (i.e., understand the sensations as part of normal/healthy body functioning) these experiences. Subsequently, their thought processes may become dysfunctional, their reasoning emotion-based or dichotomous (black and white), and catastrophic misinterpretations may be attached to these thoughts. This sequence of selective attention, dysfunctional thinking and catastrophization leads to symptom amplification and anxiety, which perpetuates a cycle and ultimately produces a chronic dysfunctional illness such as a FRD.

Efficacy of CBT for Medically Unexplained Symptoms

A number of studies have examined the efficacy of CBT for the treatment of MUS. CBT is currently considered the first line of treatment for MUS [5–9]. Six recent randomized controlled trials of good quality [10–15] provide level I evidence demonstrating CBT's effectiveness in treating MUS. (Two methodologically compromised studies [16, 17] failed to demonstrate superiority of CBT to standard care.) The literature on the value of CBT with specific application to FRDs is limited. Evidence is strongest, showing substantial and durable benefit, when applied to noncardiac chest pain (NCCP) [18–23] and to sleep disorders where it clearly is the gold standard [24–26]. The literature on CBT in dyspnea primarily addresses treatment of anxiety in patients with COPD [27–29] in which dyspnea is pathological, not functional, and is quite sparse regarding its utility in vocal cord dysfunction [30–32] and in habit cough [33].

CBT in the Primary Care Setting

There has been substantial interest in providing CBT for MUS in the primary care setting [10–14] with the goal of making it more generally available and enhancing patients' adherence to its use. There are significant individual and systemic barriers to treatment by mental health providers. A majority of patients referred for mental health services by their primary care physician (PCP) fail to seek treatment [8, 34, 35]. Patients understandably can be put off by the stigma of a psychological or psychiatric interpretation ("it's all in your head"). Communication between PCPs and mental health providers is often suboptimal, and insurance carriers often inadequately cover care by mental health providers. These factors logically place an opportunity for care of these disorders in the realm of the PCP. Nevertheless, we presume that most PCPs would initially indicate ignorance of or insecurity with CBT techniques due to lack of exposure and training. We maintain, however, that grounding in basic open-ended and motivational interviewing techniques and a patient-centered approach, ideally common to all well-trained PCPs, comprises a solid background for delivery of basic CBT in the primary care setting. Although not named as such, rudimentary "CBT" is, or should be, a part of many PCP/patient encounters in helping patients to understand and cope with medically *explained* symptoms. Extension of these logical techniques to MUS should be a short step for a motivated PCP. A "therapeutic alliance" is already established. All that is lacking is elemental instruction and training in the logical and pragmatic concepts and practices of CBT.

One might argue that PCP encounters are often brief and that remuneration for "cognitive time" is poor. We maintain that basic CBT techniques are unknowingly integral to many encounters with a thoughtful and competent PCP and that a practitioner's skill, confidence, and effectiveness in treating MUS could be enhanced significantly with modest effort at education regarding the effective utilization of these techniques. Advanced CBT techniques are clearly the domain of trained psychotherapists, and patients requiring such care are appropriately referred (see Chap. 8 for a more detailed description). Upon completion of this chapter, providers should have an understanding of basic CBT techniques appropriate for use in the primary care setting.

CBT for Medically Unexplained Symptoms: The Basics

The Therapeutic Alliance

A solid working therapeutic alliance between the health-care provider and the patient is common to all CBT approaches. This alliance is essential for the health-care provider to engage with and effect change in the patient. The ideal model requires a single consistent care provider who communicates a genuine caring for the patient and their needs and a clear understanding of their symptoms. This is most effectively accomplished through the use of open-ended interviewing, reflective and empathic listening and encouraging optimism and hope through empowerment of the patient.

Early in the therapeutic relationship, it is imperative to establish clear and honest goals with the patient. For patients with medically unexplained symptoms, this usually entails seeking practical understanding of cognitive and emotional factors that affect behavior and formulating new and improved coping skills to deal with symptoms rather than anticipating a cure. In fact, detailed thoughtful explanations of cognitive and behavioral dynamics combined with patient engagement have been shown to increase patient satisfaction and improve outcome, while brief reassurances about the benign nature of their problem generally lead to ever-increasing psychosomatic presentations [36].

Health-care providers should also encourage emotional expression and disclosure during encounters. Patient dissatisfaction and reversion to further somatic interventions and evaluations are less likely to result when patients discuss psychosocial problems openly with their care provider [36]. Recent research has suggested that exploration of the psychodynamic roots of a causal link between psychosocial stressors and the index symptom may be less important than simply providing an opportunity for patients to express these stressors [36].

Cognitive Restructuring and Reframing

Cognitive restructuring and reframing are perhaps the most important tactical elements of CBT. Seeking to challenge and replace automatic thoughts and dysfunctional beliefs, cognitive restructuring and reframing scientifically examine the patient's cognitive tendencies. Automatic thoughts refer to internalized perceptions that are often triggered by a particular situation, are quickly generated, and are not subject to detailed inquiry or logical examination (e.g., "I'm a failure"). These thoughts can be positive or negative. Dysfunctional automatic thoughts, however, are almost exclusively negative. Dysfunctional beliefs (e.g., "Nothing will ever help me") are learned patterns of thinking, which cause emotional and/or physical distress, are generally irrational, and lack objectivity.

Dysfunctional thoughts and beliefs result from various cognitive distortions. While there are many types of cognitive distortions, those most relevant to MUS involve dichotomous (black or white) or perfectionistic (all or none) thinking, catastrophizing, emotional reasoning, and negative filtering.

Dichotomous thinking is fairly self-descriptive and occurs when a patient oversimplifies a situation by seeing it as polarized between two extremes. For example, a patient (Jennifer) presents to your office with a history of cough. When asked, "what have you found that helps?" she replies "Nothing, nothing helps!" Jennifer is using dichotomous thinking. In reality, it is likely that some situations make her cough more likely to occur while others make it less likely (shades of gray). Dichotomous thinking is especially common in individuals with perfectionistic tendencies. These individuals define their performance as a success or a failure (e.g., 99% is a failure). Helping patients to identify these patterns and to recognize alternate ways of thinking can result in significant reductions in stress and negative mood.

Catastrophic thinking is often a central component of MUS and occurs when a person overestimates the possibility of a negative outcome and believes that what has happened or what will happen will be so terrible that they will be unable to handle the consequences. In functional respiratory disorders, patients can have catastrophic misinterpretations of their symptoms. For example, a patient with dyspnea may say, "I'm going to suffocate and die" despite the fact that she actually has not done so and is very unlikely to do so in the future.

Negative filtering involves selective attention to negative information while simultaneously ignoring the positive. A patient with noncardiac chest pain may continue to insist, "I just know it's my heart" despite multiple medical tests to the contrary. He fails to find reassurance in true and objective positive information.

Emotional reasoning, on the other hand, occurs when patients use their feelings or emotions as evidence for the truth, feel overwhelmed and helpless about their symptoms, and conclude that they must be impossible to solve. "I'm scared. I know this (functional dysphonia) is going to be throat cancer just like Dad's." Cognitive behavioral therapists use many techniques to dispute and restructure dysfunctional thoughts and beliefs. Most techniques begin with some type of thought monitoring that generally is combined with symptom, emotional, and behavioral monitoring. For example, in their book *Treating somatization: A cognitive behavioral approach*, Woolfolk and Allen [37] recommend having patients record their physical symptoms (including a rating of intensity), the situation in which the symptoms occur, the resulting emotion (including a rating of intensity) and their corresponding thoughts at two different times each day: during an uncomfortable moment and during a relatively comfortable moment. These records are used to elicit dysfunctional beliefs and resulting emotions and behaviors during subsequent encounters.

Cognitive restructuring subsequently proceeds through a process of scientific or Socratic investigation. Patients are encouraged to examine their beliefs from different perspectives. A common strategy involves "*examining the evidence.*" Once a dysfunctional belief is identified, the healthcare provider and patient can objectively examine the evidence for the patient's belief. Because dysfunctional thoughts and beliefs are not reality-based, they tend to appear rather distorted when compared with reality. It is often helpful to have the patient begin by identifying evidence that supports their belief followed by evidence to the contrary:

Doctor: Jennifer, have you noticed anything that makes your cough worse or more likely to occur?

Jennifer: Yes, it always seems to be the worst at bedtime.

Doctor: Hmm, that's interesting. Are there other times when you notice your cough gets worse?

Jennifer: Yes. Whenever I go over to my sister's house my cough gets really bad. I think I'm allergic to something in her house, but whenever I try to tell her anything, she just jumps down my throat. I wish I never had to go over there, but my mother would kill me if I didn't show up.

Doctor: OK, that's helpful. So you notice that your cough gets worse in the evening before bed and when you're at your sister's house.

Jennifer: Yes.

Doctor: What about the opposite? Are there ever times that your cough gets better or you just don't notice it as much?

Jennifer: Um... I don't know. I can't really think of any. I feel like it's terrible all the time.

Doctor: What about when you're doing something you really enjoy like hanging out with good friends or watching a great movie?

Jennifer: Now that you mention it, I guess it does seem a little better then, but I probably just don't notice it as much.

Doctor: That's a really good observation. I think what you're saying is that when you're distracted with fun and enjoyable activities you don't notice your cough as much. Is that true?

Jennifer: Yeah, I guess so.

Doctor: And that when there's not much going on, say at bedtime, or when your over at your sister's house it, gets worse.

Jennifer: Yup!

Doctor: Well really this is good news. We've already discovered some things that make your cough worse and more importantly some things that make it better.

While examining the evidence is an effective strategy for many patients, some patients struggle to objectively evaluate their own thoughts and actions even with the guidance of an objective care provider. For these patients, it is often useful to help them *evaluate their situation from an outside perspective*. For example, you might ask them what they would tell a friend in a similar situation with a similar belief:

A 40-year-old recently divorced mother of two experiences chronic daytime fatigue. While discussing her symptoms, she states "I can't believe I'm divorced... I'm such a failure!" In this case, you might ask the patient if she has any friends who are also divorced (she is likely to say yes). Does she believe they are a failure? You might also ask her how she would comfort a friend who felt similarly (i.e., believed she was a failure). Individuals experiencing negative affect states (e.g., anxiety and depression) are more likely to attribute personal failures to internal factors (i.e., things within themselves such as their personality) while attributing similar failures of others to external factors (e.g., the environment). Comparing and contrasting the two interpretations helps patients appreciate biases in their thinking. Patients are often much more willing to reconsider their own beliefs when examining them from someone else's perspective.

Examining the effect or function of the belief itself is another useful cognitive strategy. Patients may be asked, "What happens when you have that thought?" This question is followed with the logical opposite "What would happen if you didn't think that way?" The first question is likely to be accompanied by negative emotions and behavior while the second by more positive outcomes. Contrasting the two can be illuminating to patients.

Cognitive behavioral therapists also rely heavily on strategies of *cognitive reframing*. This straightforward process involves helping patients to restructure their thoughts and beliefs into more functional and realistic forms. For example, after discussing situations that make her cough more or less likely, Jennifer (see above) may be able to modify her previous belief that "Nothing helps" to a more realistic statement such as "I know that there are things that make my cough worse and things that make it better." The second statement not only eliminates the dichotomous thinking but also gives Jennifer an inherent sense of control over her symptom, something she noticeably lacked before. Research has shown that when given control over a negative stimulus, individuals find it significantly less distressing and less negative [38]. Reframing can also involve simple rephrasing of a negative into a positive: "I'm never going to fall asleep" to "It's inevitable that I will eventually fall asleep so there's really no sense in worrying about it."

The beauty of CBT is its logical simplicity. Many CBT interventions are quite elementary, but few untrained practitioners and even fewer patients utilize these strategies. Patients with these disorders often fail to critically examine their own thought processes. Doing so, with guidance, may be life changing.

Behavioral Interventions

In general, behavioral interventions are more diagnosis specific than cognitive strategies but share a similar investigative methodology. Determining the appropriate behavioral intervention involves an in-depth analysis of the behavior including identification of associations, antecedents, and consequences. In essence, behavioral interventions seek to manipulate the patient's environment in order to "set them up to succeed." Two learning (or conditioning) models are at the heart of behavioral interventions: classical conditioning and operant conditioning. A brief overview of each will aid in understanding behavioral interventions based on each model.

Classical conditioning is a type of learning in which a patient learns to associate a new stimulus with a reflex response. To do this, a stimulus that naturally elicits a particular reflex response (an unconditioned stimulus) is paired with a stimulus that does not naturally elicit the response (thus, a conditioned stimulus). Over time, pairing of the unconditioned stimulus with the conditioned stimulus results in the ability of the conditioned stimulus alone to elicit the response. You may recall Ivan Pavlov's dog experiments in which he described classical conditioning. In his experiments, Pavlov paired meat powder, which naturally elicited increased production of saliva in the dog's mouth with a tone of a bell, which did not. After repeated pairing of the meat powder and the tone, the tone alone came to elicit increased saliva production. Classical conditioning is thought to underlie the development of many anxiety disorders such as post traumatic stress disorder (PTSD) and specific phobias and is also the foundation of many behaviorally based treatments. A number of behavioral interventions are based upon classical conditioning.

Extinction involves the "undoing" of conditioning (i.e., elimination or suppression of the conditioned response—increased saliva production to a tone). In order for extinction of a classically conditioned behavior to occur, the conditioned stimulus (tone) must be repeatedly presented in the absence of the unconditioned stimulus (meat powder). Over time, the dog learns that the tone no longer signals the delivery of meat powder. Extinction is central to CBT treatment of anxiety disorders and occurs through the process of exposure. Exposure involves presenting a feared stimulus or situation in a graduated and controlled fashion in association with relaxation until fear and anxiety subside. In this way, the feared stimulus is repeatedly paired with relaxation instead of fear and anxiety resulting in deconditioning (extinction). Exposure can be done in vivo or through use of imagery (imaginal exposure).

Exposure has frequently been used in the treatment of dyspnea associated with anxiety (e.g., panic attacks, PTSD). These patients experience extreme anxiety typically related to a fear of suffocation during episodes. After teaching the patient relevant relaxation and coping skills, the therapist artificially induces shortness of breath by having the patient repeatedly breathe quickly in and out through a thin straw (exposure to dyspnea). The patient is encouraged to utilize coping strategies and relaxation techniques to decrease the resulting anxiety. The patient continues linking induced dyspnea with relaxation techniques until anxiety levels decrease to an acceptable level. The process of exposure accomplishes several things. By sticking with the exposure until anxiety has decreased, the patient has successfully confronted the associated fear, thereby reducing overall levels of anxiety. This allows control over symptoms through the use of relaxation strategies and reduces anxiety. In the end, dyspnea is paired with relaxation rather than anxiety, a new, healthier association.

Operant conditioning, on the other hand, uses the antecedents and/or consequences of a behavior to influence the behavior. Antecedents or consequences that make a behavior more likely to occur are referred to as reinforcers while those that make a behavior less likely to occur are called punishers. Behavioral interventions based on operant conditioning manipulate reinforcement and punishment patterns in order to influence behavior. Operant conditioning strategies are most commonly used with children since adults are able to control reinforcers and punishments.

Operant conditioning techniques are commonly used to suppress unwanted behaviors. This process also involves extinction, relevant in both classical and operant conditioning models. One of the most recognized examples of operant conditioning extinction is the process of teaching babies to sleep through the night. While each sleep method has its followers, nearly all methods involve some type of extinction. The most basic extinction methods involve placing the baby in their bed awake at bedtime and ignoring any crying until morning. More commonly, a graduated extinction program is implemented. Graduated extinction slows down the process to make it easier for the family. Parents are instructed to put their baby to bed and then check on them periodically with gradually longer waiting periods in between checks over time. The underlying model is operant conditioning. The baby has learned to associate crying with parental attention. By removing the positive reinforcer (parental attention), which makes the behavior (crying) more likely to occur, the behavior will decrease or become "extinct" over time. Also, the baby will eventually learn to associate their crib with sleeping through classical conditioning.

Operant conditioning also underlies behavioral strategies such as differential attention and reinforcement. These techniques are used most commonly in children and are relatively straightforward. Positive attention or rewards are provided for desired behaviors while no attention is given to the negative or undesired behavior. An underlying assumption of this technique is that children have an intrinsic desire for parental attention (positive or negative) and will work to get it (consciously or unconsciously). Differential attention is commonly used in the treatment of MUS. Even though these symptoms are not intentionally produced, they generally respond quite well to differential attention. For example, parents of a child with habit cough would be instructed to ignore any coughing and provide lots of positive attention to the child during times when they are not coughing.

Adult patients also can be encouraged to use similar strategies with themselves or their partners. Together with the PCP, the patient can set realistic goals and rewards for achievement. Many patients with MUS will benefit from increased physical activity. A patient may set a goal to exercise for 15–20 min three times per week for the next month. When successful, the patients should reward themselves with something reinforcing (e.g., a massage). They may also want to set up smaller rewards for successful completion of each week to keep their motivation going. PCPs can play an important role in this system by checking in (accountability) on the patient's goals during subsequent appointments and providing verbal reinforcement for successes.

A closely related behavioral technique involves *promotion of incompatible behaviors*. Incompatible behaviors and the index behavior cannot be experienced simultaneously. Relaxation is the most commonly utilized incompatible behavior in CBT. Since anxiety is such a common comorbid condition, relaxation techniques such as deep or diaphragmatic breathing often in conjunction with guided imagery are taught to patients as a component of most CBT treatments. The idea is that relaxation is incompatible with most negative affect states, especially anxiety. It is impossible to be simultaneously anxious and relaxed. A patient with dyspnea could be taught slow deep breathing techniques to use when he feels an impending episode. Encouraging patients to engage in physical and pleasurable activities in anticipation of the index symptom can also be effective. Many patients will report that their symptom seems to disappear or to be less distressing when they are spending time with friends or doing something they enjoy.

One of the most simple and effective behavioral interventions for MUS in children and adults is *distraction*. Symptoms are less likely to occur and are less distressing when the patient is engaged in a pleasurable activity. Resistant patients (those who are not receptive to or decline other types of interventions) may also be more likely to agree to an intervention that involves doing something they already enjoy. For children, distraction could be combined with strategies of differential attention. In other words, parents could be discouraged from paying attention to or inquiring about the child's symptoms (e.g., "how are you feeling?" "how's your pain?"). Instead, when a parent thinks their child may be in pain, for example, they could attempt to distract the child with an alternate activity.

Biofeedback (see Chap. 10) is an advanced behavioral technique which employs specialized instruments that provide concurrent information on various physiological functions (e.g., skin temperature, muscle tension, heart rate) in order to help individuals become more aware of these (mostly autonomic) functions and trained therapists to teach techniques to manipulate them. While there is a relatively large literature supporting the use of biofeedback in MUS [30, 39], it requires special training and equipment. A referral to a qualified biofeedback provider is essential for patients who would benefit from these techniques.

Case Studies

Case 1: Noncardiac Chest Pain and Dyspnea

Sue is a 54-year-old divorced retired teacher who reports migratory nonexertional chest pressure with associated mild dyspnea and awareness of her pulse. It is most prominent when she is alone and generally absent when distracted. (Shopping is the example she uses.) A male cousin died in his 40s this year of sudden cardiac death while shoveling snow. She has been searching the Internet and points out the medical profession's regrettable record with accurate and timely diagnosis of heart disease in women. She has no cardiac risk factors except that she has resumed smoking as she becomes more anxious and fearful that she has undiagnosed coronary disease. She fears she will die if this chest pain does not stop. She has become somewhat withdrawn socially, no longer attends exercise class with her friends, and has begun to put on a few pounds. A thorough medical evaluation including nuclear exercise testing and coronary artery CT scan is entirely negative.

1. Which of the following features is/are commonly associated with NCCP?
   (a) Increased chest pain compared with patients with ischemic heart disease
   (b) Anxiety and depression
   (c) Increased use of health-care services
   (d) Increased cardiac risk factors compared to the general population
   (e) All of the above

Answer:

1. (e): NCCP presents an illustrative, albeit complex, example of MUS. Several authors have studied these patients in RCTs and review articles [18–23]. These

are patients with chest pain who have undergone appropriate and often extensive testing (cardiac exercise testing, echocardiography, pulmonary function testing, lab work, chest imaging, and often cardiac catheterization) with negative results and a complete and presumably rigorous history and physical examination. They are generally found to manifest more anxiety and depression [18], to have more chest pain, and to utilize more health-care services than comparable patients with ischemic heart disease [40]. Of interest, as a group, they also have more cardiac risk factors than the general population. There is no consensus regarding the prognosis of these patients. Some studies indicate a benign outcome [41, 42], but others suggest that they may actually have an increased relative risk for cardiac events [43–46], emphasizing the critical importance of a thorough medical assessment and at least raising concern about its rigor in some studies. These patients present quite a difficult therapeutic challenge but one that is gratifying to approach with CBT.

2. Sue fears that she will die if her chest pain does not stop. This is an example of which type of thinking error?
   - (a) Emotional reasoning
   - (b) Catastrophic reasoning
   - (c) Negative bias
   - (d) Negative filtering
   - (e) All of the above

Answer:

2. (b): Sue's statement is a classic example of catastrophic reasoning. Her reasoning that something must be wrong with her heart because her cousin recently passed away from a cardiac event is an example of emotional reasoning. Negative bias and filtering are evident in Sue's assertion that she has a cardiac condition despite her physician providing concrete evidence to the contrary.

3. Which of the following techniques are used in the following dialogue between Sue and her doctor?

Doctor:	Sue, I see a note here in your chart that you've stopped exercising. Is that true?
Sue:	Yes, it's been a few months now.
Doctor:	And it looks like you've put on a little weight since then too. Why did you stop exercising?
Sue:	I'm afraid that I will have a heart attack.
Doctor:	Why do you think that?
Sue:	Well, exerting myself physically cannot possibly be good for my heart; we don't even know what's wrong with it.
Doctor:	That's an interesting point; let's think about it a little more. What makes you believe that exercise would be bad for your heart?
Sue:	If I exercise, my heart will have to work harder. Look at all the people who have heart attacks shoveling snow…and from stress

Doctor: So you fear that your heart may be fragile and that stressing it might make it worse.
Sue: Yes.
Doctor: OK, now that we've looked at reasons for not exercising, why don't we look at reasons for exercising. After we're finished we can compare the two.
Sue: OK.
Doctor: Exercise has been shown to help people lose weight and weight loss is good for the heart. Would you agree?
Sue: Uh huh.
Doctor: And patients are prescribed an exercise program after heart attacks to help them recover.
Sue: I guess so.
Doctor: Exercise raises endorphin levels which makes people feel better.
Sue: That wouldn't be so bad.
Doctor: Those are just a few reasons why we recommend exercise for people with and without heart disease. What do you think?
Sue: I don't know. I heard all the things you said and I believe you, but I'm still scared that something bad will happen.
Doctor: That's understandable. Why don't we try a little experiment to practice?
Sue: Uh...what do you mean?
Doctor: Why don't we test it out?
Sue: How would we do that?
Doctor: You have an appointment to see me in 2 weeks. Between now and then, why don't you try just walking for 10 min every day? I'm sure that you will be fine, but if you have any concerns, you can call me. Let's see if you can feel any endorphins! When you come back in 2 weeks, we'll see how it went.
Sue: OK.

(a) Reframing
(b) Examining the evidence
(c) Behavioral practice
(d) b and c
(e) All of the above

Answer:

3. (e): Sue's doctor employed cognitive and behavioral strategies in this interaction. First, he helped Sue examine the evidence of her belief by providing pro and con arguments. As a result, the consequence of exercise was reframed. Once Sue developed a little ambivalence, he proposed a behavioral intervention to test out her theory.

Case 2: Insomnia in an Adult

John is a 45-year-old male who reports a prolonged sleep onset latency (often 3 h or more before falling asleep) and significant daytime fatigue. He reports that he has never been a good sleeper, but his sleep has been especially bad since he started having difficulties in his marriage about 3 years ago. He reports that he often lies awake for hours, unable to fall asleep until just before his alarm goes off in the morning. While lying awake in bed at night, he says that he often is frustrated and worries about not getting enough sleep. He estimates that he gets 3–4 h of sleep per night. During the day, he struggles to stay awake at his job and has occasionally dozed while driving to and from work. He describes his mood as "terrible" and feels that his mood is becoming less predictable. He is constantly exhausted and fears that he may lose his wife and his job if things do not improve soon.

From a CBT perspective, we might conceptualize that John has a biological predisposition for insomnia (behavior) that was brought out by struggles in his marriage (life stressors) that began 3 years ago. John worries (thoughts) about not getting enough sleep, which causes him to feel anxious (emotions) and perpetuates his insomnia (behavior).

Below is a sample dialogue in which a physician inquires about John's worries.

Doctor: You've said that when you have trouble sleeping at night, you often worry. Tell me more about your worries.

John: Well, a lot of the time I worry that I'll never fall asleep.

Doctor: So you worry that you will stay awake all night.

John: Yes.

Doctor: OK, what's behind this worry? In other words, what are you worried would happen if you stayed awake all night?

John: That I would be absolutely exhausted at work and maybe even fall asleep on the job.

Doctor: And what do you worry would happen if you fell asleep at work, what's the worst that could happen?

John: I'd be fired! And then my wife would leave me for sure!

Doctor: OK, we've identified several worries related to your sleep. Now let's take a step back and examine them. You've already told me that you've always had trouble sleeping, but that it's been especially bad the past 3 years. Is that true?

John: Yes.

Doctor: Let's focus on the past 3 years when you say it's been the worst. How many nights per week do you have a really hard time falling asleep at night?

John: At least 5 nights a week, but sometimes it feels like it's every night!

Doctor: OK, for arguments sake let's say you've had insomnia on average 6 nights per week for the last year. Does that sound about right?

John: Yeah, I think so.

Doctor:	OK, now let's go back to the worries you mentioned earlier. During our conversation, you mentioned 4 specific worries; staying awake all night, falling asleep at work, losing your job, and your wife leaving you. Are those correct?
John:	Yes.
Doctor:	Great. Now I'd like you to imagine that you're lying in bed unable to fall asleep. Can you do that?
John:	I guess.
Doctor:	Good. Now while you're lying there worrying about not being able to fall asleep, how certain are you that you'll never fall asleep and you'll stay awake all night. You can give me a percent such as "I was 50% sure I would be up all night."
John:	Oh it's much worse than that. I'd say I'm 98% sure I'll never fall asleep.
Doctor:	OK, now let's do the rest. How about falling asleep at work the next day. How sure are you that you'll fall asleep at work?
John:	I don't know maybe 80%.
Doctor:	OK, great. What about losing your job? How certain are you about this?
John:	Well, things are really rough at work now so I know if I got caught falling asleep that I'd be fired so I guess 70%.
Doctor:	And what about your wife leaving you? How certain are you about this?
John:	This is the big one! I worry about it all the time. I'd say I'm 90% certain.
Doctor:	OK. Now let's do some math (gets out calculator). If you've had insomnia for 6 days a week for 3 years, that's 936 nights of insomnia and we're not even counting all the bad sleep you had before that. So that's a conservative estimate.
John:	Yeah, it's pretty bad.
Doctor:	All right, now let's determine how often your fears actually happen. In the last 3 years, how many nights have you gone without any sleep at all, staying up all night?
John:	I don't know.. That's really hard to say. I think sometimes it feels like I was up all night, but I actually fell asleep for little bits here and there. I guess I've probably only had one night that I can think of where I've gotten zero sleep.
Doctor:	Great. What about falling asleep at work?
John:	That's a little more frequent…I've probably dozed off two or three times at work.
Doctor:	Let's go with 3 just to be safe. How about getting fired? How many times in the last 3 years have you been fired?
John:	Well, none yet.
Doctor:	OK, what about your wife leaving you? How many times in the last 3 years has your wife left you?
John:	Well, she actually walked out once, but she came back a few hours later.
Doctor:	OK, we'll say one time. Now let's look at some comparisons. With a little bit of math I come up with the following: (see Table 9.1)

Table 9.1 Examining the evidence

Worry (936 nights)	Certainty (%)	Number of potential occurrences given certainty	Actual occurrences
Stay awake all night	98	917	1
Fall asleep at work	80	749	3
Get fired	70	655	0
Wife leaves	90	842	1

Doctor: Those are some pretty impressive differences aren't they?
John: Yeah, I'd say so.
Doctor: Somehow when you're trying to fall asleep at night, these seem like very reasonable and plausible outcomes. In other words, they seem quite likely to occur. However, in reality, we see that they are in fact extremely rare events all occurring less than 1% of the time. So your own experience doesn't validate your thoughts and shows you that these events are very unlikely to occur.
John: Hmm, I've never really thought about it like that.
Doctor: Most people haven't. We rarely take the time to examine the reality of our thoughts, but now that we have, you can change the way you think at night. Instead of thinking, "I'm never going to fall asleep' or 'If I don't fall asleep I'm going to lose my job," you can develop a counterthought that is based on reality. For example, "It's highly unlikely that I'm not going to sleep at all tonight" or, even better, "It's almost certain that I will fall asleep tonight!"

1. When the doctor said, "We rarely take the time to examine the reality of our thoughts, but now that we have, you can change the way you think at night. Instead of thinking, 'I'm never going to fall asleep' or 'If I don't fall asleep I'm going to lose my job,' you can develop a counterthought that is based on reality. For example, 'It's highly unlikely that I'm not going to sleep at all tonight' or, even better, 'It's almost certain that I will fall asleep tonight!'" which of the following cognitive strategies was the doctor using?

   (a) Examining the evidence
   (b) Supporting
   (c) Reframing
   (d) Refiltering
   (e) Differential attention

Answer:

1. (c): This is an example of reframing a catastrophic thought into a more objective, reality-based thought. Adopting this new way of thinking will reduce John's anxiety and likely help him fall asleep more quickly. The doctor used "examining the

evidence" when he created the chart of John's beliefs and actual occurrences. Differential attention is a behavioral intervention in which positive attention is provided for incompatible or alternate behaviors and no attention is provided for the undesired behavior.

2. John's doctor wishes to add a behavioral component to his treatment plan. Which of the following behavioral interventions would be most effective in reducing John's primary complaint of prolonged sleep onset latency?
   (a) Improve sleep hygiene factors (remove clock from bedroom, cool sleeping temperature, no electronics, etc.)
   (b) Restrict the amount of time John spends in bed
   (c) Have John go to bed earlier
   (d) Expose John to bright light early in the morning
   (e) Increase John's physical activity

Answer:

2. (b): While all of the choices except c are good recommendations, the most effective behavioral intervention for insomnia is sleep restriction. Insomnia often results from patients spending too much time awake in bed. During this time, they often become frustrated or worried. As a result, patients come to associate their bed with being awake, frustrated, and worried rather than sleep. In order to resolve their insomnia, patients gradually extend the time that they spend in bed in hope that they will have more time asleep. Unfortunately, the result is the opposite. They sleep the same amount or less and spend more time awake in bed. Sleep restriction reverses this process. To determine the amount of sleep restriction to prescribe, simply subtract the patients' current total sleep time (John estimates it is about 4 h) from their morning wake time (6 am). The resulting time will serve as their new bedtime (2 am). Patients are instructed to stay awake and out of bed until their prescribed bedtime. Once they go to bed, if they are still unable to sleep, they are told to get out of bed until they feel they can fall asleep easily. They should not spend any significant period of time awake in bed. It is critical to the process that patients not nap during the day in order to build up sleep pressure for the night. Patients are instructed to follow the sleep restriction schedule for 1 week. After a week, if their sleep onset latency is 30 min or less (on average), their sleep can be gradually extended by 15–30 min every 3–5 days of good quality sleep. This process continues until patients reach a healthy total sleep time with a normal (30 min or less) sleep onset latency and good sleep efficiency (% of time in bed spent sleeping, ideally >85%). Regardless of reported total sleep time, patients should never be prescribed less than 4 h of sleep per night. In addition, reasonable safety precautions should be taken with driving and other dangerous activities. Many patients prefer to complete the first week at a time when they do not have to work. As is common with most behavioral interventions, patients should be cautioned that things often have to get a little worse before they can get better.

3. When recommending a sleep restriction schedule, your patient says, "but I'll never be able to stay up that late!" Which of the following would be the best response(s)?
   (a) OK, let's move your bedtime an hour earlier to make it easier.
   (b) That's wonderful news, you're cured! You came to see me because you couldn't fall asleep and now you're telling me that you can't stay awake!
   (c) I understand that what I'm asking you to do is difficult, but it's very important that you try your hardest to stay up until the prescribed bedtime.
   (d) a and b.
   (e) b and c.

Answer:

3. (e): Choice "b" is a great example of *positive reframing*. The patient is expressing a sentiment that is the exact opposite of their presenting symptom. It is important to capture this and reflect it back to the patient. Choice "c" would be a good follow-up statement to "b." It honestly reflects the difficulty of the intervention while reiterating the importance of adherence.

Case 3: Behavioral Insomnia of Childhood

Timmy is a 4-year-old boy presenting with difficulty falling asleep at bedtime and frequent night wakings. His parents complain that it takes Timmy "forever" to fall asleep, and after he finally falls asleep, he wakes up 3–4 times a night and comes into his parents' room. At night, his mother brings Timmy to his bedroom and reads him a story in bed. When she tries to leave, he becomes upset and begs for another story. After three more books, his mother tires and tells him that it is time to go to sleep. Timmy begins to cry when his mother tries to leave the room so she sits back down with him and rubs his back to try to get him to fall asleep. After 5 min, she attempts to leave the room again, but this time he throws an all-out temper tantrum. Timmy's mother is extremely frustrated with his behavior but realizes that over an hour has gone by and now Timmy really needs to fall asleep. Ultimately, his mother lies down with him until he falls asleep (usually in about 15 min). Timmy will typically sleep for 1–2 h before he wakes up and comes into his parents' room. Each time he wakes up, his mother has to bring him back to his room and lay with him until he returns to sleep. She reports that she is often so tired in the middle of the night that she falls asleep in Timmy's bed and wakes up there in the morning. She is not sure why, but Timmy never seems to wake up when she falls asleep in his bed.

1. What should you recommend?
   (a) Timmy's mother should sleep with him from the beginning of the night so that everyone will get more sleep
   (b) Provide differential attention for desired sleep behaviors

(c) Begin a program of gradual extinction
(d) a and b.
(e) b and c.

Answer:

1. (e): Four-year-old Timmy has behavioral insomnia of childhood. His trouble sleeping stems from two primary behavioral problems: first, his parents struggle to set appropriate limits at bedtime, and second, Timmy has learned to associate his mother with falling and returning to sleep. Treatment would involve differential attention for positive sleep-related behaviors and gradual extinction for the learned association of parental presence at bedtime. Timmy's parents should institute a consistent bedtime routine. It might be helpful to make pictures of each step for Timmy so that he knows what to expect. A formal bedtime routine with pictures can also help parents to set limits. For example, if Timmy's bedtime routine included a picture of 2 books, his parents can tell him, "I'm sorry honey, but the picture only has two books so we can't read any more tonight. We can read that book tomorrow night." Timmy should be provided lots of positive reinforcement for good bedtime behavior (stickers or hand stamps are often useful). In addition, any negative behaviors such as crying or temper tantrums should be ignored. A gradual extinction plan should be created to help Timmy's mother slowly transition out of his room at bedtime. As a reasonable first step, you might suggest that she sit on the edge of the bed while he falls asleep instead of lying next to him. Once Timmy gets used to that, she can move to a chair that can gradually be moved across the room, to the doorway, and ultimately out of the room. Consistency is key with this type of intervention, but resisting a child's cries for attention is difficult. Therefore, it is imperative to anticipate complications and potential hurdles ahead of time.

2. What should Timmy's parents expect to happen the first night they institute the new bedtime program?

   (a) Timmy will fall asleep faster.
   (b) Timmy's negative behaviors (screaming, crying, etc.) will get worse.
   (c) Timmy will sleep through the night.
   (d) Timmy will stay up all night and never fall asleep.
   (e) None of the above.

Answer:

2. (b): When recommending any type of behavioral extinction program, parents should be warned about the "extinction burst." The extinction burst occurs when the child's behavior temporarily escalates before ultimately improving. The burst occurs based on the child's prior learning. Timmy has learned that bad bedtime behavior results in a later bedtime and more time with his parents. In operant conditioning terms, we would say that Timmy's bad behavior has been reinforced and is therefore likely to recur. When Timmy's parents attempt to set new limits, Timmy will most likely respond with negative behavior since it has worked well in the past. If Timmy's

parents ignore this behavior, Timmy is likely to escalate in a further attempt to get his parents attention. Over time, when Timmy's parents consistently ignore his bad behavior and reward his good behavior, he will learn that the negative behaviors are not worthwhile. Parents can be told to expect 2–3 days of decreasing escalation followed by significant behavioral improvement.

3. Timmy's parents tell you that they've had it with Timmy's behavior and they want to go "cold turkey" with the extinction program rather than taking a gradual approach. If they do, which of the following is (are) likely to occur?
   (a) If Timmy's parents are consistent, his sleep will improve more quickly than it would with gradual extinction
   (b) Timmy will display more negative behavior for a longer period of time compared with gradual extinction
   (c) Timmy's parents are less likely to be successful
   (d) All of the above.
   (e) None of the above.

Answer:

3. (d): "All or none" extinction or standard extinction will eliminate an undesired behavior more quickly *IF* it is instituted consistently. Unfortunately, the vast majority of families are unable to do this due to increased negative behaviors from the child. It is not uncommon for children undergoing standard extinction to scream, cry, and throw temper tantrums for hours at a time. Most parents, understandably, find this challenging and ultimately give in to their child's demands, thereby unintentionally reinforcing the child's bad behavior. Therefore, we almost always recommend gradual extinction.

Case 4: Habit Cough

Alex is an 11-year-old boy with a 5-month history of persistent cough. His parents report that initially he had a respiratory infection, which resolved, but the cough has never gone away. Alex coughs frequently with two or three coughs per episode. The cough is not exertional. It is nonproductive and not accompanied by rhinorrhea, wheezing, dyspnea, or chest pain. Alex does not cough during sleep or pleasurable activities. An extensive medical workup is negative. Alex reports very little distress associated with the symptom, but his teachers have expressed concern and his parents are frustrated.

1. What factor(s) are most suggestive in Alex's case are most suggestive of a psychological explanation?
   (a) The medical workup is negative
   (b) Alex is not distressed by his symptoms

(c) The school has expressed concern
(d) Symptoms are not present during sleep or pleasurable activities
(e) The symptoms have lasted 5 months

Answer:

1. (d): While a negative medical workup and concerns from multiple systems (e.g., home and school) are certainly supportive of a psychological underpinning, the fact that Alex's symptoms remit during sleep and pleasurable activities is much more telling. Psychologically based symptoms are very sensitive to environmental changes, whereas most medical symptoms are not. It would be difficult to explain why Alex's cough disappears during sleep and pleasurable activities from a medical perspective. Psychologically, however, it makes sense that Alex's cough disappears when he is distracted or unconscious. Another common presentation in children involves symptoms that are either present or absent depending upon parental presence. For example, an anxious child may not be able to fall asleep at night unless her mother is present, but falls asleep easily when she is there. The opposite pattern may be evident in children who have been abused. The key observation in either case is that the "symptom" is environmentally dependent.

2. Which domain(s) would be the most appropriate target for intervention in Alex's case?

   (a) Cognitive
   (b) Behavioral
   (c) Physiologic
   (d) Both a and b
   (e) Both b and c

Answer:

2. (e): Alex is likely experiencing habit cough, which is thought to be psychogenic in nature. Since the patient (Alex) is not experiencing significant distress from the symptom, behavioral and physiological interventions are more likely to be effective than cognitive-based strategies. Habit cough can be described as a dissociative disorder. Individuals with dissociative disorders are usually unaware of the psychological stressor that creates the somatic symptom. The psychological conflict is "converted" into a somatic symptom and "solves" an intrapsychic conflict that would otherwise be causing distress. While uncovering and resolving the psychic conflict would likely result in rapid symptom resolution, discovering unconscious processes takes time and is often met with resistance by patients and families (due to the "it's all in your head" implication).

   A CBT approach to habit cough would likely involve differential reinforcement for incompatible and/or low rates of behaviors, relaxation training, and possibly biofeedback. The goal of differential reinforcement is to decrease attention to the symptom and provide an alternate response for the cough. Relaxation training is used to help the patient improve coping skills with stress.

3. Which of the following would be useful recommendations to make to Alex's parents?
   (a) When you hear Alex cough, try to ignore it.
   (b) Since we know Alex is faking, each time he coughs take away 5 min of TV or video game time.
   (c) Provide Alex with lots of praise for practicing his relaxation skills and during times when he is not coughing.
   (d) a and c.
   (e) a, b, and c.

Answer:

3. (d): The most helpful advice you can offer to parents in this situation is genuine reassurance combined with a recommendation for differential attention. Differential attention simply means that the parents should avoid providing Alex with any type of attention for his symptom both positive and negative (e.g., "Stop it!" "Are you OK?" or "Just don't think about it"). Attention to the symptom will only serve to increase it. Praise for alternate behaviors is also recommended. In this way, Alex will receive attention for incompatible behaviors and will therefore be more likely to engage in them. Choice b is not recommended, as Alex is not faking. Children with habit cough or other functional disorders are not intentionally producing their symptoms. They are occurring on an unconscious level. Punishing Alex for coughing would not be expected to improve the symptom and may in fact reinforce it.

Case 5: Paradoxical Vocal Cord Dysfunction

Kathy is a 16-year-old high school junior, third in her class, and a star on the volleyball team. Her parents are each well educated and successful in their professions. She is in the process of applying to colleges and expectations are high for her to enter a prestigious university. Kathy has carried a diagnosis of asthma since early childhood that for years has been controlled easily with use of a daily inhaled steroid. However, recently, she has developed distressing episodes of dyspnea, chest tightness and stridor of sudden onset, lasting 5–15 min. These occur most frequently during volleyball matches, and have led to Kathy having to be taken out of half of her games during the past season. There have been several ER visits where oxygen saturation was found to be normal and usual emergent asthma treatment was only of marginal benefit. Subcutaneous epinephrine was associated with an anxiety reaction, which worsened her symptoms and nearly resulted in endotracheal intubation. Her parents and family doctor have presumed that her asthma has worsened. Her dosage of inhaled steroid has been doubled. Inhaled albuterol and ipratropium and oral montelukast and omeprazole have been added, all with no improvement. Pulmonary function testing when she was asymptomatic was normal. Her family doctor referred her to an otolaryngologist who had the occasion to examine her during an episode. He observed paradoxical adduction of the vocal cords during inspiration on direct laryngoscopy. The inspiratory portion of the flow/volume loop on a pulmonary function study during her episode was blunted consistent with extrathoracic airway obstruction.

1. Which one or more of the following statements is/are true?
   (a) The presence of asthma excludes the diagnosis of PVCD.
   (b) Conventional asthma treatments are usually effective in the treatment of PVCD.
   (c) Failure to recognize PVCD results in unnecessary use of medical resources.
   (d) PVCD is exclusively a psychogenic disorder.
   (e) The gold standard for diagnosis of PVCD is laryngoscopy.

Answer:

1. (c and e): This patient's presentation is typical of paradoxical vocal cord dysfunction (PVCD), a somewhat rare disorder seen predominantly in high functioning adolescents or young adults with a 2 : 1 female predominance and symptoms often precipitated by exercise, irritants or emotional stress and anxiety. It is commonly misdiagnosed as asthma but is successfully treated only if recognized as a distinct entity. It can be seen in patients with or without underlying asthma. Treatment modalities successful in the management of asthma are unsuccessful in the management of PVCD. Until properly diagnosed, these patients often experience repeated ER visits and can be subjected to endotracheal intubation and even emergency tracheostomy.

2. Which one or more of the following studies is appropriate for inclusion in the medical evaluation of patients with suspected PVCD?
   (a) PFT with flow volume loop
   (b) Laryngoscopy
   (c) CBC for eosinophils
   (d) PA and lateral chest X-ray
   (e) Peripheral oxygen saturation

Answer:

2. (a, b, c, d, and e): A fairly straightforward medical evaluation can help to define the condition and exclude other possible diagnoses: Oxygen saturation is normal during an episode. Pulmonary function testing can show characteristic blunting of the inspiratory portion of the flow volume loop only during an episode and is otherwise normal. The eosinophil count generally is normal. Gastroesophageal reflux and tracheal aspiration can be excluded by appropriate contrast studies and/or a trial of a PPI or H2 blocker. Acute epiglottitis is excluded by clinical context and lateral neck X-ray. The gold standard for diagnosis is direct visualization of paradoxical inspiratory and sometimes expiratory adduction of the vocal cords during an episode.

3. Effective components of management of PVCD may include:
   (a) Hypnosis
   (b) Speech therapy
   (c) Psychotherapy
   (d) Inhaled ipratropium
   (e) All of the above

Answer:

3. (e): Simple reassurance, avoidance of obvious precipitants, and a straightforward explanation of PVCD will often improve and sometimes resolve PVCD. Most patients, however, will require further treatment. While PVCD is not purely psychogenic in nature, anxiety plays a substantial role in the precipitation of many episodes. The most consistently effective treatments involve teaching patients relaxation skills and addressing associated psychological stressors. Hypnosis can be very effective for PCVD, although relaxation strategies from CBT such as progressive muscle relaxation may also be helpful. Speech therapy can also be very useful in teaching patients some control of laryngeal function to favor an open airway during respiration. Biofeedback using hand warming techniques has been shown to be effective in eliminating vocal cord dysfunction while simultaneously providing an alternate behavior and relaxation [30]. Use of inhaled ipratropium for exercise-induced PVCD has been reported as beneficial. If episodes do not resolve with the aforementioned interventions, psychotherapy and rarely pharmacotherapy for anxiety may be indicated. Psychotherapy such as CBT can help to resolve complex psychological issues, which require more in-depth examination and understanding.

4. In CBT, relaxation training can involve which one or more of the following:
   (a) Deep breathing
   (b) Progressive muscle relaxation
   (c) A mind body connection
   (d) Use of medications
   (e) Guided imagery

Answer:

4. (a, b, c, and e): When individuals experience stress, they generate multiple thoughts and memories that feedback into and often amplify their distress. Relaxation training (a behavioral intervention of CBT) can often cut through these cognitive and emotional complexities, thereby reducing the patient's distress without necessarily resolving the underlying issue. Relaxation training is considered a psychophysiological intervention in that it involves both the mind and the body. The goal of relaxation training is to induce a psychophysiological state of relaxation that is incompatible with stress and arousal. Stress and arousal are associated with increased heart rate, blood pressure, respiration, and adrenaline while relaxation is essentially the opposite. Common components of relaxation training include deep breathing, progressive muscle relaxation, and guided

imagery. Most relaxation sessions begin with slow diaphragmatic breathing and then progress to either progressive muscle relaxation or guided imagery. Progressive muscle relaxation involves a two-part sequence of tensing and relaxing, which is repeated for each part of the body. Patients often find the contrast between tension and relaxation helpful in learning to gain control over these physical changes. Guided imagery (which is a form of hypnosis) takes the client on an imaginal journey to a special place of their choosing. The special place can be a place the patient has been to before, one they wish to visit, or one they create in their mind. As the patient relaxes using deep breathing, the therapist guides the patient to their special place by encouraging the patient to engage all five of their senses ("take a minute to look around your special place, notice the sounds that are there, the smell of the air, etc."). Throughout the relaxation process, messages of safety, self-control, and security should be conveyed to the patient. For example, during deep breathing, the therapist might convey, "with each breath you feel more and more in control of your anxiety." After the initial relaxation training session, patients should be encouraged to practice their relaxation daily. Many patients find it helpful to have an audio recording of their relaxation session to use during practice. Once the patient is comfortable using the relaxation techniques, they can be abbreviated for use in stressful situations.

Conclusions

The full range of CBT is one of the most effective tools available to the trained mental health professional for the treatment of medically unexplained symptoms. However, basic cognitive behavioral strategies have the potential to provide the primary care physician with a model for understanding and a technique for effective intervention with a wide variety of these disorders. Interventions can occur within the context of a standard medical encounter. Interventions in one domain (cognitive or behavioral) often result in cascading improvements in the physical and emotional domains. Integrating basic cognitive behavioral approaches during patient encounters results in improved outcomes and increased patient and physician satisfaction [36].

References

1. Chambless DL, Ollendick TH. Empirically supported psychological interventions: controversies and evidence. Annu Rev Psychol. 2001;52:685–716.
2. Butler AC, Chapman JE, Forman EM, Beck AT. The empirical status of cognitive-behavioral therapy: a review of meta-analyses. Clin Psychol Rev. 2006;26(1):17–31.
3. Kazdin AE, Weisz JR, editors. Evidence-based psychotherapies for children and adolescents. New York: Guilford; 2003.

4. Norcross JC, Beutler LE, Levant RF, editors. Evidence-based practices in mental health: debate and dialogue on the fundamental questions. Washington: American Psychological Association; 2005.
5. Witthoft M, Hiller W. Psychological approaches to origins and treatments of somatoform disorders. Annu Rev Clin Psychol. 2010;6:257–83.
6. Deary V, Chadler T, Sharpe M. The cognitive behavioral model of medically unexplained symptoms: a theoretical and empirical review. Clin Psychol Rev. 2007;27(7):781–97.
7. Sumathipala A. What is the evidence for the efficacy of treatments for somatoform disorders? A critical review of previous intervention studies. Psychosom Med. 2007;69(9):889–900.
8. Allen LA, Woolfolk RL. Cognitive behavioral therapy for somatoform disorders. Psychiatr Clin N Am. 2010;33(3):579–93.
9. Dimsdale JE, Xin Y, Kleinman A, et al., editors. Somatic Presentations of Mental Disorders: refining the Research Agenda for DSM-V. Arlington, VA: American Psychological Association; 2009.
10. Smith RC, Lyles JS, Gardiner JC, et al. Primary care clinicians treat patients with medically unexplained symptoms. J Gen Intern Med. 2006;21(7):671–7.
11. Martin A, Rauh E, Fichter M, Reif W. A one-session treatment for patients suffering from medically unexplained symptoms in primary care: a randomized clinical trial. Psychosomatics. 2007;48(4):294–303.
12. Magallon R, Gili M, et al. Cognitive-behaviour therapy for patients with abridged somatization disorder (SSI 4,6) in primary care: a randomized, controlled study. BMC Psychiatry. 2008;8:47.
13. Smith RC, Gardiner JC, Luo Z, Schooley S, Lamerato L, Rost K. Primary care physicians treat somatization. J Gen Intern Med. 2009;24(7):829–32.
14. Escobar JI, Gara MA, Diaz-Martinez AM, et al. Effectiveness of a time-limited cognitive behavior therapy-type intervention among primary care patients with medically unexplained symptoms. Ann Fam Med. 2007;5(4):328–35.
15. Allen LA, Woolfolk RL, Escobar JI, Gara MA, Hamer RM. Cognitive-behavioral therapy for somatization disorder. Arch Intern Med. 2006;166(14):1512–8.
16. Sumathipala A, Siribaddana S, Abeysingha MR, et al. Cognitive-behavioural therapy vs. structured care for medically unexplained symptoms: randomised controlled trial. Br J Psychiatry. 2008;193(1):51–9.
17. Arnold IA, Waal MW, Eekhof JA, Assendelft WJ, Spinhoven P, Van Hemert AM. Medically unexplained physical symptoms in primary care: a controlled study of the effectiveness of cognitive behavioral treatment by the family physician. Psychosomatics. 2009;50(5):515–24.
18. White KS. Assessment and treatment of psychological causes of chest pain. Med Clin N Am. 2010;94(2):291–318.
19. van Peski-Oosterbaan AS, Spinhoven P, van Rood Y, van der Does JW, Bruschke AV, Rooijmans HG. Cognitive-behavioral therapy for noncardiac chest pain: a randomized trial. Am J Med. 1999;106(4):424–9.
20. Van Peski-Oosterbaan AS, Spinhoven P, Van der Does AJ, Bruschke AV, Rooijmans HG. Cognitive change following cognitive behavioural therapy for non-cardiac chest pain. Psychother Psychosom. 1999;68(4):214–20.
21. Mayou RA, Bass CM, Bryant BM. Management of non-cardiac chest pain: from research to clinical practice. Heart. 1999;81(4):387–92.
22. Mayou RA, Bryant BM, Sanders D, Bass C, Klimes I, Forfar C. A controlled trial of cognitive behavioural therapy for non-cardiac chest pain. Psychol Med. 1997;27(5):1021–31.
23. Klimes I, Mayou RA, Pearce MJ, Coles L, Fagg JR. Psychological treatment for atypical non-cardiac chest pain: a controlled evaluation. Psychol Med. 1990;20(3):605–11.
24. Morgenthaler TI, Owens J, Alessi C, et al. American academy of sleep medicine. Practice parameters for behavioral treatment of bedtime problems and night wakings in infants and young children. Sleep. 2006;29(1):1277–81.
25. Morin CM, Culbert JP, Schwartz SM. Nonpharmacological interventions for insomnia: a meta analysis of treatment efficacy. Am J Psychiatry. 1994;151(8):1172–80.

26. Perlis ML, Jungquist C, Smith MT, Posner D, editors. Cognitive behavioral treatment of insomnia. New York: Springer; 2004.
27. Nguyen HQ, Kohlman-Carpieri V. Dyspnea self-management in patients with chronic obstructive pulmonary disease: moderating effects of depressed mood. Psychosomatics. 2005;46(5):402–10.
28. Livermore N, Sharpe L, McKenzie D. Prevention of panic attacks and panic disorder in COPD. Eur Respir J. 2010;36(2):457–8.
29. Hallenbeck J. The pathophysiology and treatment of dyspnea. Accessed 10 Feb 2011. http://www.chestnet.org/accp/pccsu/pathophysiology-and-treatment-dyspnea?page=0,3.
30. Earles J, Kerr B, Kellar M. Psychophysiologic treatment of vocal cord dysfunction. Ann Allergy Asthma Immunol. 2003;90(6):669–71.
31. Noyes BE, Kemp JS. Vocal cord dysfunction in children. Paediatr Respir Rev. 2007;8(2):155–63.
32. Thurston NL, Fiedorowicz JG. Improvement of paradoxical vocal cord dysfunction with integrated psychiatric care. Psychosomatics. 2009;50(3):282–4.
33. Labbe EE. Biofeedback and cognitive coping in the treatment of pediatric habit cough. App Psychophysiol Biofeedback. 2006;31(2):167–72.
34. Kroenke K. Efficacy of treatment for somatoform disorders: a review of randomized controlled trials. Psychosom Med. 2007;69(9):881–8.
35. Escobar JI, Waitzkin H, Silver RC, Gara M, Homan A. Abridged somatization: a study in primary care. Psychosom Med. 1998;60(4):466–72.
36. Salmon P, Humphris GM, Ring A, Davies JC, Dowrick CF. Primary care consultation about medically unexplained symptoms: patient presentations and doctor responses that influence the probability of somatic intervention. Psychosom Med. 2007;69(6):571–7.
37. Woolfolk RL, Allen LA, editors. Treating somatization: a cognitive-behavioral approach. New York: The Guilford Press; 2007.
38. Lazarus RS, Folkman S, editors. Stress, appraisal, and coping. New York: Springer; 1984.
39. Astin JA, Shapiro SL, Eisenberg DM, Forys KL. Mind-body medicine: state of the science, implications for practice. J Am Board Family Pract. 2002;16(2):131–47.
40. Eifert GH, Hodson SE, Tracey DR, Seville JL, Gunawardane K. Heart-focused anxiety, illness beliefs, and behavioral impairment: comparing healthy heart-anxious patients with cardiac and surgical inpatients. J Behav Med. 1996;19(4):385–99.
41. Kemp HG, Kronmal RA, Vliestra RE, Frye RL. Seven year survival of patients with normal or near normal coronary arteriograms: a CASS registry study. J Am Coll Cardiol. 1986;7(3):479–83.
42. Lichtlen PR, Bargheer K, Wenzlaff P. Long-term prognosis of patients with anginalike chest pain and normal coronary angiographic findings. J Am Coll Cardiol. 1995;25(5):1013–8.
43. Eslick GD, Talley NJ. Natural history and predictors of outcome for non-cardiac chest pain: a prospective 4-year cohort study. Neurogastroenterol Motil. 2008;20(9):989–97.
44. Robinson JG, Wallace R, Limacher M, et al. Cardiovascular risk in women with non-specific chest pain (from the WHI hormone trials). Am J Cardiol. 2008;102(6):693–9.
45. Robinson JG, Wallace R, Limacher M, et al. Elderly women diagnosed with nonspecific chest pain may be at increased cardiovascular risk. J Womens Health. 2006;15(10):1151–60.
46. Bodegard J, Erikssen G, Bjornhold JV, Thelle D, Erikssen J. Possible angina detected by the WHO angina questionnaire in apparently healthy men with a normal exercise ECG: coronary heart disease or not? A 26 year follow up study. Heart. 2004;90(6):627–32.

Chapter 10
Biofeedback Therapy for Asthma

Paul M. Lehrer

This chapter contains videos, please download from
http://www.springerimages.com/videos/10.1007/978-1-61779-857-3_10

Abstract Many asthma sufferers refuse to take prescribed levels of asthma medication, because of their concerns about its costs and possible side effects, and turn instead to various herbal and mind-body treatments. Biofeedback is one of the better documented of these approaches. Biofeedback involves using information from various electrophysiological measures as a means of exercising voluntary control over the measured functions. This chapter reviews several biofeedback approaches, including biofeedback training to reduce respiratory resistance, surface electromyographic biofeedback to achieve relaxation of the skeletal muscles of the face, neurofeedback to control electroencephalographic activity, and heart rate variability biofeedback to increase respiratory sinus arrhythmia. The best documented effects are for heart rate variability biofeedback, wherein people learn to breathe at a particular slow frequency for each individual that is the resonance frequency of the cardiovascular system. This technique has large autonomic and psychological effects, which produce increases in baroreflex gain, modulation of blood pressure, and decreases in anxiety and depression. There is evidence that it also produces both acute and chronic decreases in airway resistance in asthma patients, and in one well-controlled single blind study, it appeared to have 100% effectiveness in preventing asthma exacerbations requiring increased doses of controller medications. Symptoms, medication consumption, and airway resistance all decreased, with fewer exacerbations. However, the mechanism of action is still poorly understood.

Keywords Resonance frequency • Forced oscillation • Psychological stress • Baroreflex • Vagal trigeminal reflex loop • Alternative and complementary medicine • Applied psychophysiology

P.M. Lehrer (✉)
Department of Psychiatry, University of Medicine & Dentistry of New Jersey, Robert Wood Johnson Medical School, 671 Hoes Lane, Piscataway, NJ 08854, USA
e-mail: lehrer@umdnj.edu

R.D. Anbar (ed.), *Functional Respiratory Disorders: When Respiratory Symptoms Do Not Respond to Pulmonary Treatment*, Respiratory Medicine,
DOI 10.1007/978-1-61779-857-3_10,

Background

Biofeedback involves use of bioelectronic instruments to record physiological data and provide real-time information to an individual that is then used for the person to control his or her own physiology. The technique has been applied to many physiological functions, most frequently skin conductance, finger temperature, the surface electromyogram, various electroencephalographic variables, heart rate, and heart rate variability [1]. In the biofeedback procedure, the patient receives continuous information about a target physiological function (e.g., heart rate, surface muscle tension, palmar skin conductance) and uses this information to control that function. Although functions such as muscle tension and breathing can usually easily be controlled by this method in a relatively few sessions of training with close to 100% success, people appear also able to develop the coordination necessary to control various autonomic and neural functions, e.g., EEG rhythms at particular brain sites, finger temperature, skin sweating, blood pressure, and heart rate. The latter functions are more difficult to control, however, and require longer training, with more variable results. Although an autonomic function, however, heart rate variability is also easy to learn to control, because it can be directly manipulated by altering breathing patterns.

In principle, almost any physiological function that can be measured continuously can be used for biofeedback, and people can learn to use the feedback information to voluntarily control various physiological functions. Continuous measurement is necessary because most physiological functions continuously change, so the patient needs information about exactly when a particular function is heading in the "right" direction. Also, in the literature of operant conditioning, wherever positive reinforcement is given to "shape" a behavior by reinforcement for successive approximations, the procedure only is effective when reinforcement is delivered within seconds of the response. Delayed reinforcement usually impairs learning of new behavioral patterns [2, 3], although some learning with delayed reinforcement can take place, usually with less effectiveness [4, 5], thus demonstrating the positive but limited effects of such health care behaviors as frequent weighing to control obesity as components in behavior modification programs for overeating [6, 7].

Using biofeedback, people often are able to produce profound changes in most physiological parameters, within certain physiological limits. The method has been successfully applied to a number of disorders, most prominently including anxiety [8–11], Raynaud's disease [12], headache [13], incontinence [14–16], depression [17–21], and attention deficit disorder [22–24]. In some respects, biofeedback is a component in various devices used medically and in daily life, without necessarily being identified as such. For example, biofeedback for respiratory behavior is built into almost all devices measuring exhaled nitric oxide, to insure that proper force of exhalation is achieved. Similarly, calibration of various spirometry devices often involves feedback to the operator of force applied to the plunger of a three-liter syringe. Even automobiles give biofeedback to the driver, by giving information about the force applied to the gas pedal (in the form of engine RPM's).

Biofeedback may be particularly helpful for asthma, both because it can effectively alter important parameters of airway function and because many asthma patients would prefer this type of therapy to standard drug treatment. Current guidelines define asthma as a chronic inflammatory disorder of the airways associated with reversible airways obstruction and increased airways responsiveness to a variety of stimuli [25]. Accordingly, early and aggressive treatment with anti-inflammatory agents, particularly inhaled steroids, is recommended by all existing guidelines for persistent asthma. An extensive literature supports the efficacy and effectiveness of inhaled corticosteroids to improve asthma outcomes and reduce asthma morbidity and mortality [26–28].

Unfortunately, adherence to prescribed inhaled steroids in real-world settings is poor in all patient groups, with average adherence rate estimated at about 50% [29–32]. Solid evidence exists linking poor adherence to adverse asthma outcomes [31, 32]. Interventions to improve adherence have shown, at best, limited success in improving patient behavior in clinically relevant and/or sustainable fashions [33–37], although ongoing efforts are justifiably encouraged and necessary. The reasons for such poor adherence to prescribed inhaled corticosteroids are complex and largely unknown. However, a recent literature review found that the most common reasons given by patients include concerns about medication cost and safety (with particular concern about steroids), beliefs that asthma severity is not sufficient to require daily treatment, worry about dependence or diminished effectiveness from long-term use of medication, and a general distrust of the medical establishment [38]. There is indeed reason to believe that fears of long-term side effects, such as osteoporosis, are not unfounded [39].

Many patients seek non-medication treatments for asthma [40]. A survey of 4,741 asthmatic patients from the United Kingdom showed that 59% of these patients tried non-pharmaceutical treatments [41]. The most common techniques used were breathing-based therapies (30%), homeopathy (12%), herbalism (11%), Yoga (9%), and acupuncture (7%). Similarly, in an interview study of 601 adult asthmatics, 8% reported reliance on herbal remedies, 6% on use of tea and coffee, and 6% on OTC epinephrine or ephedrine at some point in the prior year to control their asthma [42]. In the long run, most of these alternative treatments are much cheaper than inhaled steroids.

Several biofeedback modalities have been attempted for asthma, including biofeedback for facial muscle tension via surface electromyography, neurofeedback of EEG waves, biofeedback of respiratory resistance from the forced oscillation method, and biofeedback for increasing heart rate variability. Of them, only heart rate variability biofeedback (HRV BF) has consistently shown positive and clinically significant effects.

In addition to possible effects on physiological processes underlying asthma, biofeedback may impact on functional aspects of the disease. Because of its substantial effects on anxiety and depression, biofeedback may directly impact on emotional factors that often interact with asthma. It is known that prevalence of anxiety disorders and depression is higher among asthma patients than in the general population [43, 44]. There is some evidence that life stress may contribute to incidence of asthma [45–48] as well as severity and, additionally, that stress or emotional reactions may contribute to asthma exacerbations [49]. There also is evidence that experimental inducement of sadness can do likewise [50]. Additionally, comorbidity has been particularly high for asthma and panic disorder, where some of the symptoms overlap, and symptom confusion often occurs [45–48]. This can lead to inappropriate treatment for both disorders, often leading to overuse or underuse of albuterol, occasionally with fatal results [51–53]. Also, stress, anxiety, and depression often are accompanied by subjective overperception of the severity of various physical problems [54–56]. This inaccurate perception perhaps is due to greater mental focus on unpleasant sensations, probably accompanied by changes in the brain that could exaggerate such symptoms [57–59]. Perception of dyspnea, a common asthma symptom, is known to have an emotional component, which is only partially related to *intensity* of the sensation, and even less related to changes in pulmonary function [60–62].

There also is evidence that many asthma patients tend to respond to stress with elevated parasympathetic activity and consequent bronchoconstriction [49, 63]. This may reflect a characteristic of "individual response stereotypy," [63] whereby some people respond to many kinds of stressors with a specific physiological response [64–67]. This occurs with many diseases that are affected by stress and has been measured among individuals with headache [68], back pain [69–72], and hypertension [73, 74]. A related disorder that may be related to stress is paradoxical vocal cord dysfunction, where constriction of the vocal cords can produce asthma-like symptoms [75, 76]. It is known that various relaxation techniques can improve vocal cord function among individuals with functional dysphonias and other vocal problems [77–79] and are commonly used among actors, singers, and orators to improve vocal production [80, 81]. Although biofeedback has not been specifically applied to this condition, it may have great unexplored potential for treating this condition.

Surface Electromyographic (sEMG) Biofeedback

Kotses and his colleagues [82] noted the known relationships between the trigeminal and vagal systems, where increased trigeminal efferents produce increases in vagus nerve activity. They noted that facial muscle tension may play a particular role in stress-induced asthma, since facial muscle tension is affected by emotion, and asthma is exacerbated by vagus nerve activity. They observed experimentally induced decreases in pulmonary function in response to induced facial muscle tension, and improved pulmonary function with decreased tension [82–84]. Stress is known to play a role in asthma exacerbations in a large minority of asthma patients [49, 85, 86], and stress usually produces increases in muscle tension, often in emotion-specific patterns in the face [87–90]. However, although small but statistically significant improvements in asthma have been noted in response to general muscle relaxation [91], the method has not been found to produce clinically significant improvements in the disease [91–93]. Initial studies of relaxation training using frontal surface EMG (sEMG) found that decreases in facial muscle tension produced improvements in pulmonary function in asthma, while a comparison procedure involving training to *increase* tension in this area had the opposite effect [84]. These studies also found that sEMG biofeedback training to the forearm muscles had no effects. However, several recent studies from other laboratories have failed to replicate the initial positive findings [91, 94–96].

Another sEMG biofeedback strategy for asthma treatment has involved instruction in relaxed breathing, using sEMG feedback to skeletal muscles of the neck and thorax [97], to help relax some of the accessory breathing muscles in the chest, neck, and shoulders. Simultaneously, biofeedback was provided to increase force, volume, and smoothness of inhalation, using an incentive inspirometer as a biofeedback instrument. These studies also included psychological treatment targeted at anxiety about asthma symptoms and training in slow diaphragmatic breathing. At follow-up, all subjects significantly reduced their sEMG tension levels while simultaneously increasing their inhalation volumes. In an uncontrolled study, subjects reported reductions in their asthma symptoms, medication use, emergency room visits, and episodes of dyspnea. A subsequent controlled study from our laboratory did not show significant effects for this method [94], but it did show large and significant effects of HRV BF (see below). Although this study was based on too small a sample to prove the relaxed breathing method ineffective, it indicated that HRV BF may be a more promising approach, although more research on the sEMG method may be warranted.

Biofeedback of Respiratory Resistance

Several studies have provided biofeedback of respiratory resistance to asthma patients, using forced oscillation. In this method, oscillations of air molecules in the airways are produced using a loudspeaker, playing a sound with particular multifrequency characteristics into the lung. The instrument then measures resistance of the lung to oscillations at each frequency. This method is particularly useful for biofeedback because it can provide immediate and continuous feedback. Unlike in spirometry, this method does not involve forced expiratory maneuvers, which cannot be done continuously, and which can cause fatigue and bronchoconstriction when done repeatedly [98]. Although small studies have found that forced oscillation biofeedback may be useful, equipment is not easily commercially available to deliver this type of feedback, and necessary larger scale trials have not been done. Mass and his colleagues [99] trained subjects to decrease respiratory resistance by providing continuous biofeedback of this measure. In an uncontrolled trial, this feedback technique decreased average respiratory resistance within sessions but not between sessions [100]. It did not increase forced expiratory volume in 1 s (FEV_1) [99]. They concluded that respiratory resistance biofeedback is not an effective technique for the treatment of bronchial asthma in adults. However, they did not assess whether subjects were able to abort asthma exacerbations using training derived from this method, so the clinical utility of the method has not been fully assessed.

Neurofeedback

Biofeedback of electroencephalographic rhythms has been reported in one case study of a child with asthma [101]. The 6-year-old child had been having frequent asthma exacerbations and was trained to increase sensorimotor EEG (approximately 14 Hz). Asthma exacerbations ceased and the patient remained symptom-free throughout a 1-year follow-up period. In another study, however, we used biofeedback to increase frontal-to-occipital EEG alpha rhythms and found a borderline significant improvement in asthma symptoms, but not in pulmonary function [102]. These findings parallel those obtained from medication placebos [103] and suggest that this method of neurofeedback is ineffective as an asthma treatment over that obtainable by suggestion. The rationale for neurofeedback is not clear. Presumably, it decreases general physiological reactivity by stabilizing some aspect of neural control. This may decrease susceptibility to stress-induced asthma exacerbations. The relationship between EEG activity and airways reactivity has not been explored, nor has neurofeedback as an asthma treatment been fully evaluated.

Heart Rate Variability Biofeedback

HRV BF [104] can be easily learned and has large and clinically significant effects on asthma. The pathway for its effects is not understood. The technique may, as explained below, trigger a number of salutary mechanisms, including decreased autonomic reactivity to stimulation (including airway reactivity to irritants and emotionally based autonomic reactivity, which may indirectly affect the airways), mechanical stretching of the airways, and decreased inflammation in tissues of the airways.

In a study involving 94 patients, we compared HRV BF with EEG alpha biofeedback (which was considered to be an active placebo treatment) and a waiting list control. We found that HRV BF was 100% effective in preventing asthma exacerbations over a period of approximately 4 months in a population with varying levels of asthma severity, from mild to severe [102]. This effect was accompanied by a significant decrease in use of controller medications, as prescribed by a cadre of pulmonologists who were blinded to experimental condition, an improvement in pulmonary function as assessed by forced oscillation, and a decrease in asthma symptoms. All these effects were significantly greater than in two control conditions. These findings replicate those in a smaller similarly controlled trial [94] and in systematically documented but uncontrolled multiple case observations [105].

The method appears to be useful in children [105] as well as in adults [102], although controlled investigations among children have not been done.

HRV BF and the Baroreflex

One possible mechanism for the therapeutic effects is stabilization of autonomic reactivity, through strengthening of the baroreflex. One of the mechanisms for asthma exacerbation is constriction of the smooth muscles of the airways [25]. These muscles are mediated by the parasympathetic nervous system, which may be related to other mechanisms of asthma exacerbations as well, including increased irritability and inflammation of the airways [106–108]. Parasympathetic innervation of the lung is via the vagus nerve [109]. Vagus nerve output is a component in the baroreflex system [110–113], which is specifically targeted by HRV BF [114]. The baroreflexes are triggered by changes in blood pressure that are detected by stretch receptors in the aorta and carotid artery ("baroreceptors"), which sense changes in blood pressure and trigger reflexes that modulate these changes. When blood pressure rises, the baroreflexes increase vagus nerve outflow and decrease heart rate, which, after a brief (about 5-s) delay, decreases blood pressure [115]. The opposite happens when blood pressure then falls.

The baroreflex modulates fluctuations in blood pressure, such that it causes heart rate to fall when blood pressure rises and to rise when blood pressure falls. Decreases in heart rate cause an eventual decrease in blood pressure by mechanical action (less blood flowing through a vessel of the same size) after a delay averaging about 5 s, caused by inertia in blood flow, plasticity in the blood vessels, and perhaps other cardiovascular characteristics. The baroreflex thus stabilizes blood pressure fluctuations. It also may similarly modulate emotional and general physiological oscillations, through rhythms induced at the same frequency throughout the body, particularly in the brain [116]. Baroreflex control centers in the nucleus tractus solitarius are known to interact with the limbic system [117], and controlled studies have found that HRV BF (which directly increase baroreflex amplitude) can produce substantial improvements in anxiety disorders [118, 119] and depression [119], with several uncontrolled studies showing similar results [20, 21, 120]. Both anxiety and depression can play a role in stimulating asthma exacerbations in some people [121]. The method also may be helpful for treating other functional disorders.

Resonance, the Baroreflex System, and HRV BF

The mechanism for high HRV fluctuations in HRV BF is stimulation of resonance characteristics in the baroreflex system. The baroreflex-induced interaction between heart rate and blood pressure produces a rhythm in heart rate and blood pressure of

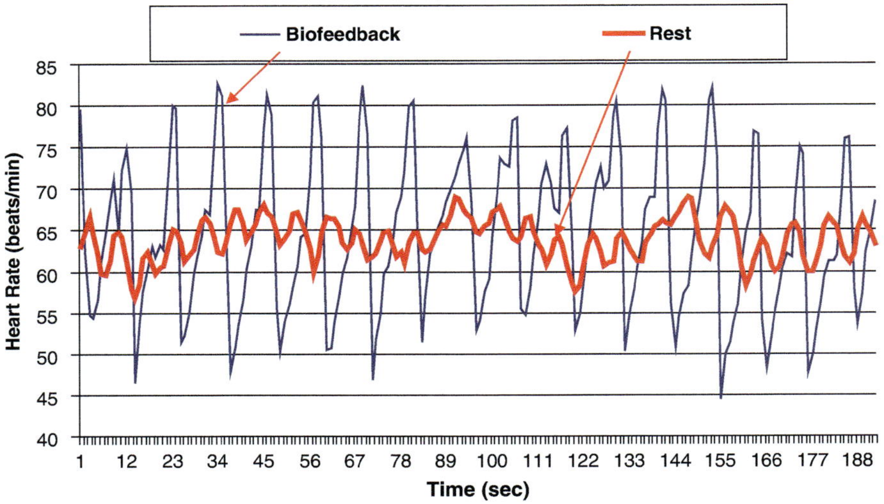

Fig. 10.1 *Example of resonance effects in heart rate when stimulated at its resonance frequency.* This figure illustrates heart rate at rest and when breathing at about 5.5 times per minute. Note the small and irregular heart rate oscillations at rest, but regular and very high-amplitude oscillations when breathing 5.5 times per minute

about 10 s and underlies resonance characteristics in the cardiovascular system at about this frequency.

The resonance properties of any resonant system can be activated by an external stimulus applied the resonance frequency, producing oscillations with very high amplitudes at that frequency, obliterating traces of oscillations that may occur at other frequencies [122]. All of us have experienced this effect when we push a child in a swing. When we push the swing at its resonance frequency (determined mostly by the length of the cords), the swing goes higher and higher at the frequency of the push. If we push at another frequency, the swing may stop or oscillate irregularly. Other sources of swing movement (e.g., the child's wriggling, effects of a breeze) become so small in comparison with the resonance frequency oscillations that they become unnoticeable. High amplitude resonance frequency oscillations in heart rate can easily be obtained by breathing at that frequency, but other sources of resonance frequency stimulation also can cause this effect. Figure 10.1 shows a cardiotachometer recording of heart rate oscillations without external stimulation, and when stimulated by breathing at the individual's resonance frequency (approximately one breath every 11 s). Oscillations are small and irregular at rest, but regular with amplitudes much higher when breathing at resonance frequency. Figure 10.2 shows a respiration tracing, heart rate oscillations, and a spectral analysis of heart rate when a person breathes at resonance frequency and at other frequencies. Notice

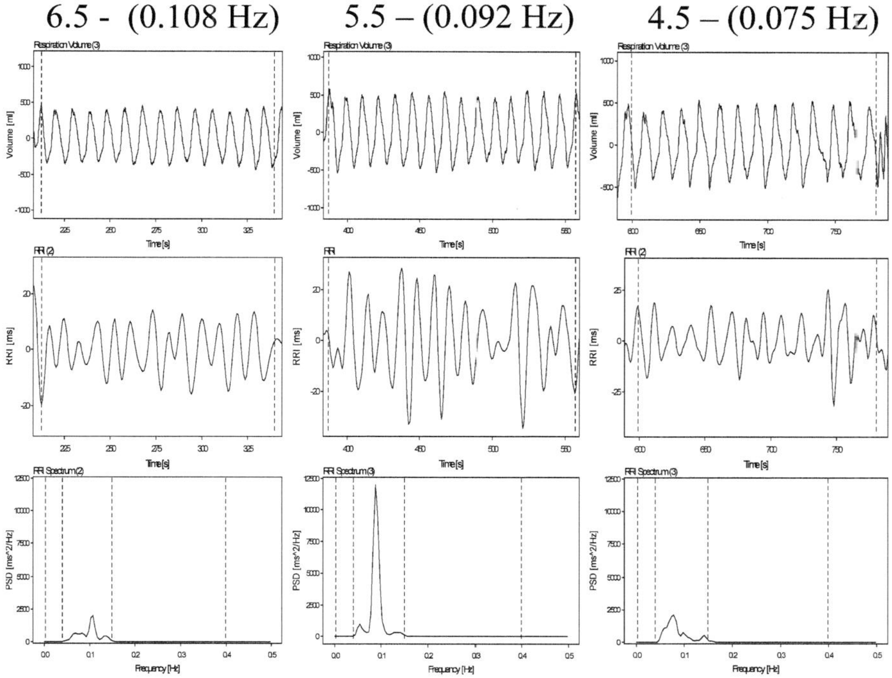

Fig. 10.2 *Respiration, heart rate, and spectral analysis of heart rate when breathing at three frequencies*. The top charts in this figure show respiration, as assessed by a strain gauge placed around the abdomen. An upward direction reflects inhalation, a downward exhalation. The middle charts reflect beat-to-beat heart rate recorded every beat and shown as a cardiotachometer tracing. The *bottom* charts show a spectral (Fourier) analysis of heart rate. Notice a high spectral peak at about 0.09 Hz when the individual breathes at this frequency (5.5 times/min), but lower spectral peaks at other respiratory frequencies

high-amplitude regular oscillations in heart rate at respiratory frequency when the individual breathes 5.5 times per minute, but lower-amplitude and more irregular oscillations when the individual breathes 6.5 or 4.5 times per minute.

Resonance is a characteristic of any feedback system with a constant delay in it [122]. In the case of the cardiovascular system, the delay is caused by the effect of heart rate changes on blood pressure. When the baroreflex causes heart rate to fall, the decreased blood flow eventually causes blood pressure to fall, from mechanical action, but with a delay of about 5 s, apparently caused by inertia in the blood supply [117]. It is a constant within individuals, whose length is probably determined by blood volume. In adults, the resonance frequency of the baroreflex system usually varies around 6 breaths/min, or 0.1 Hz (i.e., 0.1 cycles/s, obtained by dividing 6 [breaths/min] by 60 [s/min]).

In the case of HRV BF, the external stimulus is provided by respiratory sinus arrhythmia (RSA), i.e., increases and decreases in heart rate that accompany breathing, such that heart rate rises in response to inhalation and decreases in response to exhalation. When people breathe at the baroreflex rhythm, the resonance characteristics of the system produce huge oscillations in heart rate (approximately tenfold, as seen in Fig. 10.1) as well as in baroreflex gain (assessed by the number of beats per minute change in heart rate per millimeter of mercury change in blood pressure in each oscillation) [117, 123]. In this process, the baroreflex and RSA stimulate each other, thereby producing large increases in both oscillations.

The baroreflex is an important modulator of blood pressure [115]. Similarly, RSA plays a role in internal regulation by influencing gas exchange efficiency at the lung [124], although its effect in *modulating* changes in physiological activity, if any, is not understood. In theory, the technique of HRV BF may improve asthma by stimulating and strengthening two regulatory reflex systems affecting the cardiorespiratory system.

Mechanisms for HRF BF Effects on Asthma

There is no direct evidence that baroreflex stimulation mediates the effects of HRV BF on asthma. Levels of pulmonary function have not been found to be related to changes in levels of baroreflex control, either acutely or chronically [102, 125]. It is nevertheless possible that changes in autonomic activity contributed to the effects when the technique is not used during asthma exacerbations outside of the laboratory, where use of the method nor physiological effects were monitored.

There is indirect evidence that modulation of the autonomic dampening effect of inflammation may be specifically affected by biofeedback. This is relevant to asthma, because airway reactivity to parasympathetic stimulation in asthma is thought to result from inflammation [126, 127]. The specific effects of HRV BF on inflammation of the airways have not been investigated. However, we have investigated the effect of HRV BF on inflammatory effects produced by experimental exposure to lipopolysaccharide, a potent inflammatory cytokine [128]. Although brief training in biofeedback did not affect various markers of inflammation, it did partially reverse the inflammation-induced suppression of autonomic function. This and other studies of lipopolysaccharide exposure show a pattern of general autonomic withdrawal and decreased heart rate variability at all frequencies, indicating decreased general adaptability [129]. A similar mechanism of autonomic modulation in response to inflammation may occur in asthma. Possible contributions of these mechanisms to HRV BF effects on asthma deserve further evaluation.

Another possible mechanism for the beneficial effects of HRV BF is stretching of the airways by slow deep breathing. Deep inhalations during methacholine challenge tests are known to substantially dampen airway reactivity in this situation [130]. Informal observations supplied to us by M Goldman in one patient showed that slow deep breathing can produce large effects in reversing the effects of an asthma exacerbation that are similar to effects of albuterol and, indeed, augment

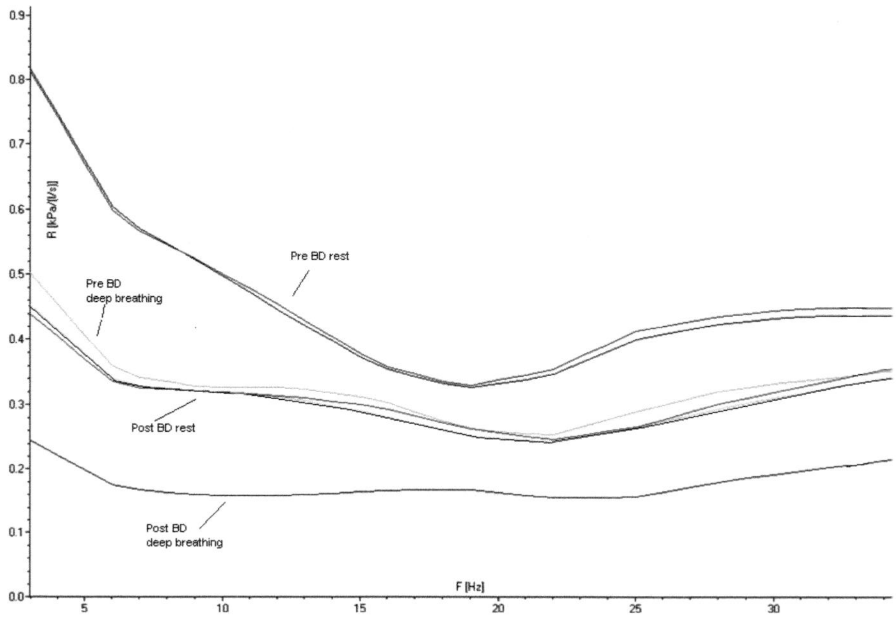

Fig. 10.3 Forced oscillation resistance of asthma patient measured before and after bronchodilator (BD) during rest and during deep breathing

albuterol effects (Fig. 10.3). It is possible that deep inhalations during initial phase of an asthma exacerbation may dampen the bronchoconstriction, and acting similarly to albuterol, the technique may thus prevent the cascade of events, including coughing, further bronchoconstriction, and inflammation, which can lead to more severe asthma events.

A third possible mechanism for HRV BF effects on asthma is through increased efficiency of gas exchange. When people breathe at their resonance frequency, RSA and breathing occur *in phase* with each other, such that heart rate begins rising as inhalation begins and begins decreasing exactly when exhalation starts [131]. During normal breathing, the phase relationship is closer to 90°, such that resting heart rate begins rising during mid-inspiration and begins falling during mid-exhalation. Animal studies have found that gas exchange efficiency at the alveoli is maximized when the organism breathes in phase with heart rate [124]. Similarly, respiratory gas exchange in humans appears to be maximized when people breathe at 6 times per minute [132], which is approximately the baroreflex resonance frequency for most people, compared with uninstructed breathing. This may explain the apparent beneficial effects of HRV BF among patients with emphysema, as suggested by the results of one uncontrolled study [133].

Cost of HRV BF

HRV BF may be useful even among those individuals who decline to take inhaled steroids because of cost. Ten sessions of HRV BF can be provided for approximately $1,000–1,500, with four sessions proportionately less expensive. After training, many patients can continue to use this technique for years, although further research will be needed to establish the "half-life" of HRV BF training. Based on the current costs of the major inhaled steroid agents now on the market, the HRV BF training is equivalent to less than 1 year of medication costs, which now average about $200/month. Therefore, if controlling asthma and preventing serious exacerbations, or in reducing the need for controller medications, biofeedback could be a very reasonable alternative or complement to conventional medical treatment.

Procedure for HRV BF

We have found that the technique for HRV BF can be mastered in approximately four sessions of treatment, of about ½h each, slightly longer in the first session [104, 134]. A more complete explanation with details for the procedure has been published elsewhere [104]. HRV BF can easily be mastered by most people, with the possible exception of those with frequent cardiac arrhythmias (e.g., frequent missed beats or extra systoles), where it becomes difficult to assess the patient's resonance frequency. While adults usually prefer software that shows actual heart rate, and find this signal easiest to follow, special software is available that is appealing to children, where "games" have been constructed that provide incentives and feedback for increasing the amplitude of heart rate variability.

The following video is available:

An example of how to teach a patient about HRV BF (Video 10.1).

At the outset of treatment, the therapist introduces the purpose of HRV BF. This description presupposes that the patient has already been given preliminary asthma education, including use of an asthma action plan, and proper use of a home pulmonary function monitor assessing peak flow and/or FEV_1, and of proper controller and rescue medication use. Although use of a biofeedback device measuring the EKG and respiration (through a strain gauge belt consisting of a waistband whose electrical resistance changes as the individual breathes, or similar device) is the preferable training method, it also can effectively be carried out by a simpler and less expensive device that measures only heart rate, taken from the pulse in the finger or ear. Although the second hand of a clock can be used as a signal for pacing breathing, it is more effectively done with one of the many respiration pacers available on line for various computer devices. Most HRV BF units provide both a cardiotachometer display and a graph representing frequency components of HRV, known as a Fourier transformation analysis, as shown in Fig. 10.2. Figure 10.4

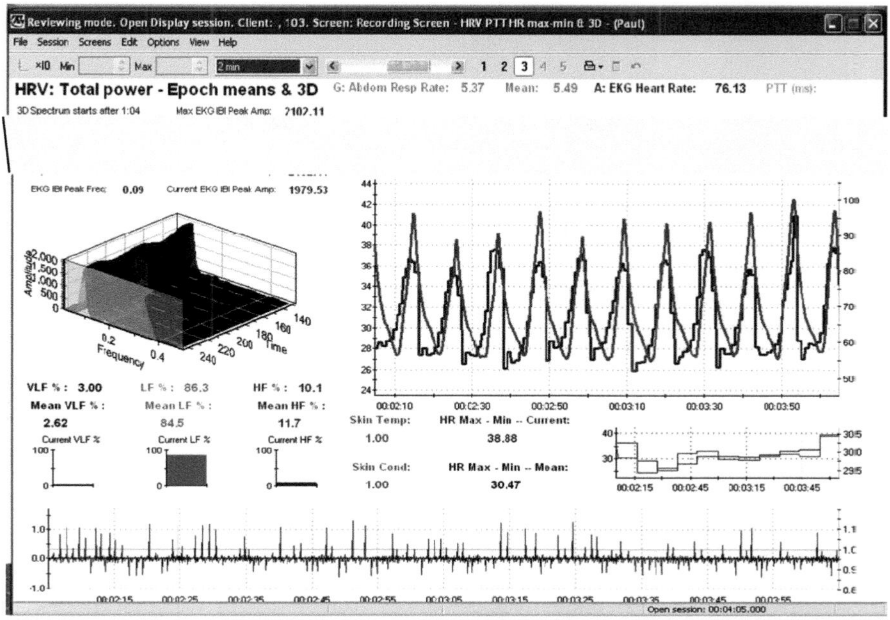

Fig. 10.4 Example of a typical heart rate variability biofeedback display

shows a typical biofeedback display, showing a cardiotachometer, phase relationship between heart rate and respiration, a Fourier analysis, and a graph showing peak-to-trough changes in heart rate with each breath.

Patients may be instructed regarding HRV BF as follows: *I am going to teach you a technique to help you control your asthma. People with asthma are able to use it both to reverse and prevent asthma symptoms. The technique involves learning to do slow breathing at a specific rate. When you practice the technique for two times each day, about* 20 min *each, some reflexes in your body called the "baroreflexes" are stimulated, which help to regulate your heart and breathing and make asthma exacerbations less likely. It also may "stretch" the airways and provide some immediate relief from your symptoms. You can also use the technique if you start experiencing asthma symptoms, but if your symptoms persist for more than a few minutes, take albuterol as you usually do. Although HRV BF might sometimes substitute for albuterol, this has not definitively been proven yet. For your safety, do not let your symptoms persist too long. HRV BF may also help to prevent asthma exacerbations and allow you to take less steroid medication. However, do not change your dose of controller medication without consulting your doctor first.*

This machine will measure your heart rate variability. (Attach electrodes to measure heart rate with a continuous cardiotachometer display and, where possible, respiration. Show how the signal goes up when heart rate increases, and down when it decreases.) *Look how your heart rate goes up and down. Notice that it tends to go along with your breathing, although not necessarily at exactly the same time.* (Point out phase relationships between breathing and heart rate on the computer display, or from the patient's observation of his/her own breathing.)

Now please try breathing along with this respiration pacer. (Point to a respiration pacer displayed on the computer screen.) *Inhale through your nose when the signal goes up and exhale through pursed lips when the signal goes down. Try to breathe low down in your body, about* 2 in. *below your navel. But do not breathe too deeply, or you will hyperventilate and feel lightheaded. If this happens, just breathe more shallowly, although continue breathing along with the pacer.* (Demonstrate the breathing technique.)

We will now try to find the respiration rate that makes your heart rate go up and down the most in phase with your breathing. When you inhale, the graph showing your heart rate should rise. When you exhale, it should fall. I will set this pacer at several different rates, and ask you to breathe at each rate for a few minutes. (Set the heart rate for 6 breaths/min.)

Now start breathing at this rate. If you feel uncomfortable, just stop, and we can start over later.

Monitor the patient's breathing, be sure that the patient is breathing at the assigned rate, coach the patient accordingly, and compliment the patient for doing the task correctly. Coach the patient to breathe abdominally, exhaling through pursed lips. Once the patient has been breathing at the assigned rate for 2 min, record the following values, where available: (1) the patient's respiration rate, (2) the amplitude of the low-frequency spectral peak from the Fourier analysis at the assigned respiration rate (i.e., the height of the spectral power peak that will occur in the spectral analysis graph at the respiratory frequency), (3) the average peak-to-trough amplitude of heart rate fluctuations with breathing (i.e., the number of beats per minute between minimum and maximum heart rate for each breath), and (4) the phase relationship between heart rate and respiration, noting whether the two fluctuate together, whether heart rate changes precede breathing or vice versa, and whether the heart rate values show a smooth high-amplitude curve of RSA. The oscillations in heart rate on the cardiotachometer tracing should rise and fall the greatest number of beats per minute with each breath, and the amplitude should be about the same in succeeding breaths, with no other sources of variation intruding on the smooth curve. If the program provides an average value for low-frequency heart rate variability (approximately 0.05–0.15 Hz), record this value as well. Resonance characteristics of the cardiovascular system will produce the maximum heart rate variations in this frequency range, all at a single frequency, that is, the frequency at which the individual is breathing. Allow the patient to breathe at this rate until all of the above measures become relatively stable over time, where possible. This usually occurs within a minute or two.

After recording this information, invite the patient to relax and breathe naturally for a few minutes. Then reset the respiration rate for 6.5 breaths per minute, and repeat the entire process. Then repeat the process for 5.5, 5, and 4.5 breaths per minute. Almost all adults have resonance frequencies within this range. It is probable that some children may have higher rates, since resonance frequency tends to be inversely associated with blood volume, but this has not been studied empirically.

Compare the patient's profile on each of the criteria above for each respiration rate, and tell the patient that his/her "resonance frequency" is the one that shows the highest spectral peak at respiratory frequency. Confidence in this value will be greatest if it also is the value where heart rate and respiration vary synchronously (without a phase lag), where the low-frequency HRV values and peak-to-trough amplitudes are greatest, and where the heart rate tracing appears like a smooth sine wave. Where there is a discrepancy among these values, choose the one meeting the most criteria, and repeat the process in the following session for frequencies varying 0.5 breaths/min from the resonance frequency calculated in the first session. The error in calculating this frequency is rarely greater than this amount.

When the resonance frequency has been determined or estimated, tell the patient to breathe at this rate at home, either following the second hand of a clock or watch, or using a respiration pacer downloaded from the Internet. Several are available commercially, including AZ Air Plus (from the Biofeedback Foundation of Europe, http://www.bfe.org), the Breath Pacer (an iPhone application from Larva Labs http://www.larvalabs.com/product_detail.php?app=12), My Calm Beat (www.mycalmbeat.com) and others that are increasingly becoming available.

Note that the value for resonance frequency often cannot accurately be estimated in the first session of training. Paced breathing is an unfamiliar activity for many people, and their emotional reaction to it may change during the session. Some people may initially find it uncomfortable and may feel anxious performing the paced breathing task. Usually, people become more comfortable within a few minutes. As emotional state changes, so will the amplitude of HRV, so the highest amplitude of HRV may represent the frequency at which the patient felt most relaxed at the time, rather than the physical characteristic of the cardiovascular system's resonance frequency. After a week of home practice, the patients usually find the procedure to be more comfortable, and a more reliable estimate of resonance frequency often can be made.

Subsequent training sessions should be partially devoted to training in abdominal pursed lips breathing, which appears to augment the effect of HRV BF in preventing asthma exacerbations [102], and to strategies for using the technique when experiencing asthma symptoms. Abdominal breathing often is a challenge for some patients. It most often is absent when patients are anxious or under stress. It is often helpful to explain that the diaphragm *always* pushes the lower abdomen out during inhalation, unless the muscles of the abdomen, back, and pelvis are tense and prevent this action. Encourage the patient to relax the lower abdomen, back, and pelvis, and to breathe into these areas. When these areas are deeply relaxed, respiratory action can also often be felt in the thighs. Sometimes, it helps for the patient to place one hand on the lower abdomen and one on the chest and to try to breathe so that only the hand on the abdomen moves during inhalation.

Also, during the third or fourth session, it may be worthwhile to turn off the pacing signal and to have the patient breathe at the rate where the cardiotachometer tracing shows maximum fluctuations during breathing. This will ordinarily be very close to the previously determined resonance frequency. The rate at which the patient breathes during this exercise often is a more accurate representation of resonance frequency than can be obtained with paced breathing. Instruct the patient to breathe at this rate at home.

Many patients find it useful to have a biofeedback device to use at home. Both free-standing and computer-assisted devices are available at moderate cost from any of several companies that produce these devices, e.g., Stress-eraser at www.stresseraser.com, the HeartMath Institute at www.heartmath.org, Thought Technology Ltd. at www.thoughttechnology.com, and J&J Engineering at www.jjengineering.com.

Side effects from this procedure are rare. Frequently, patients hyperventilate during early sessions, producing symptoms mostly of lightheadedness, sometimes also anxiety, palpitations, headache, and mental cloudiness. When this happens, they should be coached to breathe more shallowly, even while breathing slowly. No instances of increased asthma symptomatology have been reported with this technique.

HRV Biofeedback Therapy in the Office of the Primary Physician

Many primary care physicians hire biofeedback specialists to provide this treatment in their offices, billed with CPT codes either for "biofeedback" or "psychophysiological therapy with psychotherapy," depending on the competencies of the provider and the complete content of the patient visits. Competence in biofeedback is assured by the clinician's attainment of certification by the Biofeedback Certification International Alliance (BCIA) (www.bcia.org). Certification is available both for unlicensed technicians, who must practice under supervision of the physician, for licensed health care providers, often a nurse, social worker, or psychologist, who can work within a physician's practice, and for academicians who primarily use biofeedback in research and education. Some physicians obtain BCIA certification and offer biofeedback treatment themselves. Certification ordinarily requires taking a course in biofeedback and having a required number of hours of supervised practice with the technique. The specific blueprint of training requirements is available at www.bcia.org. Forty-eight hours of didactic biofeedback and psychophysiology training are required, most of which will already have been obtained by prior professional education. Additionally, 20 contact hours with a BCIA-approved mentor are required to review 10 sessions of personal biofeedback demonstrating self-regulation, 50 sessions of patient/client treatment, and 10 h of case conference presentations.

Case Studies

Below, we report clinically significant treatment results in three patients with varying levels of asthma severity, who participated in a 10 weekly session clinical trial of HRV biofeedback, with a 1-to-2-month follow-up on two of the

Table 10.1 Patient 1 asthma severity

Session	Symptoms	Pulmonary function	Medication	Overall
1	Moderate	Mild intermittent	Moderate	Moderate
4	Moderate	Mild persistent	Moderate	Moderate
7	Mild intermittent	Mild intermittent	Mild persistent	Mild persistent
10	Mild intermittent	Mild intermittent	Mild persistent	Mild persistent
Follow-up	Mild intermittent	Mild intermittent	Mild persistent	Mild persistent

In this table, normal pulmonary function ($FEV_1 > 80\%$) is labeled as "mild intermittent"
After session 1(8/31/2000): Flovent 44 2 puffs (p) twice daily (BID) and Serevent 50 1 p BID, FEV_1 95%, AM peak flow—465 L/min. This is the patient's baseline value
After session 4 (9/28/2000): Flovent 44 2 p BID, FEV_1 96%, AM peak flow—490 L/min
After session 7 (10/26/2000): Flovent 44 2 p BID, FEV_1 99%, AM peak flow—510 L/min
After session 10 (11/16/2000): Flovent 44 1 p BID, FEV_1 94%, AM peak flow—500 L/min
After BFB treatment (11/30/2000): Flovent 44 1 p daily, AM peak flow—490 L/min

patients. In this trial, levels of asthma controller medication were adjusted every 2 weeks by a cadre of pulmonologists who did not know whether the patients were receiving HRV biofeedback or were assigned to a control condition. Medication was given using a 13-step medication protocol including, where necessary, use of fluticasone, salmeterol, montelukast, and prednisone, as well as prn albuterol, as detailed in the publication reporting this study. Adjustments were made according to symptomatology, albuterol use, and weekly pulmonary function test results.

Improvement included decreases in asthma symptom severity, decreases in medication consumption, and increases in pulmonary function. In all three cases, treatment results began to appear after the first session. Peak flow gradually increased, and asthma symptom severity decreased during the first month from first to the fourth session. After the fourth session, treatment results stabilized and the physicians began to decrease medications. In two cases, after 3 months of treatment, the patients no longer took any asthma medication and remained symptom-free with improved pulmonary function. Positive results were maintained during the follow-up month. Overall asthma severity was scored based on the 1997 NHLBI *Guidelines* [135]. Severity was scored separately for symptoms, pulmonary function, and medication use. The domain showing greatest severity level was used to determine overall asthma severity.

Note that Patient 1 (Table 10.1 and Fig. 10.5), who improved from moderate to mild persistent asthma, showed improvements in symptoms with less medication, while pulmonary function remained at the mild intermittent level. Patient 2 (Table 10.2) showed improvement in all three areas, with overall severity improving from severe to mild intermittent. Patient 3 (Table 10.3) showed improvements in pulmonary function with less medication, but continued to have severe symptoms. This patient appeared to overperceive asthma symptoms, a perhaps hypochondriacal tendency that was not improved by biofeedback. All patients showed a pronounced decrease in home peak flow variability and an increase in peak flow values over the course of the study.

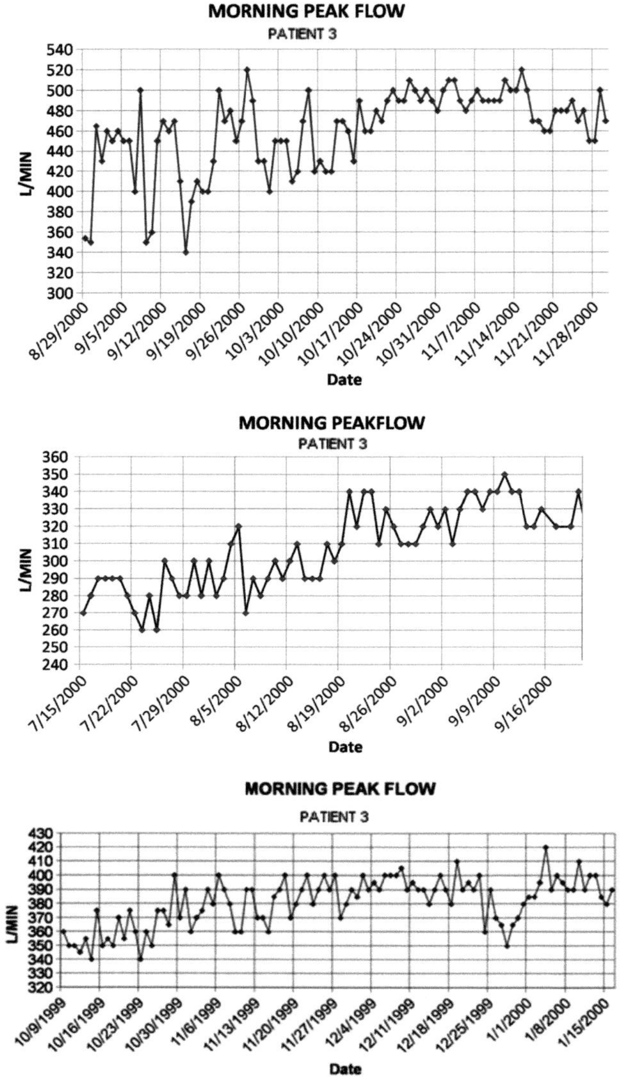

Fig. 10.5 Home morning peak flow values for three patients

Table 10.2 Patient 2 asthma severity

Session	Symptoms	Pulmonary function	Medication	Overall
1	Moderate	Severe	Moderate	Severe
4	Mild persistent	Moderate	Moderate	Moderate
7	Mild intermittent	Moderate	Moderate	Moderate
10	Mild intermittent	Moderate	Mild persistent	Moderate
Follow-up	Mild intermittent	Mild intermittent	Mild intermittent	Mild intermittent

In this table, normal pulmonary function ($FEV_1 > 80\%$) is labeled as "mild intermittent"
After session 1 (baseline) (7/19/2000): Flovent 110 2 p BID, FEV_1 62%, AM peak flow—290 L/min
After session 4 (8/8/2000): Flovent 110 1 p BID, FEV_1 65%, AM peak flow—280 L/min
After session 7 (9/12/2000): Flovent 44 2 p BID, FEV_1 67%, AM peak flow—340 L/min
After session 10 (10/02/2000): Flovent 44 1 p BID, FEV_1 67%, AM peak flow—320 L/min
After BFB treatment (10/05/2000): no medications, average AM peak flow—330 L/min
Follow-up (11/5/2000): no medications, AM peak flow—320 L/min (FEV_1 not measured)

Table 10.3 Patient 3 asthma severity

Session	Symptoms	Pulmonary function	Medication	Overall
1	Severe	Moderate	Moderate	Severe
4	Severe	Mild intermittent	Moderate	Severe
7	Severe	Moderate	Mild persistent	Severe
10	Moderate	Mild intermittent	Mild persistent	Severe
Follow-up	Severe	Mild intermittent	Mild intermittent	Severe

In this table, normal pulmonary function ($FEV_1 > 80\%$) is labeled as "mild intermittent"
After session 1 (10/13/1999) (baseline): Azmacort 3 p BID, FEV_1 77%, AM peak flow—340 L/min
After session 4 (11/04/1999): Azmacort 3 p BID, FEV_1 85%, AM peak flow—390 L/min
After session 7 (11/24/1999): Azmacort 2 p BID, FEV_1 79%, AM peak flow—390 L/min
After session 10 (12/16/1999): Azmacort 1 p BID, FEV_1 80%, AM peak flow—400 L/min
After BFB treatment (01/06/2000): no medications, AM peak flow—400 L/min. In the physician's judgment, the patient's symptoms did not reflect asthma
Follow-up (01/21/2000): no medications, AM peak flow—400 L/min (FEV_1 not measured)

Questions:

1. In order to do biofeedback:
   (a) An instrument must be capable of recording an EKG.
   (b) An instrument must provide instant information to the patient.
   (c) An instrument must have resonance capabilities.
   (d) An instrument must be capable of performing classical conditioning.
   (e) The patient must be in the physician's office.

2. HRV BF has been shown to:
   (a) Affect airway inflammation
   (b) Affect baroreflex interaction with the lung
   (c) Decrease the probability of asthma exacerbations
   (d) Increase respiratory sinus arrhythmia in asthma patients
   (e) Decrease depression in asthma patients

3. Which of the following biofeedback modalities has *not* been studied as a treatment for asthma?
   (a) EEG
   (b) Finger temperature
   (c) Heart rate variability
   (d) sEMG
   (e) Respiratory resistance
4. Resonance characteristics of the baroreflex system can be stimulated by:
   (a) Breathing
   (b) Emotional thoughts
   (c) Muscle tension
   (d) (a) and (c) above
   (e) (a), (b), and (c) above
5. When a person breathes about six times a minute, which effects have been proven to occur (pick all that apply)?
   (a) Respiratory gas exchange efficiency increases'/
   (b) The baroreflexes are stimulated.
   (c) Respiratory sinus arrhythmia increases.
   (d) Heart rate varies in phase with breathing.
   (e) Airway inflammation decreases.

Answers:

1. (b): Immediate feedback (b) is needed in order to be useful for physiological control. Delayed feedback (or reinforcement of any operant response) is not effective. HRV biofeedback can be given from cardiotachometer readings derived from the finger or ear pulse, so (a) is incorrect. Item (c) is incorrect because there is no such thing as "resonance capabilities" in an instrument. Resonance is a characteristic of a particular kind of feedback system. Item (d) is incorrect because biofeedback involves operant conditioning, not classical conditioning. Item (e) is incorrect because home trainer devices are effective and easily available.
2. (c): Lehrer et al. [102] found that HRV biofeedback was 100% effective in preventing asthma exacerbations. No interactions were found with baroreflex activity (b) or resting respiratory sinus arrhythmia (d). No data were reported on airway inflammation (a) or depression (d).
3. (b): Other applications are discussed in the chapter. Of these, only heart rate variability has been definitively found to be effective. EMG biofeedback has statistically significant but small positive effects. There is contradictory evidence for respiratory resistance biofeedback and very little evidence about EEG biofeedback.

4. (e): Any stimulus that perturbs the system at resonance frequency will stimulate resonance characteristics of a system.
5. (a), (b), (c), (d): Item (e) has not been studied.

Conclusions

Of the biofeedback methods, only HRV BF has been demonstrated to have reliable and clinically significant effects on improving asthma condition. The role of this technique in asthma therapeutics remains to be evaluated, i.e., whether it should best be used as a complementary treatment to standard steroid therapy or whether it may serve as a viable alternative.

Acknowledgments Preparation of this chapter was partially supported by Grant # 1R01HL089495-01A2 from the National Heart, Lung, and Blood Institute, of the National Institutes of Health.

References

1. Schwartz MD, Andrasik F, editors. Biofeedback: a practitioner's guide. 3rd ed. New York: Guilford Publications; 2003.
2. Reeve L, Reeve KF, Brown AK, Brown JL, Poulson CL. Effects of delayed reinforcement on infant vocalization rate. J Exp Anal Behav. 1992;58(1):1–8.
3. Sutphin G, Byrne T, Poling A. Response acquisition with delayed reinforcement: a comparison of two-lever procedures. J Exp Anal Behav. 1998;69(1):17–28.
4. Okouchi H. Response acquisition by humans with delayed reinforcement. J Exp Anal Behav. 2009;91(3):377–90.
5. Lattal KA. Delayed reinforcement of operant behavior. J Exp Anal Behav. 2010;93(1): 129–39.
6. DePue JD, Clark MM, Ruggiero L, Medeiros ML, Pera Jr V. Maintenance of weight loss: a needs assessment. Obes Res. 1995;3(3):241–8.
7. Qi BB, Dennis KE. The adoption of eating behaviors conducive to weight loss. Eat Behav. 2000;1(1):23–31.
8. Mikosch P, Hadrawa T, Laubreiter K, et al. Effectiveness of respiratory-sinus-arrhythmia biofeedback on state-anxiety in patients undergoing coronary angiography. J Adv Nurs. 2010;66(5):1365–2648.
9. Moore NC. A review of EEG biofeedback treatment of anxiety disorders. Clin Electroencephalogr. 2000;31(1):1–6.
10. Pallavicini F, Algeri D, Repetto C, Gorini A, Riva G. Biofeedback, virtual reality and mobile phones in the treatment of generalized anxiety disorder (GAD): a phase-2 controlled clinical trial. J Cyber Ther Rehabil. 2009;2:315–27.
11. Wenck LS, Leu PW, D'Amato RC. Evaluating the efficacy of a biofeedback intervention to reduce children's anxiety. J Clin Psychol. 1996;52(4):469–73.
12. Karavidas MK, Tsai P-S, Yucha C, McGrady A, Lehrer PM. Thermal biofeedback for primary Raynaud's phenomenon: a review of the literature. Appl Psychophysiol Biofeedback. 2006;31(3):203–16.
13. Andrasik F. Biofeedback in headache: an overview of approaches and evidence. Cleve Clin J Med. 2010;77 Suppl 3:S72–6.
14. Enck P, Van der Voort IR, Klosterhalfen S. Biofeedback therapy in fecal incontinence and constipation. Neurogastroenterol Motil. 2009;21(11):1133–41.

15. Glazer HI, Laine CD. Pelvic floor muscle biofeedback in the treatment of urinary incontinence: a literature review. Appl Psychophysiol Biofeed. 2006;31(3):187–201.
16. Norton C. Fecal incontinence and biofeedback therapy. Gastroenterol Clin North Am. 2008;37(3):587–604.
17. Uhlmann C, Fröscher W. Biofeedback treatment in patients with refractory epilepsy: changes in depression and control orientation. Seizure. 2001;10(1):34–8.
18. Nazarian M. An alternative treatment for depression using EEG biofeedback to alter frontal alpha asymmetry and improve mood, Nazarian, Maria: U Arizona, US; 2005
19. Klee S, Meyer RG. Alleviation of performance deficits of depression through thermal biofeedback training. J Clin Psychol. 1981;37(3):515–8.
20. Karavidas MK, Lehrer PM, Vaschillo E, et al. Preliminary results of an open label study of heart rate variability biofeedback for the treatment of major depression. Appl Psychophysiol Biofeedback. 2007;32(1):19–30.
21. Siepmann M, Aykac V, Unterd J, et al. A pilot study on the effects of heart rate variability biofeedback in patients with depression and in healthy subjects. Appl Psychophysiol Biofeedback. 2008;33(4):195–201.
22. Friel PN. EEG biofeedback in the treatment of attention deficit hyperactivity disorder. Altern Med Rev. 2007;12(2):146–51.
23. Hirshberg LM. Place of electroencephalographic biofeedback for attention-deficit/hyperactivity disorder. Expert rev. 2007;7(4):315–9.
24. Monastra VJ, Lynn S, Linden M, Lubar JF, Gruzelier J, LaVaque TJ. Electroencephalographic biofeedback in the treatment of attention-deficit/hyperactivity disorder. Appl Psychophysiol Biofeed. 2005;30(2):95–114.
25. National Heart Lung and Blood Institute (NHLBI). Expert panel report 3: guidelines for the diagnosis and management of asthma: full report. Washington, DC: National Asthma Education and Prevention Program, Department of Health and Human Services; 2007.
26. Barnes PJ, Pedersen S, Busse WW. Efficacy and safety of inhaled corticosteroids. New developments. Am J Respir Crit Care Med. 1998;157(3 Pt 2):S1–53.
27. Jackson LD, Polygenis D, McIvor RA, Worthington I. Comparative efficacy and safety of inhaled corticosteroids in asthma. Can J Clin Pharmacol. 1999;6(1):26–37.
28. Pedersen S, O'Byrne P. A comparison of the efficacy and safety of inhaled corticosteroids in asthma. Allergy. 1997;52(39 Suppl):1–34.
29. World Health Organization. Adherence to long-term therapies: Evidence for action. 2003.
30. Strunk RC, Ford JG, Taggart V. Reducing disparities in asthma care: priorities for research–National heart, lung, and blood institute workshop report. J Allergy Clin Immunol. 2002;109(2):229–37.
31. Williams LK, Pladevall M, Xi H, et al. Relationship between adherence to inhaled corticosteroids and poor outcomes among adults with asthma. J Allergy Clin Immunol. 2004;114(6):1288–93.
32. Milgrom H, Bender B, Ackerson L, Bowry P, Smith B, Rand C. Noncompliance and treatment failure in children with asthma. J Allergy Clin Immunol. 1996;98(6 Pt 1):1051–7.
33. Bender B, Milgrom H, Apter A. Adherence intervention research: what have we learned and what do we do next? J Allergy Clin Immunol. 2003;112(3):489–94.
34. Haynes RB, McDonald H, Garg AX, Montague P. Interventions for helping patients to follow prescriptions for medications. Cochrane Database Syst Rev. 2002;CD000011.
35. McDonald HP, Garg AX, Haynes RB. Interventions to enhance patient adherence to medication prescriptions: scientific review. JAMA. 2002;288(22):2868–79.
36. Toelle BG, Ram FS. Individualised management plans for asthma in children and adults. Cochrane Database Syst Rev. 2004;CD002171.
37. Lemanek KL, Kamps J, Chung NB. Empirically supported treatments in pediatric psychology: regimen adherence. J Pediatr Psychol. 2001;26(5):253–75.
38. Bender BG, Bender SE. Patient-identified barriers to asthma treatment adherence: responses to interviews, focus groups, and questionnaires. Immunol Allergy Clin North Am. 2005;25(1):107–30.

39. Ip M, Lam K, Yam L, Kung A, Ng M. Decreased bone mineral density in premenopausal asthma patients receiving long-term inhaled steroids. Chest. 1994;105(6):1722–7.
40. Langmack EL. Complementary and alternative therapies for asthma. In: Szefler SJ, Leung DYM, editors. Severe asthma, pathogenesis and clinical management. 2nd ed. New York: Marcel Dekker; 2001. p. 221–38.
41. Ernst E. Complementary therapies for asthma: what patients use. J Asthma. 1998;35(8): 667–71.
42. Blanc PD, Kuschner WG, Katz PP, Smith S, Yelin EH. Use of herbal products, coffee or black tea, and over-the-counter medications as self-treatments among adults with asthma. J Allergy Clin Immunol. 1997;100(6 Pt 1):789–91.
43. Jonas BS, Wagener DK, Lando JF, Feldman JJ. Symptoms of anxiety and depression as risk factors for development of asthma. J Appl Biobehav Res. 1999;4(2):91–110.
44. Ortega AN, McQuaid EL, Canino G, Goodwin RD, Fritz GK. Comorbidity of asthma and anxiety and depression in Puerto Rican children. Psychosomatics. 2004;45(2):93–9.
45. Chen E, Hanson MD, Paterson LQ, Griffin MJ, Walker HA, Miller GE. Socioeconomic status and inflammatory processes in childhood asthma: the role of psychological stress. J Allergy Clin Immunol. 2006;117(5):1014–20.
46. Marin TJ, Chen E, Munch JA, Miller GE. Double-exposure to acute stress and chronic family stress is associated with immune changes in children with asthma. Psychosom Med. 2009;71(4):378–84.
47. Weil CM, Wade SL, Bauman LJ, Lynn H, Mitchell H, Lavigne J. The relationship between psychosocial factors and asthma morbidity in inner-city children with asthma. Pediatrics. 1999;104(6):1274–80.
48. Wright RJ, Rodriguez M, Cohen S. Review of psychosocial stress and asthma: an integrated biopsychosocial approach. Thorax. 1998;53(12):1066–74.
49. Isenberg S, Lehrer PM, Hochron S. The effects of suggestion and emotional arousal on pulmonary function in asthma: a review. Psychosom Med. 1992;54(2):192–216.
50. Miller BD, Wood BL. Influence of specific emotional states on autonomic reactivity and pulmonary function in asthmatic children. J Am Acad Child Adolesc Psychiatry. 1997;36(5): 669–77.
51. Dirks JF, Kinsman RA. Death in asthma: a psychosomatic autopsy. J Asthma. 1982;19(3): 177–87.
52. Friedman MS. Psychological factors associated with pediatric asthma death: a review. J Asthma. 1984;21(2):97–117.
53. Tietz W, Kahlstrom E, Cardiff M. Relationship of psychopathology to death in asthmatic adolescents. J Asthma Res. 1975;12(4):199–206.
54. Betrus PA, Elmore SK, Hamilton PA. Women and somatization: unrecognized depression. Health Care Women Int. 1995;16(4):287–97.
55. Ebert D, Martus P. Somatization as a core symptom of melancholic type depression. Evidence from a cross-cultural study. J Affect Disord. 1994;32(4):253–6.
56. Lipsanen T, Saarijärvi S, Lauerma H. Exploring the relations between depression, somatization, dissociation and alexithymia–overlapping or independent constructs? Psychopathology. 2004;37(4):200–6.
57. Howren M, Suls J, Martin R. Depressive symptomatology, rather than neuroticism, predicts inflated physical symptom reports in community-residing women. Psychosom Med. 2009;71(9):951–7.
58. Rosenkranz MA, Davidson RJ. Affective neural circuitry and mind-body influences in asthma. Neuroimage. 2009;47(3):972–80.
59. Skotzko CE. Symptom perception in CHF: (Why mind matters). Heart Fail Rev. 2009;14(1): 29–34.
60. Peiffer C. Dyspnea and emotion: what can we learn from functional brain imaging? Am J Respir Crit Care Med. 2008;177(9):937–9.
61. von Leupoldt A, Sommer T, Kegat S, et al. Dyspnea and pain share emotion-related brain network. Neuroimage. 2009;48(1):200–6.
62. Lehrer PM, Hochron SM, Isenberg S, Rausch L, Carr R. The asthma symptom profile: a psychophysically based scale for assessment of asthma symptoms. J Psychosom Res. 1993;37(5):515–21.

63. Feldman JM, Lehrer PM, Hochron SM, Schwartz GE. Defensiveness and individual response stereotypy in asthma. Psychosom Med. 2002;64(2):294–301.
64. Arena JG, Goldberg SJ, Saul DL, Hobbs SH. Temporal stability of psychophysiological response profiles: analysis of individual response stereotypy and stimulus response specificity. Behav Ther. 1989;20(4):609–18.
65. Robinson JW, Whitsett SF, Kaplan BJ. The stability of physiological reactivity over multiple sessions. Biol Psychol. 1987;24(2):129–39.
66. Salomon K, Matthews KA, Allen MT. Patterns of sympathetic and parasympathetic reactivity in a sample of children and adolescents. Psychophysiology. 2000;37(6):842–9.
67. Sersen EA, Clausen J, Lidsky A. Autonomic specificity and stereotypy revisited. Psychophysiology. 1978;15(1):60–7.
68. Lehrer PM, Murphy AI. Stress reactivity and perception of pain among tension headache sufferers. Behav Res Ther. 1991;29(1):61–9.
69. Lariviere C, Forget R, Vadeboncoeur R, Bilodeau M, Mecheri H. The effect of sex and chronic low back pain on back muscle reflex responses. Eur J Appl Physiol. 2010;109(4): 577–90.
70. Silfies SP, Squillante D, Maurer P, Westcott S, Karduna AR. Trunk muscle recruitment patterns in specific chronic low back pain populations. Clin Biomech. 2005;20(5):465–73.
71. Mitchell T, O'Sullivan PB, Smith A, et al. Biopsychosocial factors are associated with low back pain in female nursing students: a cross-sectional study. Int J Nurs Stud. 2009;46(5): 678–88.
72. Schneider S, Schmitt H, Zoller S, Schiltenwolf M. Workplace stress, lifestyle and social factors as correlates of back pain: a representative study of the German working population. Int Arch Occup Environ Health. 2005;78(4):253–69.
73. Anderson DE. Respiratory psychophysiology in hypertension research. Behav Modif. 2001;25(4):606–20.
74. Schwartz AR, Gerin W, Davidson KW, et al. Toward a causal model of cardiovascular responses to stress and the development of cardiovascular disease. Psychosom Med. 2003;65(1):22–35.
75. Deckert J, Deckert L. Vocal cord dysfunction. Am Fam Physician. 2010;81(2):156–9.
76. Weinberger M, Abu-Hasan M. Pseudo-asthma: when cough, wheezing, and dyspnea are not asthma. Pediatrics. 2007;120(4):855–64.
77. Fischer MJ, Gutenbrunner C, Ptok M. Intensified voice therapy: a new model for the rehabilitation of patients suffering from functional dysphonias. Int J Rehabil Res. 2009;32(4): 348–55.
78. Lee E-K, Son Y-I. Muscle tension dysphonia in children: voice characteristics and outcome of voice therapy. Int J Pediatr Otorhinolaryngol. 2005;69(7):911–7.
79. Emerich KA. Nontraditional tools helpful in the treatment of certain types of voice disturbances. Curr Opin Otolaryngol Head Neck Surg. 2003;11(3):149–53.
80. Chabora PD. A descriptive study of the application of research in neuropsychology to self-use training for actors. Dissertation Abstracts International Section A: Humanities and Social Sciences. Jun 1995;55(12-A):3686
81. Wilson GD. Psychology and performing arts. Lisse: Swets & Zeitlinger Publishers; 1991. p. 32.
82. Glaus KD, Kotses H. Facial muscle tension influences lung airway resistance; limb muscle tension does not. Biol Psychol. 1983;17(2–3):105–20.
83. Kotses H, Glaus KD, Bricel SK, Edwards JE, Crawford PL. Operant muscular relaxation and peak expiratory flow rate in asthmatic children. J Psychosom Res. 1978;22(1):17–23.
84. Kotses H, Harver A, Segreto J, et al. Long-term effects of biofeedback-induced facial relaxation on measures of asthma severity in children. Biofeedback Self Regul. 1991;16(1): 1–21.
85. Wright RJ. Stress and atopic disorders. J Allergy Clin Immunol. 2005;116(6):1301–6.
86. Wright RJ, Subramanian SV. Advancing a multilevel framework for epidemiologic research on asthma disparities. Chest. 2007;132(5 Suppl):757S–69S.

87. Cacioppo JT, Petty RE, Losch ME, Kim HS. Electromyographic activity over facial muscle regions can differentiate the valence and intensity of affective reactions. New York: Psychology Press; 2008.
88. Kukde MP, Neufeld RW. Facial electromyographic measures distinguish covert coping from stress response to stimulus threat. Pers Indiv Differ. 1994;16(2):211–28.
89. Sato W, Fujimura T, Suzuki N. Enhanced facial EMG activity in response to dynamic facial expressions. Int J Psychophysiol. 2008;70(1):70–4.
90. Witvliet CV, Vrana SR. Psychophysiological responses as indices of affective dimensions. Psychophysiology. 1995;32(5):436–43.
91. Lehrer PM, Hochron SM, Mayne T, et al. Relaxation and music therapies for asthma among patients prestabilized on asthma medication. J Behav Med. 1994;17(1):1–24.
92. Richter R, Dahme B. Bronchial asthma in adults: there is little evidence for the effectiveness of behavioral therapy and relaxation. J Psychosom Res. 1982;26(5):533–40.
93. Lehrer P, Generelli P, Hochron S. The effect of facial and trapezius muscle tension on respiratory impedance in asthma. Appl Psychophysiol Biofeedback. 1997;22(1):43–54.
94. Lehrer P, Carr RE, Smetankine A, et al. Respiratory sinus arrhythmia versus neck/trapezius EMG and incentive inspirometry biofeedback for asthma: A pilot study. Appl Psychophysiol Biofeedback. 1997;22(2):95–109.
95. Mass R, Wais R, Ramm M, et al. Frontal muscles activity: a mediator in operant reduction of respiratory resistance? J Psychophysiol. 1992;6(2):167–74.
96. Ritz T, Dahme B, Wagner C. Effects of static forehead and forearm muscle tension on total respiratory resistance in healthy and asthmatic participants. Psychophysiology. 1998;35(5): 549–62.
97. Peper E, Tibbetts V. Fifteen-month follow-up with asthmatics utilizing EMG/incentive inspirometer feedback. Biofeedback Self Regul. 1992;17(2):143–51.
98. Mackay AD, Mustchin CP, Sterling GM. The response of asthmatic patients and normal subjects to maximum respiratory manoeuvres. Spirometry-induced bronchoconstriction. Eur J Respir Dis Suppl. 1980;106:35–40.
99. Mass R, Richter R, Dahme B. Biofeedback-induced voluntary reduction of respiratory resistance in severe bronchial asthma. Behav Res Ther. 1996;34(10):815–9.
100. Mass R, Dahme B, Richter R. Clinical evaluation of a respiratory resistance biofeedback training. Biofeedback Self Regul. 1993;18(4):211–23.
101. Tansey MA. EEG sensorimotor biofeedback training and the treatment of a six-year-old asthmatic child. Am J Clin Biofeedback. 1982;5:145–9.
102. Lehrer PM, Vaschillo E, Vaschillo B, et al. Biofeedback treatment for asthma. Chest. 2004;126(2):352–61.
103. Wise RA, Bartlett SJ, Brown ED, et al. Randomized trial of the effect of drug presentation on asthma outcomes: The American lung association asthma clinical research centers. J Allergy Clin Immunol. 2009;124(3):436–44.
104. Lehrer PM. Biofeedback training to increase heart rate variability [References]. Principles and practice of stress management. 3rd ed. New York: Guilford Press; 2007. p. 227–48.
105. Lehrer P, Smetankin A, Potapova T. Respiratory sinus arrhythmia biofeedback therapy for asthma: a report of 20 unmedicated pediatric cases using the Smetankin method. Appl Psychophysiol Biofeedback. 2000;25(3):193–200.
106. Goyal M, Jaseja H, Verma N. Increased parasympathetic tone as the underlying cause of asthma: A hypothesis. *Medical Hypotheses*. 2010;74(4):661–664.
107. Hashimoto A, Maeda H, Yokoyama M. Augmentation of parasympathetic nerve function in patients with extrinsic bronchial asthma–evaluation by coefficiency of variance of R–R interval with modified long-term ECG monitoring system. Kobe J Med Sci. 1996;42(6):347–59.
108. Morrison JF, Pearson SB. The parasympathetic nervous system and the diurnal variation of lung mechanics in asthma. Respir Med. 1991;85(4):285–9.
109. Undem B, Canning B. Neuronal control of airway function in allergy. In: Yunginger J, Adkinson NJ, Busse W, Bochner B, Holgate S, Simons F, editors. Middleton's allergy principles & practice. Philadelphia: Mosby; 2003. p. 231–41.

110. Deley G, Picard G, Taylor JA. Arterial baroreflex control of cardiac vagal outflow in older individuals can be enhanced by aerobic exercise training. Hypertension. 2009;53(5): 826–32.
111. Drew RC, Bell MPD, White MJ. Modulation of spontaneous baroreflex control of heart rate and indexes of vagal tone by passive calf muscle stretch during graded metaboreflex activation in humans. J Appl Physiol. 2008;104(3):716–23.
112. Sapoznikov D, Backenroth R, Rubinger D. Baroreflex sensitivity and sympatho-vagal balance during intradialytic hypotensive episodes. J Hypertens. 2009;28(2):314–24.
113. Tanaka G, Sawada Y, Fujii R. Cardiac vagal withdrawal during stressful tasks estimated by the baroreflex sensitivity and respiratory sinus arrhythmia. Jpn J Psychol. 1994;65(1):9–17.
114. Lehrer PM, Vaschillo E, Vaschillo B, et al. Heart rate variability biofeedback increases baroreflex gain and peak expiratory flow. Psychosom Med. 2003;65(5):796–805.
115. Eckberg DL, Sleight P. Human baroreflexes in health and disease. Oxford: Clarendon; 1992.
116. Mayhew JW, Askew S, Zheng Y, et al. Cerebral vasomotion: a 0.1-Hz oscillation in reflected light imaging of neural activity. Neuroimage. 1996;4(3 Pt 1):183–93.
117. Vaschillo EG, Vaschillo B, Lehrer PM. Characteristics of resonance in heart rate variability stimulated by biofeedback. Appl Psychophysiol Biofeedback. 2006;31(2):129–42.
118. Thurber MR. Effects of heart-rate variability biofeedback training and emotional regulation on music performance anxiety in university students, Thurber, Myron Ross: U North Texas, US; 2007
119. Zucker TL, Samuelson KW, Muench F, Greenberg MA, Gevirtz RN. The effects of respiratory sinus arrhythmia biofeedback on heart rate variability and posttraumatic stress disorder symptoms: a pilot study. Appl Psychophysiol Biofeedback. 2009;34(2):135–43.
120. Hassett AL, Radvanski DC, Vaschillo EG, et al. A pilot study of the efficacy of heart rate variability (hrv) biofeedback in patients with fibromyalgia syndrome. Appl Psychophysiol Biofeedback. 2007;32(1):1–10.
121. Alvarez GG, Fitzgerald JM. A systematic review of the psychological risk factors associated with near fatal asthma or fatal asthma. Respiration. 2007;74(2):228–36.
122. Grodins FS. Control theory and biological systems. New York: Columbia University Press; 1963.
123. Vaschillo EG, Lehrer P, Rishe N, Konstantinov M. Heart rate variability biofeedback as a method for assessing baroreflex function: a preliminary study of resonance in the cardiovascular system. Appl Psychophysiol Biofeedback. 2002;27(1):1–27.
124. Yasuma F, Hayano J. Respiratory sinus arrhythmia: why does the heartbeat synchronize with respiratory rhythm? Chest. 2004;125(2):683–90.
125. Lehrer P, Vaschillo E, Lu S-E, et al. Heart rate variability biofeedback: effects of age on heart rate variability, baroreflex gain, and asthma. Chest. 2006;129(2):278–84.
126. Brannon JD. Bronchial hyperresponsiveness in the assessment of asthma control: airway hyperresponsiveness in asthma: Its measurement and clinical significance. Chest. 2010; 138(2 Suppl):11S–7S.
127. Anderson SD. Indirect challenge tests: airway hyperresponsiveness in asthma: Its measurement and clinical significance. Chest. 2010;138(2 Suppl):25S–30S.
128. Lehrer P, Karavidas MK, Lu S-E, et al. Voluntarily produced increases in heart rate variability modulate autonomic effects of endotoxin induced systemic inflammation: an exploratory study. Appl Psychophysiol Biofeed. 2010;35(4):303–15.
129. Jan BU, Coyle SM, Oikawa LO, et al. Influence of acute epinephrine infusion on endotoxin-induced parameters of heart rate variability: a randomized controlled trial. Ann Surg. 2009;249(5):750–6.
130. Cockcroft DW, Davis BE. Deep inhalation bronchoprotection in asthma: correlation with airway responsiveness. J Allergy Clin Immunol. 2006;117(4):951–2.
131. Vaschillo E, Vaschillo B, Lehrer P. Heartbeat synchronizes with respiratory rhythm only under specific circumstances. Chest. 2004;126(4):1385–6.
132. Bernardi L, Spadacini G, Bellwon J, Hajric R, Roskamm H, Frey AW. Influence of breathing frequency and pattern on oxygen saturation and exercise performance. Lancet. 1998; 351(9112):1308–11.

133. Giardino ND, Chan L, Borson S. Combined heart rate variability and pulse oximetry biofeedback for chronic obstructive pulmonary disease: preliminary findings. Appl Psychophysiol. 2004;29(2):121–33.
134. Lehrer P, Vaschillo E. Heart rate variability biofeedback: a new tool for improving autonomic homeostasis and treating emotional and psychosomatic disorders. Jpn J Biofeedback Res. 2003;30:7–16.
135. National Heart Lung and Blood Institute (NHLBI). Expert panel report 2: Guidelines for the diagnosis and management of asthma. Washington, DC: National Asthma Education and Prevention Program, U.S. Department of Health and Human Services; 1997.

Chapter 11
Breathing Techniques for Asthma and Other Respiratory Diseases

Christine R. Jenkins

Abstract Since the evolution of understanding of asthma as an inflammatory airways disease, maintenance of effective anti-inflammatory medications has been the mainstay of management. With the recognition of the many contributors to breathlessness and the role of anxiety in some patients, behavioral strategies, including breathing techniques, have again attracted interest. Breathing techniques can help to improve symptoms and quality of life in patients with asthma, but do not modify characteristics of the underlying disease, particularly airway inflammation and airway hyperresponsiveness. However, there is strong evidence that breathing techniques can assist in controlling asthma symptoms and in reducing dependence on short-acting reliever medications. The evidence for this will be discussed along with specific approaches that have been studied in randomized controlled trials. Many of these studies have been conducted in primary care and the community, making the findings applicable to this context and enabling the approach to teaching breathing techniques to be readily translated into general practice. The importance of anxiety and panic in patients with chronic obstructive pulmonary disease (COPD) has prompted interest in breathing techniques for controlling symptoms in this disease although the evidence for their benefit is not yet well established.

Keywords Breathing techniques • Breathing exercises • Dysfunctional breathing • Asthma symptoms • Asthma management • Asthma symptom control

---

C.R. Jenkins (✉)
Clinical Professor, University of Sydney, Co-operative Research Centre for Asthma and Woolcock Institute of Medical Research, Thoracic Physician, Concord Hospital, Australia

Department of Thoracic Medicine, Concord Hospital, Hospital Road, Concord, NSW 2137, Australia
e-mail: christine.jenkins@sydney.edu.au

R.D. Anbar (ed.), *Functional Respiratory Disorders: When Respiratory Symptoms Do Not Respond to Pulmonary Treatment*, Respiratory Medicine,
DOI 10.1007/978-1-61779-857-3_11,

Background

Breathing techniques for asthma and other respiratory disorders go back a long way. Preceding our current understanding of the inflammation that underlies many lung conditions characterized by breathlessness, it was thought that conscious attempts to reduce the rate and depth of breathing could reduce distress from lung disease. Further, often it is difficult to distinguish between breathlessness due to underlying lung disease and that due to anxiety, because of the similar associated symptoms such as chest tightness, apprehension, and light headedness, as well as the observation that anxiety can amplify a sense of difficulty breathing. This led people to believe that controlling the rate and depth of breathing could reduce the impact of lung disease.

In ancient times, asthma was believed to be a condition of nervous breathing, and it has taken centuries for that view to be replaced by our current understanding that asthma is an inflammatory disease of the airways in which they are prone to narrowing too easily and too much in response to a range of triggers. Nevertheless, there is some physiologic rationale to consider that breathing techniques can make an important contribution to symptom management for patients with asthma [1]. The most commonly advocated approach of reducing depth and rate of breathing in people with asthma is likely to be beneficial through its associated reduction in cooling and drying of the airways. Heat and water loss from the airways in the context of increased ventilation, such as occurs with exercise, can induce bronchoconstriction. Conversely, preventing this by warming and humidifying air, such as through encouragement of a nasal route of breathing, can ameliorate bronchoconstriction. Further, increased ventilatory rates can result in hypocapnia, which is another factor which can contribute to bronchoconstriction. Hence, techniques which focus on nasal route of breathing, and reduced depth and rate of breathing, have been the focus of particular interest in relation to symptom control in asthma. Other techniques, such as abdominal breathing, while not having an obvious physiologic rationale, may confer benefit, suggesting that there are several different aspects of breathlessness that can be influenced by breathing techniques.

Asthma and Dysfunctional Breathing

Evidence links dysfunctional breathing with asthma and respiratory disorders, and hyperventilation disorder is commonly seen in patients presenting to specialist respiratory clinics [2, 3]. In several studies, a link has been demonstrated between asthma and symptomatic hyperventilation [2, 4]. In a hospital clinic, 42% of patients showed evidence of hyperventilation disorder, and it is well known that hyperventilation may complicate and compound asthma presentations [4].

To explore this further, Thomas et al. undertook a study of dysfunctional breathing in patients with asthma, identified through practice records as receiving treatment in the previous year in a primary care setting in the UK [5]. The Nijmegen questionnaire (Table 4.4) was used to assess the prevalence of dysfunctional breathing in patients aged between 17 and 65 with a diagnosis of asthma. This questionnaire assesses 16 symptoms associated with abnormal breathing on a five-point scale, and scores $\geq$23 have been reported as showing high sensitivity and specificity (greater than 90%) as a screening instrument in patients diagnosed with hyperventilation syndrome. The questionnaire however explores a range of symptoms beyond documenting the classical "overbreathing" manifestations of air hunger, breathlessness, light headedness, paresthesia, and sweating. Although it has been assumed that many of these symptoms are due to hypocapnia, most do not require a fall in pCO_2.

About one third of women and one fifth of men with asthma in this practice had symptom scores on the Nijmegen questionnaire, suggestive of dysfunctional breathing when this questionnaire was administered during a period of apparent stability between consultations. Affected patients were more likely to be younger, but there was no correlation between the severity of asthma and dysfunctional breathing score. In a follow-up study [6], the questionnaire was administered to a random sample of 300 people aged 16–65 without any evidence of asthma in practice records. Positive screening scores were more common in women (14%) than men (2%), and higher scores were more prevalent in those with current asthma than those without. Comparing these two populations that resided in the same primary health care region, the prevalence of positive screening scores in those treated for asthma (29%) was significantly higher than in those with no diagnosis of asthma (8%), $P<0.001$.

Work undertaken a decade ago by Osborne et al. [1] studied patterns of breathing in 23 currently asymptomatic people with stable asthma, normal lung function, and only occasional reliever use, comparing them to 17 matched control subjects without asthma. Although the patients with asthma had no clinical evidence of hyperventilation and normal lung function, their arterial blood gas measurements revealed a lower pCO_2, lower end-tidal CO_2, and higher anxiety scores, suggesting possible subclinical hyperventilation.

However, although hyperventilation syndrome has been well observed in patients with asthma, when strict criteria are applied, it does not appear to be more prevalent than in the general population [7, 8]. In acute asthma, hyperventilation may be difficult to distinguish from tachypnea, which is a frequent characteristic when patients present for emergency care. This is particularly so when anxiety is present [9, 10]. The observation that asthma patients have slightly lower than normal pCO_2 when breathing at rest along with a mildly elevated respiratory rate has prompted some investigators to propose that hyperventilation underlies asthma and contributes to bronchoconstriction. The Russian physician Buteyko proposed that hyperventilation is the cause of asthma and that breathing retraining, which reduces the rate and depth of breathing, may be effective in reducing the symptoms and reversing the pathology of the disease [11, 12]. Buteyko believed that an incorrect breathing pattern caused asthma, primarily through hyperventilation resulting in hypocapnia and consequently bronchoconstriction. Others have suggested that hyperventilation does not inevitably occur in asthma [7, 8]. Nonetheless, when present, hyperventilation can aggravate symptoms, increase beta-agonist use, and amplify anxiety, thus creating a vicious cycle that worsens the manifestations of the disease [13, 14]. Breaking into this vicious cycle by using breathing techniques that reduce the rate and depth of breathing can have beneficial effects on symptom control and overuse of short-acting reliever medications.

Asthma and Breathing Techniques

There are many different approaches to modifying the rate, depth, and route of breathing, in people with asthma. Historically, breathing techniques for asthma have focused on relaxation, diaphragmatic breathing, nasal route of breathing, and reduced depth and rate of breathing. Research into breathing retraining needs to consider not only whether breathing techniques can influence symptoms or features of the underlying airways disease but also the particular techniques that are most useful in this regard. Although there is theoretical evidence, as cited above, to support the potential role for breathing techniques in reducing breathlessness, early studies lacked rigorous methodology, left the question of benefit unresolved, and failed to identify the crucial components of the intervention [4, 15]. A Cochrane review of many studies concluded that breathing exercises, such as Buteyko, yoga, and diaphragmatic breathing, led to a reduction in short-acting beta-agonist use and a trend toward improvement in quality of life in patients with asthma [16]. However, there was no consistent evidence of improved disease control, such as reduced requirement for anti-inflammatory medication, reduced airway hyperresponsiveness, or improved lung function. Critics of these findings have suggested that several studies failed to demonstrate benefit in lung function and airway hyperresponsiveness because of the deep inspirations and forced expirations required for monitoring peak expiratory flow and clinic spirometry. Several investigators highlighted the need for further studies addressing these concerns and several other methodological weaknesses in the trials published up to 2004 [16–18]. These include more rigorously evaluating the impact of breathing techniques on symptom-free days, asthma control, and control of the underlying inflammatory process.

Although research in breathing techniques dates back to the 1960s, small studies with poorly defined interventions and subjective outcomes led to a poor appreciation of the potential benefit and applicability of these techniques. Additionally, a wide range of strategies and approaches have been included under the banner of "breathing techniques" without a clear body of evidence to support them. Over the last 10–15 years, however, several large randomized controlled trials with standardized interventions and validated outcome measures have made a major contribution to our understanding of the role of these techniques in asthma management (Table 11.1). It is clear that it is possible to objectively define the nature of the intervention, to apply it across a range of different contexts with patients whose symptoms vary in severity, and to measure the benefits with a variety of measures that

Table 11.1 Summary characteristics of major randomized controlled trials of breathing techniques

First author (Reference)	Active intervention	Control or passive intervention	Subjects completed/ duration	Mean pre BD FEV_1 % pred.	Asthma severity/control	Outcome
Bowler [26]	Buteyko breathing	Asthma education and relaxation techniques	39/3 months	74%	Moderate/poorly controlled	Improved: markedly reduced reliever use
Cooper [20]	Buteyko breathing or Pranayama, using PCLE[a]	PCLE placebo device	69/6 months	80%	Mild–moderate/ suboptimal control	Improved: reduced reliever use and symptoms
Thomas [29]	Physiotherapist, breathing retraining	Asthma education, asthma nurse	28/6 months	Not stated	Mild/suboptimal control	Improved: AQLQ[b] and symptoms
Holloway [32]	Papworth method 5 components	Usual medical care	72/12 months	89%	Mild, control not stated	Improved: HADS[c], SGRQ[d], and symptoms
Slader [33]	Hypoventilation, pause, and nasal route of breathing, video	Abdominal exercises and relaxation, video	48/32 weeks	79%	Mild–moderate, suboptimal–poor control	Improved both arms: reduced reliever use and symptoms
Cowie [34]	Buteyko breathing	Paced breathing, physiotherapist	119/6 months	81%	Moderate, suboptimal control	Improved asthma control and reduced ICS[e]
Thomas [31]	Physiotherapist, diaphragmatic, and nasal breathing techniques similar to Papworth	Asthma education, nurse provided	129/6 months	89%	Moderate, suboptimal–poor control	Improved AQLQ[b] and HADS[c]

[a] *PCLE* pink city lung exerciser, see reference
[b] *AQLQ* asthma quality-of-life questionnaire
[c] *HADS* hospital anxiety and depression score
[d] *SGRQ* St. George's respiratory questionnaire
[e] *ICS* inhaled corticosteroids

assess symptoms, reliever use, quality of life, and well-established objective criteria reflecting the underlying inflammatory process.

Singh et al. [19] undertook a small study in India over a 6-week period randomizing patients to regular breathing exercises using a pink city lung exerciser (PCLE, a cylinder with resistance to expiration designed to mimic pranayama yoga) or a placebo, which was a mouthpiece with no attachment and thus no resistance to breathing. Pranayama is a yoga breathing exercise that promotes reduction in breathing frequency through increased duration of exhalation. Patients received each of these therapies in a crossover study for 2 weeks following a 2-week placebo period. In the active intervention period using the PCLE, there was a significant increase in forced expiratory volume in 1 s (FEV_1) and a reduction in nighttime wheezing. Subsequently, a larger study was performed in the UK comparing the same yoga breathing technique with a sham intervention [20], showing some improvement in airway hyperresponsiveness but no other change in lung function despite symptomatic benefit.

In a larger Canadian study [21], 67 patients with mild asthma were randomized to receive a 16-week exercise program aimed at developing respiratory muscles and diaphragmatic breathing. This group was compared to patients receiving an exercise program that did not focus on the respiratory muscles and a wait-list group which acted as a control. The group receiving diaphragmatic and respiratory muscle training experienced a reduction in their asthma medication use and an improvement in asthma symptoms, but this benefit was not sustained 2 months following the end of their treatment period.

The methodology for breathing techniques studies and the difficulty of blinding the interventions and investigators have plagued the development of an evidence body regarding the efficacy of breathing techniques. Nevertheless, several studies have contributed to refinements in these techniques that ultimately resulted in the clear demonstration of their benefit [22].

To pursue the possible role of yoga breathing and compare it to Buteyko breathing, Cooper et al. [20] randomized 90 patients with asthma requiring inhaled corticosteroids for asthma control, to Buteyko breathing or use of a PCLE. There was no significant difference in airway hyperresponsiveness at 3 or 6 months, and symptoms remained relatively stable in the placebo and lung exerciser groups but were reduced in the Buteyko group. The study suggested that Buteyko breathing technique improves symptoms and reduces reliever use, but it does not modify the underlying physiological characteristics of the disease.

Yoga has been studied in a number of randomized controlled trials showing varying benefits in symptom control and some underlying markers of asthma. A trial of Iyengar yoga (stretching) resulted in symptomatic improvement to a similar extent in the intervention group compared to those undertaking stretching in the control group [23]. Finally, in a study of lifestyle modification based on yoga, nutrition counseling, and self-monitoring versus a wait-list approach in 57 adults with asthma, lung function, quality of life, and reduced exercise-induced bronchoconstriction was observed in the lifestyle modification group [24]. There was reduced reliever medication use in both groups but no change in inflammatory markers in either group. In a study of Sahaja yoga ("mental silence") Manocha et al. [25] demonstrated improved airway hyperresponsiveness and mood in 59 patients with mild asthma over a 4-month treatment period.

In a further study of the Buteyko technique, Bowler et al. [26] undertook a prospective blinded randomized study comparing Buteyko breathing with asthma education and relaxation techniques, in 39 patients taking high doses of reliever bronchodilators. Patients underwent extensive physiological testing and measurements of asthma control over a 3-month period following participation in these interventions. There was no difference between the groups in measures of airway function, including morning peak flow readings, spirometry, end-tidal CO_2, and minute volume. Three months after the intervention, the Buteyko group showed a mean reduction in daily beta-agonist use of 904 μg compared to 57 μg in the control group. There was a trend in reduction of inhaled corticosteroids use, but this did not reach statistical significance. This study provided persuasive evidence that a technique incorporating strategies to reduce the depth and frequency of breathing could significantly reduce reliever use and improve symptom control.

Relaxation exercises and therapies have been used widely as control interventions in breathing techniques studies, as relaxation has not been shown to have significant therapeutic benefit. In contrast, rather than using relaxation for the control group, in a study teaching the Buteyko technique by video, the control involved viewing a video of landscape scenery [27]. Thirty-six patients were randomly allocated to either the Buteyko intervention or landscape video, and again, the Buteyko breathing group experienced significant reductions in symptoms, improvement in quality of life, and a marked reduction in beta-agonist use, in this case, by more than 60% over the 4-week intervention period. Again, there were no significant changes in inhaled corticosteroids use.

A Cochrane review published in 2002 [16] and revised in 2006 [28] assessed the evidence for the efficacy of breathing retraining. This review identified 42 full-text papers regarding the topic, but excluded 35 papers as they did not satisfy basic methodological criteria in regard to randomization or blinding. The reviewers noted that most studies were of small size, used multiple interventions, and unvalidated outcomes. They were unable to draw reliable conclusions from the body of data: Even though a number of trends and improvement were noted, these were not of statistical significance as a result of poor study design. They strongly recommended that large-scale trials with good-quality methodology were needed to assess the impact of breathing retraining in the management of asthma.

Thomas et al. [29] recruited patients aged 17–65 years with a diagnosis of asthma, who had received at least one prescription for an inhaled or oral asthma medication in the previous year. The patients completed a Nijmegen questionnaire that they received by mail, and if they qualified with a score suggestive of dysfunctional breathing (>23), they were invited to participate in a controlled trial. The subjects were randomized to receive breathing retraining with a physiotherapist or asthma education with an asthma nurse. An hour-long retraining session took place in small groups followed by two individual short sessions. The sessions involved explanations by the physiotherapist regarding abnormal breathing patterns, including hyperventilation, and instruction in diaphragmatic breathing exercises using an established physiotherapy methodology that emphasized slow regular breathing and dominant diaphragmatic effort. Subjects were encouraged to practice these techniques for at least 10 min every day over the 6 months of the study. The primary endpoint was measured by the Juniper asthma quality-of-life questionnaire (AQLQ) [30]. There was a statistically significant improvement in the AQLQ score after 1 month, along with improvements in the activity and symptom domains. At 6 months, there was a trend to improvement in the overall AQLQ score, but this was no longer statistically significant. Improvement in asthma quality-of-life score and the Nijmegen dysfunctional breathing questionnaire showed a moderate correlation. There were no significant changes in lung function, the doses of inhaled corticosteroids, or bronchodilator medications. The authors concluded that breathing retraining could result in an improvement in health-related quality-of-life score of patients with asthma who demonstrate dysfunctional breathing abnormalities, based on their Nijmegen questionnaire. However, the lack of sustained statistically significant changes left some unanswered questions about these techniques.

Subsequently, the authors undertook a larger prospective parallel group randomized controlled trial comparing asthma education and breathing retraining [31]. In addition to asthma quality of life, they studied a range of physiologic outcomes including airway hyperresponsiveness, exhaled nitric oxide, induced sputum cell count, and the asthma control questionnaire. In this study, dysfunctional breathing was not a requirement, but rather, patients were recruited if they had an abnormal AQLQ score. Patients received either three sessions of physiotherapist-directed breathing exercises or three sessions of nurse-provided asthma education. 183 subjects were randomized, and 152 subjects completed the intervention and follow-up period. Significant improvements in the asthma quality-of-life score occurred after both interventions with no significant difference between groups at 1 month. However, by 6 months, a higher proportion of the breathing techniques group showed clinically important improvements in asthma quality-of-life score. Hospital and anxiety depression score (HADS) improved in the intervention group, but breathing training was not associated with significant changes in airway physiology, inflammation, or airway hyperresponsiveness.

Holloway and West [32] undertook a randomized controlled trial of integrated breathing and relaxation techniques in 85 patients with asthma from a rural UK practice. Patients included in this study were between 16 and 70 years old, and the majority had a long duration of asthma and normal lung function. Symptom burden and treatment requirements are not provided, but the authors indicate that the majority of patients had either mild asthma or symptoms well controlled with medication. The primary outcome measure was the St. George's Respiratory Questionnaire (SGRQ) assessing health status over 6 and 12 months after the intervention. Patients were randomized to either usual care or usual care plus the Papworth method. This involved breathing training to reduce dysfunctional breathing with a focus on diaphragmatic breathing and nasal expiration, education focused on recognizing and managing stress responses, relaxation training and home exercises with an audiotape containing reminders of the breathing and relaxation techniques. The intervention group received five 60-min individual sessions with a respiratory physiotherapist. Symptom scores were lower in the Papworth group immediately after the intervention and at

12 months. The posttreatment and 12-month quality-of-life scores were significantly lower (improved) in the treatment group as were the Nijmegen and HADS scores compared to the control group. Objective measures of respiratory function did not differ across the groups. The effect sizes on symptoms were statistically and clinically significant, and the intervention achieved important reductions in anxiety and depression scores. Nonetheless, the study again failed to demonstrate that breathing techniques can affect underlying physiologic measures of asthma.

In summary, early studies of breathing techniques in asthma were hampered by poor study design, inadequately validated endpoints, and poorly described interventions. Despite this, symptomatic benefits were observed, although it was difficult to conclude that these benefits could be reproduced in other settings or sustained longterm.

It was in this context that we undertook a double-blind randomized control trial of two different breathing techniques for the management of asthma [33]. Several of the studies had suggested that nasal route of breathing, slow exhalation and avoidance of hyperventilation were important aspects of the effectiveness of breathing techniques. We designed a study to test the hypothesis that techniques aimed at reducing tidal volume and rate of breathing, including encouraging a nasal route of breathing, would result in greater improvements in asthma symptoms and measures of disease control than nonspecific upper body exercises. As supporters of Buteyko breathing techniques had criticized studies that incorporated peak flow monitoring because of the requirement for a deep inspiration, a secondary hypothesis was that twice daily peak flow monitoring did not have a detrimental effect that masked the benefit of the breathing techniques intervention.

Fifty-seven subjects were randomized to receive instruction in (1) exercises that incorporated techniques to achieve hypoventilation, prolonged exhalation, nasal route of breathing, and controlled breathing, or (2) alternative breathing techniques that involved shoulder rotations, forward curls, and control of breathing focusing on good posture and relaxation. Participants learned their breathing techniques by video instruction and were asked to practice their routine exercises twice daily. The study was carefully blinded, using an unblinded research assistant to instruct the patients, be available for assistance, and who reviewed the outcome measures including physiologic asthma endpoints such as airway responsiveness to mannitol, clinic spirometry, and end-tidal CO_2. The primary route of breathing was assessed during questionnaire completion, while the subjects were wearing a thermistor with small probes sitting at nose and mouth, attached to a lightweight headpiece.

The study included a 12-week initial period with daily video review and use of the exercises, and a 12-week inhaled corticosteroids reduction period, separated by a 2-week peak flow monitoring period and a 2-week washout period. Subjects again monitored peak flow readings over the 2 weeks at the end of the study. The primary outcome was asthma quality of life and daily symptom scores between groups at weeks 12 and 28. Both groups had a dramatic reduction in reliever use, commencing from week one after randomization, with no significant differences between the groups at week 12. The mean reduction in short-acting beta-agonist use was 86% from baseline. There was no significant difference in ACQ scores at week 12, as significant improvements occurred in both groups. There were small differences between the groups in physician global assessments, but no consistent differences at week 12 for physiologic outcomes, specifically airway responsiveness, end-tidal CO_2, and lung function or asthma control measurements. Inhaled corticosteroid dose was reduced by about 50% in each group. Hence, the study showed marked benefits in symptom control and reduced bronchodilator use, with a trend to reduce inhaled corticosteroid use and no difference between the two treatment interventions with respect to these improvements.

Finally, in a university-based asthma program [34], a randomized controlled trial of the Buteyko technique was compared to instruction in two physiotherapy-guided breathing and relaxation techniques. Participants were aged between 18 and 50 with a diagnosis of asthma and current use of asthma medications. The patients received instruction on the Buteyko technique on five consecutive evenings, and the "control" group was instructed with a series of exercises designed to develop slow, controlled exhalation and paced breathing. Both groups received education about asthma. Subjects were followed up at 3 months and 6 months after completion of the intervention. 129 subjects were randomized, and 119 subjects were studied 6 months. Subjects in both groups improved significantly in asthma control, with the proportion of patients achieving good control almost doubling in both groups. The inhaled corticosteroid doses were reduced by both interventions, to a greater extent in the Buteyko group. It is of interest that this study achieved similar benefits with both interventions, as occurred in the previously described study [33]. While this might be attributed to a placebo effect, it is more likely that some of the symptoms experienced by these patients were not due to their asthma per se, and that some patients were overtreated at baseline.

Clinical trials of inhaled corticosteroids have tended to emphasize the importance of achieving good control by stepping up doses, without necessarily offering strategies for dose reduction. Non-pharmacological interventions are one mechanism by which patients can be enabled to progressively reduce their inhaled corticosteroid doses under medical supervision, while maintaining good symptom control. Many times, patients use their reliever for prevention ("in case I get symptoms") rather than for actual relief of symptoms. We suspect that any effective technique—such as breathing exercises—which delays the taking of reliever will reduce some of this unnecessary use. So, although breathing exercises may not have any *particular* physiological benefit, the process of using breathing techniques may allow people to substantially reduce their use of reliever bronchodilators.

Given the magnitude of the differences in *content* of the two breathing techniques that were used in our study, it appears likely that the observed clinical improvements were not due to the use of a particular type of exercise, but due to the *process* of both routine and as-required exercises that reinforce a message of relaxation and self-efficacy. There are several possible reasons why these breathing techniques were successful:

- Participants felt in control, calm and relaxed, and less reliant on medication.
- They are likely to have experienced fewer side effects as a result of reduced reliever use.

- Clinical trial participation—regular monitoring, increased awareness of asthma, and increased adherence to prescribed medication (inhaled corticosteroids)—is usually valued by patients and beneficial to them.
- Patients felt comfortable about using a nondrug method, which was supported by health professionals.
- The techniques offered a distraction from the symptoms and a focus on performing a task.
- Continued use of the exercises was reinforced by patients experiencing the benefits for themselves.

Reduced use of reliever may have several benefits, including a greater sense of freedom and control over asthma symptoms. We asked the participants in this study, which aspects of it they found helpful.

At the end of the study, patients reported:

- "I feel relaxed, confident in controlling the asthma, relieved."
- "I am no longer worried about my asthma. I no longer have daily symptoms."
- "I am certain the whole thing has helped me."
- "The exercises were outstandingly effective in making me feel better than any other time in 30 years."

In summary, breathing techniques improve asthma symptoms and reduce reliever use but do not alter underlying airway physiology or lung function. Participants describe having a sense of control over their breathing pattern and symptom evolution. Anxiety levels are reduced through this mechanism as well as through avoidance of the overuse of short-acting beta-agonists. It appears that these techniques are effective in patients with mild-to-moderate symptomatic asthma, but whether they are effective in a more severe group has not been studied.

Should Breathing Techniques Be Taught to Patients with Asthma?

The results of breathing techniques studies over the last 5 years provide high-quality evidence that breathing techniques can assist symptom control and reduce reliever use in patients with asthma. Additionally, breathing techniques appear to assist in reducing inhaled corticosteroid doses when coupled with regular medical review and assessment of asthma control. Breathing techniques, therefore, offer the potential to reduce unnecessary doses of controller medication as well as confer benefits in reducing symptom frequency and use of reliever medication. Since these are goals of good asthma management, breathing techniques could be incorporated into a multidisciplinary approach to achieving asthma control, which as proposed by current asthma management guidelines includes minimizing medication. The cost effectiveness of breathing techniques has not been assessed in the randomized controlled trials so far, but avoidance of side effects and reduced doses of inhaled corticosteroids and bronchodilators over a lifetime of asthma would be expected to have significant cost benefit.

Can Breathing Techniques Be Taught in Primary Care?

Most of the recent randomized double-blind controlled trials described above were undertaken in primary care settings. Patients were selected because they had asthma, and no specific procedures were undertaken to determine whether they would be likely to respond to an intervention in which they learned breathing techniques for symptom control. The patients generally are representative of those usually seen in primary care. The studies include a range of patients with mild-to-moderate asthma, as well as some who were very high users of short-acting reliever medication and others with high scores on the dysfunctional breathing questionnaire. The only patients not represented in these studies are those with generally more persistent asthma that is poorly responsive to medication despite good adherence and device technique. Thus, breathing techniques appear to be applicable to a wide group of patients with asthma and not specifically those who are anxious or prone to hyperventilation.

Teaching breathing techniques can be undertaken in a variety of ways. Several studies used a physiotherapist with skills and knowledge in breathing training, specifically teaching diaphragmatic breathing, nasal route of breathing, and prolonged exhalation, as well as good posture and relaxation. Other studies have used video teaching that patients watch in their own time, including at home, and which enables them to access a real-life demonstration of the necessary maneuvers and encourages them to practice these on a daily basis. At least one of these videos is available as a free download on the Cooperative Research Center (CRC) for asthma website: *www.woolcock.org.au.* This DVD provides accessible free information to patients and also enables practitioners to learn the evidence as well as the skills in order to teach them effectively. Primary care physicians may not have time to teach these techniques, but the availability of videos and DVDs enables practice nurses and physiotherapists to acquire the expertise. Several studies enabled patients to contact the physiotherapist throughout the study or an investigator to discuss the techniques to ensure they were following them appropriately. This is probably an important component and should be made available in practices where these techniques are promoted.

Components of Breathing Techniques Studies: What Is Crucial?

The study we undertook is described here briefly, but can be seen in more detail on the CRC web site *www.woolcock.org.au.* The participants practiced these twice daily, including once daily while watching the video, as well as using a briefer set of exercises whenever they experienced asthma symptoms.

We used two different techniques which we termed "Group A" and "Group B." Our results showed both were effective, and so we suggest that patients can select the group of exercises they wish.

Group A exercises involved:

- Breathing through the nose “nasal route of breathing”
- Breathing more shallowly, “relaxed breathing”
- Breathe hold after a normal breath out while sitting “extended delay”

The daily exercise routine consisted of these components performed in 2-min cycles accompanied by footage of scenery. The same exercises were used when symptoms occurred.

Group B exercises involved:

- Focus on good posture and relaxation (“control of breathing”).
- Shoulder rotations, forward curls and arm raises repeated in sets of four while seated.
- Route of breathing was not specified, and both nasal and mouth breathing were demonstrated.

For symptom relief, subjects used techniques we named “Control of breathing” exercises with focus on good posture and relaxation, without the physical maneuvers.

All subjects were provided with two videos. An “instruction” video that demonstrated and explained the exercise components, outlined as-needed use of the exercises for symptoms, and went through the daily exercise routine, and a “daily exercises” video that demonstrated the daily exercise routine. Participants were asked to practice their exercises twice daily and to watch the video at least once daily. The “instruction” video could be used again at any time. We told both groups of participants that they could use the techniques instead of their reliever at any time, but we advised them to use their reliever if they did not gain benefit from the exercises or their asthma symptoms persisted.

Who Should Receive Breathing Techniques Instruction?

Essentially, the studies so far do not suggest there is any particular subgroup of asthma patients who might be unlikely to respond to the use of breathing techniques to control asthma symptoms. There are limited data in patients with unstable asthma and in patients with moderately severe asthma. Hence, the use of breathing techniques in these groups should be undertaken very cautiously after maximum attention has been paid to achieving better asthma control with appropriate pharmacotherapy, device use training, and self-management education.

Can Breathing Techniques Be Used for COPD?

There are many fewer studies examining the role of breathing techniques in chronic obstructive pulmonary disease (COPD). The pathophysiology of dyspnea in COPD is complex, and multiple factors contribute to it. Hence, it has been more difficult to demonstrate that specific strategies targeted at depth or rate of breathing can make a difference to dyspnea in COPD patients. In these patients, breathlessness results from varying contributions including functional respiratory muscle weakness, increased ventilatory demand, gas exchange abnormalities, increased mechanical loading of inspiratory muscles, dynamic airway compression, and distortions of the thoracic cage resulting in mechanical disadvantage and increased work of breathing. Considerable controversy surrounds the value of techniques such as pursed lip breathing, diaphragmatic breathing, and respiratory muscle training in COPD [35]. The latter has been thoroughly researched, particularly inspiratory muscle training which in addition to exercise training has been shown to improve exercise capacity and reduce dyspnea [36]. Controlled exhalation, prolonging the time for lung emptying while maintaining positive end expiratory pressure, is likely to reduce pulmonary hyperinflation and sensation of dyspnea [37]. Slow breathing reduces sympathetic excitation and thus through incorporation into a training program has the potential to improve exercise tolerance and reduce dyspnea [38]. Both yoga and singing have been shown to be associated with improved quality of life, reduced dyspnea, and anxiety levels in patients with COPD [39, 40]. As with asthma, no changes in lung function have been demonstrated with breathing techniques and COPD [35].

Case Studies

Case 1

A 19-year-old woman with asthma is referred for consideration of additional treatment to control her asthma. She takes regular inhaled corticosteroids and long-acting bronchodilator medication (fluticasone/salmeterol 250/50 mcg twice daily) but has been using reliever medication more frequently, up to four times daily and not experiencing complete relief of symptoms. No obvious trigger for these symptoms is identified in her home or occupational setting, but she describes the sensation of difficulty achieving a full inspiration, persistent breathlessness after exercise, and lack of relief from her usual medications.

Questions:

1. The next steps in management should include:
   (a) Assessment of asthma control using a standardized questionnaire and spirometry
   (b) Discussion of the circumstances in which she takes more reliever medication
   (c) Referral to an asthma educator to assess her inhaler technique
   (d) A dialogue regarding the possible benefits, and training in breathing techniques
   (e) All of the above

2. Patients studied in the larger randomized controlled trials of breathing techniques generally have:

   (a) Been taking excessive doses of short-acting beta-agonists
   (b) Been long-standing patients of respiratory specialists
   (c) Been representative of patients with mild-to-moderate asthma in the community
   (d) Had symptoms of, but not confirmed asthma
   (e) Included children and adults aged between 8 and 65 years.

Answers:

1. (e): All patients with symptomatic persistent asthma should have their asthma control and spirometry assessed regularly at medical review. This will help to guide treatment and ensure that patients are not inappropriately prescribed excessive doses of inhaled corticosteroids. Symptoms or reliever use that are out of keeping with objective measures of control should not be treated with higher doses of medication. Inhaler technique should be checked to ensure that the pulmonary deposition of the intended doses is being achieved. Breathing techniques may be helpful for all patients, as there is an opportunity to substitute an approach to managing symptoms that will help reduce reliever use and manage day-to-day symptoms more effectively.
2. (c): Most of the methodologically sound studies described in this chapter have recruited adult patients aged 18–65 years, from the community or primary care. A few studies have recruited patients from specialist clinics. Generally, the patients have not been selected for high dependence on reliever medication even though some studies have specifically recruited symptomatic patients, patients using high doses of short-acting beta-agonists, or patients with high scores on the Nijmegen questionnaire.

Case 2

A 65-year-old man whose COPD was diagnosed 8 years earlier is now experiencing marked exercise limitation. His spirometry reveals an FEV_1 of 33% of predicted, and an FEV_1/FVC ratio of 35%. His 6-min walk distance is moderately reduced at 320 m (usual normal 6 MWD>450 m). He is taking appropriate doses of combination long-acting bronchodilator and inhaled corticosteroid, long-acting anticholinergic medication, and short-acting beta-agonist as needed. He has had two hospital admissions for acute exacerbations of his COPD in the last 6 months. He relates feeling frightened when he becomes breathless and is aware that this anxiety worsens his dyspnea not only when he is experiencing an exacerbation but also during more stable periods, especially when he exerts himself suddenly or tries to exercise.

Questions:

1. This patient would most likely be helped by:

   (a) A higher dose of combination inhaled corticosteroid and long-acting bronchodilator
   (b) Oxygen therapy
   (c) Pulmonary rehabilitation
   (d) Cognitive behavior therapy
   (e) Breathing techniques

2. In relation to the benefit of breathing techniques for people with asthma identified in randomized controlled trials:

   (a) Only techniques promoting nasal route of breathing confer improvements in symptom control.
   (b) The benefit does not last any longer than the first few weeks of the intervention.
   (c) The intervention must be delivered by a physiotherapist.
   (d) Significant improvements in lung function have been demonstrated.
   (e) A variety of different interventions have been effective in improving symptoms and reducing reliever use.

Answers:

1. (c): This patient has severe COPD but has had frequent exacerbations recently and reports anxiety as a significant contributor to his worsening breathlessness. Although he may be helped by cognitive behavior therapy and breathing techniques, the intervention most likely to be beneficial for him is pulmonary rehabilitation. Pulmonary rehabilitation has been shown to improve quality of life, reduce hospital admissions, reduce symptoms, and improve exercise capacity. It is a multidisciplinary program which offers patients a supervised exercise program tailored to specific activity levels, along with education to achieve optimal medication use, diet, and self-management.
2. (e): Several different breathing techniques have been shown to be effective in reducing reliever use, improving symptom control, and quality of life in people with asthma. Although there are plausible physiologic explanations for the benefits of nasal breathing, reduced depth, and frequency of breathing, other interventions have been successful, particularly those promoting diaphragmatic breathing and relaxation. The benefits of these techniques extend beyond the first few weeks of the intervention, but are best maintained when patients are consistently practicing them and using them in an appropriate way. Education in these techniques has been undertaken by a variety of health professionals and does not appear to require the skilled expertise of a physiotherapist in all circumstances, even though most of the techniques have their basis in well-established physiotherapy methodology.

Case 3

A 40-year-old man with asthma presents for review following an exacerbation that triggered his admission to hospital. The patient had attended a Buteyko breathing course 5 years earlier and had gained considerable improvement in his asthma symptoms, to the point that he no longer needed his reliever medication. He ran out of inhaled corticosteroids medication and noting that he no longer seemed to be symptomatic, decided not to recommence this, about 12 months earlier than his recent presentation. He had not been particularly conscientious about practicing his breathing techniques over the last year although he did try them during his recent exacerbation and found they were not effective in controlling his symptoms. He now seeks your confirmation that he should return to the Buteyko breathing course without recommencing inhaled corticosteroids but applying himself to be more conscientious with his breathing exercises.

Question:

1. In these circumstances, this patient should:
   (a) Pursue the course of action he has outlined and only return for review if the exercises are not successful in completely controlling his symptoms.
   (b) Carry his reliever with him at all times, but be reassured that there is no need to recommence inhaled corticosteroids.
   (c) Be given a written action plan and a reserve course of oral corticosteroids in case he has another exacerbation, but be reassured he does not need regular inhaled corticosteroids.
   (d) Continue on inhaled corticosteroids and be provided with a written action plan and a reserve course oral corticosteroids, as well as being booked to return to see you for regular review. The Buteyko breathing exercises should be discouraged as they did not work for him.
   (e) Be encouraged to use the Buteyko breathing exercises whenever he feels the need for reliever medication, but to maintain inhaled corticosteroids under your ongoing guidance.

Answer:

1. (e): Patients who present with an asthma exacerbation and require hospital admission have been shown to be at high risk for recurrent exacerbations and life-threatening asthma. No matter how well they recover from these episodes, they require regular review until optimal asthma control is achieved. It is highly unlikely that such patients will remain well controlled without regular controller medication (most often inhaled corticosteroids), which significantly reduces their risk of exacerbations, hospital presentations, and life-threatening asthma

attacks. All patients with asthma who have a history of exacerbations should have a written action plan and receive education to help them identify their triggers, signs of worsening asthma, and the steps they need to take to optimally self-manage an evolving exacerbation, as well as guidance as to when to seek medical attention. This patient may gain benefit from recommencing breathing techniques, but will require regular medical review as well, in order to determine the minimal dose of inhaled corticosteroid he requires to maintain his asthma control.

Conclusions

Breathing techniques have been consistently shown to improve symptom control, reduce short-acting reliever use, and improve well-being as measured by a variety of quality-of-life instruments, in patients with asthma. It is unclear whether specific components of breathing techniques are crucial for achieving the observed effects, and more work is needed to define the optimal exercises, the extent to which these should be practiced, and the circumstances in which they are likely to be most helpful to patients. Although some studies suggest that a combination of diaphragmatic breathing, nasal route of breathing, slow exhalation, and hyperventilation are important, other studies have shown benefit from techniques that do not employ these particular exercises.

References

1. Osborne CA, O'Connor BJ, Lewis AE, Kanabar V, Gardner WN. Hyperventilation and asymptomatic chronic asthma. Thorax. 2000;55(12):1016–22.
2. Jack S, Rossiter HB, Pearson MG, Ward SA, Warburton CJ, Whipp BJ. Ventilatory responses to inhaled carbon dioxide, hypoxic and exercise in idiopathic hyperventilation. Am J Respir Crit Care Med. 2004;170(2):118–25.
3. Gardner WN. The pathophysiology of hyperventilation disorders. Chest. 1996;109(2):516–34.
4. Ringsberg KC, Akerlind I. Presence of hyperventilation in patients with asthma-like symptoms but negative asthma test responses: provocation with voluntary hyperventilation and mental stress. J Allergy Clin Immunol. 1999;103(4):601–8.
5. Thomas M, McKinley RK, Freeman E, Foy C. Prevalence of dysfunctional breathing in patients treated asthma in primary care: cross-sectional survey. Br Med J. 2001;322(7294):1098–100.
6. Thomas M, McKinley RK, Freeman E, Foy C, Price D. The prevalence of dysfunctional breathing in adults in the community with and without asthma. Prim Care Respir J. 2005;14(2):78–82.
7. Demeter SL, Cordasco EM. Hyperventilation syndrome and asthma. Am J Med. 1986;81(6):989–94.
8. Howell JB. The hyperventilation syndrome: a syndrome under threat? Thorax. 1997;52 Suppl 3:S30–4.

9. Bass C, Gardner WN. Respiratory and psychiatric abnormalities in chronic symptomatic hyperventilation. Br Med J. 1985;290(6479):1387–90.
10. Afari N, Barnhart S, Buchwald D. Psychiatric comorbidity and functional status in adult patients with asthma. J Clin Psychol Med. 2001;8(4):245–52.
11. Karazinov VA. Buteyko method: the experience of implementation in medical practice. In: Buteyko KP, editor. The biochemical basis of KP Buteyko's theory of the diseases of deep respiration. Moscow: Patriot Press; 1990.
12. Stalmatski A. Freedom from asthma: Buteyko's revolutionary treatment. London: Kyle Cathie Limited; 1997.
13. Jones K, Cleary R, Hyland M. Associations between asthma morbidity index and ideas of fright and bother in a community population. Respir Med. 1999;93(7):515–9.
14. Busse WW, Kielcolt-Glaser JK, Coe C, Martin RJ, Parker SR. NHLBI Workshop summary. Stress and asthma. Am J Respir Crit Care Med. 1995;151(1):249–52.
15. Mendes FA, Gonçalves RC, Nunes MP, et al. Effects of aerobic training on psychosocial morbidity and symptoms in patients with asthma. A randomized clinical trial. Chest. 2010;138(2): 331–7.
16. Holloway E, Ram FS. Breathing exercises for asthma. Cochrane Database Syst Rev. 2000;3: CD001277.
17. Bruton A, Lewth GT. The Buteyko breathing technique for asthma: a review. Complement Ther Med. 2005;13(1):41–6.
18. Ram FS, Holloway EA, Jones PW. Breathing retraining for asthma. Respir Med. 2003;97(5): 501–7.
19. Singh V, Wisniewski A, Britton J, Tattersfield A. Effect of breathing exercise (pranayama) on airways reactivity in subjects with asthma. Lancet. 1990;335(8702):1381–3.
20. Cooper S, Oborne J, Newton S, et al. Effects of two breathing exercises (Buteyko and pranayama) in asthma: a randomized controlled trial. Thorax. 2003;58(8):674–9.
21. Girodo M, Ekstrand KA, Metivier GJ. Deep diaphragmatic breathing: rehabilitation exercises to the asthmatic patient. Arch Phys Med Rehabil. 1992;73(8):717–20.
22. Bruton A, Thomas M. The role of breathing training in asthma management. Curr Opin Allergy Clin Immununol. 2011;11(1):53–7.
23. Nagarathna R, Nagendra H. Yoga for bronchial asthma: a controlled study. Br Med J. 1985;291(6502):1077–9.
24. Vempati R, Bijlani RL, Deepak KK. The efficacy of a comprehensive lifestyle modification programme based on yoga in the management of bronchial asthma: a randomized controlled trial. BMC Pulm Med. 2009;9:37.
25. Manocha R, Marks GB, Kenchington P, Peters D, Salome CM. Sahaja yoga in the management of moderate to severe asthma: a randomized controlled trial. Thorax. 2002;57(2):110–5.
26. Bowler SD, Green A, Mitchell CA. Buteyko breathing techniques in asthma: a blinded randomized controlled trial. Med J Aust. 1998;169(11–12):575–8.
27. Opat A, Cohen M, Bailey M, Abramson M. A clinical trial of the Buteyko breathing technique in asthma as taught by a video. J Asthma. 2000;37(7):557–64.
28. Holloway E, Ram FS. Breathing exercises for asthma. Cochrane Database Syst Rev. 2004;1:CD001277.
29. Thomas M, McKinley R, Freeman E, Foy C, Prodger P, Price D. Breathing retraining for dysfunctional breathing in asthma: a randomized controlled trial. Thorax. 2003;58(2):110–5.
30. Juniper EF, Guyatt GH, Cox FM, Ferrie PJ, King DR. Development and validation of the mini asthma quality of life questionnaire. Eur Respir J. 1999;14(1):32–8.
31. Thomas M, McKinley RK, Mellor S, et al. Breathing exercises for asthma: a randomized controlled trial. Thorax. 2009;64(1):55–61.
32. Holloway EA, West RJ. Integrated breathing and relaxation training (the Papworth Method) for adults with asthma in primary care: a randomized controlled trial. Thorax. 2007;62(12): 1039–42.
33. Slader CA, Reddel HK, Spencer LM, et al. To find randomized controlled trial of the two different breathing techniques in the management of asthma. Thorax. 2006;61(8):651–6.

34. Cowie RL, Conley DP, Underwood MF, Reader PG. A randomized controlled trial of the Buteyko technique as an adjunct to conventional management of asthma. Respir Med. 2008;102(5):726–32.
35. Gosselink R. Breathing techniques in patients with chronic obstructive pulmonary disease (COPD). Chron Respir Dis. 2004;1(3):163–72.
36. Lotters F, van Tol B, Kwakkel G, Gosselink R. Effects of controlled inspiratory muscle training in patients with COPD: a meta-analysis. Eur Respir J. 2002;20(3):570–6.
37. Raupach T, Bahr F, Herrmann P, et al. Slow breathing reduces sympathoexcitation in COPD. Eur Respir J. 2008;32(2):387–92.
38. Livermore N, Butler JE, Sharpe L, McBain RA, Gandevia SC, McKenzie DK. Panic attacks and perception of inspiratory resistive loads in chronic obstructive pulmonary disease. Am J Respir Crit Care Med. 2008;178(1):7–12.
39. Lord VM, Cave P, Hume VJ, et al. Singing teaching as a therapy for chronic respiratory disease—A randomised controlled trial and qualitative evaluation. BMC Pulm Med. 2010;10:41.
40. Livermore N, Sharpe L, McKenzie D. Prevention of panic attacks and panic disorder and COPD. Eur Respir J. 2010;35(3):557–63.

Chapter 12
Hypnosis for the Treatment of Functional Respiratory Disorders

Ran D. Anbar

This chapter contains videos, please download from
http://www.springerimages.com/videos/10.1007/978-1-61779-857-3_12

Abstract Clinical hypnosis is an efficient and effective tool for addressing the mind/body connection for many patients with functional respiratory disorders. Such patients can benefit from learning self-hypnosis techniques in as little as 10 min, which can help them rapidly improve or resolve their symptoms altogether, as demonstrated in several published case series. Asthma sometimes has been shown to improve with the use of hypnosis perhaps because of the large number of patients who have a functional component as part of their presentation. Keys to successful hypnosis include establishment of rapport with patients and their families, facilitating patients' self-mastery, and following patients' expectations, motivation, lead, and interests. Clinicians who have completed 3- to 4-day hypnosis training workshops learn to appreciate better the power of communication and usually find that their language and nonverbal interactions with patients improve, even when they are not employing formal hypnosis. Practical considerations regarding provision of clinical hypnosis in a primary care setting are discussed in this chapter; a sample text of an hypnotic encounter intended to achieve relaxation is provided; and case studies are presented that include links to videos demonstrating instruction in hypnosis to children and adults, with accompanying quiz questions and explanatory material regarding patients with chest pain, dyspnea, habit cough, vocal cord dysfunction, and insomnia.

Keywords Asthma • Chest pain • Cystic fibrosis • Dyspnea • Habit cough • Hypnosis • Insomnia • Vocal cord dysfunction

---

R.D. Anbar (✉)
Department of Pediatrics, SUNY Upstate Medical University, 750 East Adams St., 13210-1834, Syracuse, NY, USA
e-mail: anbarr@upstate.edu

R.D. Anbar (ed.), *Functional Respiratory Disorders: When Respiratory Symptoms Do Not Respond to Pulmonary Treatment*, Respiratory Medicine,
DOI 10.1007/978-1-61779-857-3_12,

Background

Clinical hypnosis is an efficient and effective tool for addressing the mind/body connection for many patients with functional respiratory disorders [1]. Such patients can benefit from learning self-hypnosis techniques in as little as 10 min, which can help them rapidly improve or resolve their symptoms altogether [2]. Interested clinicians can learn how to teach their patients hypnosis through participation in 3- or 4-day training workshops [3].

While experts in hypnosis have not come up with a consensus definition for clinical hypnosis, many agree that hypnosis involves focused attention, dissociation from the usual state of awareness, and heightened responsiveness to suggestions. When hypnosis is used in the treatment of medical conditions, a state of inward attention can be focused on ideas of therapeutic value that can potentiate physiologic change. The ideas can be suggested by a health care provider, or can be self-suggested by the patient [4–6].

Hypnosis can be introduced to patients as follows: [1] "Hypnosis is a way of using your imagination in order to help yourself. If you do not want to use hypnosis, I cannot and would not force you to do so and neither can anyone else. On the other hand, if you choose to follow my suggestions, you will go into hypnosis because you tell yourself to do so. Hypnosis is not an unusual state of mind. For example, when some people are bored, they begin to daydream. That is spontaneous hypnosis. Other people can imagine what music sounds like. That also is hypnosis. Have you ever driven on the highway for three miles and suddenly become startled and ask yourself, 'How did I get here?' Where has your mind been? Who's been driving the car? That is yet another example of hypnosis."

Other therapeutic modalities with hypnotic features of inward attention include biofeedback (see Chap. 10), breathing techniques (Chap. 11), meditation (Chap. 16), speech therapy (Chap. 13), and suggestion therapy (Chap. 5). Guided imagery is a form of hypnosis in which clinicians encourage patients to visualize imagery intended to promote therapeutic change [7]. Guided imagery frequently depends on the use of scripts, which do not allow for modification of the therapeutic suggestions based on the responsiveness of the patients, and thus limits its effectiveness. The advantages of self-hypnosis instruction for medical purposes as compared to these other modalities include that it can and should be modified based on individual patient requirements, its rapid effect, relative simplicity, and the ability of the patient to utilize the technique independently and without need for special equipment [1].

Many forms of psychological therapy can be utilized more effectively during a hypnotic state because during hypnosis patients are less apt to be distracted by interfering thoughts. For example, patients who are treated with cognitive behavioral therapy (Chap. 9) for anxiety-associated respiratory symptoms such as dyspnea (Chap. 4) may be able to control their anxious feelings better while in hypnosis, which allows them to be more receptive to a discussion regarding possible triggers and solutions for their anxiety.

Evidence for the Efficacy of Hypnosis for Functional Respiratory Disorders

There have been no published randomized clinical trials regarding the use of hypnosis for patients with functional respiratory disorders. However, several case series have been published regarding children using hypnosis for functional respiratory disorders at the SUNY Upstate Medical University Pediatric Pulmonary Center. At this center, hypnosis was reported to be helpful in achieving improvement or resolution of chest pain or pressure in nine out of ten children who utilized hypnosis [2]. Chronic dyspnea thought to be related to functional disorders, which occurred with or without exercise, resolved in 81% and improved in the remaining 19% of 16 children who had normal lung function at rest, following one or two sessions of hypnosis instruction [8]. Habit cough resolved following the use of hypnosis in 90% of 51 children [9]. Two case series demonstrated that vocal cord dysfunction resolved in 54% and improved in 38% of 37/51 children who returned for follow-up after the pediatric pulmonologist or the social worker at the Pediatric Pulmonary Center instructed them in hypnosis [2, 10]. Difficulty with sleep onset was reported to improve in 90% of 75 children following hypnosis and counseling. In the same study, nighttime awakenings were reported to resolve in 52% and improve in 38% of 21 children [11]. Notably, at this center, instruction in hypnosis was offered to 36% of 6- to 11-year-old and 55% of 12- to 18-year-old children who were newly referred for evaluation of pulmonary symptoms during an 18-month period of study. This was done because it was felt that there was a significant psychological or functional component in their presentation [12]. Thus, hypnosis appears to be applicable to a large number of pediatric patients with respiratory disorders.

Asthma sometimes also has been shown to improve with the use of hypnosis perhaps because a large number of patients with asthma have a functional component as part of their presentation. In a multicenter year-long trial, 252 children and adults with moderate or severe asthma were randomized to monthly hypnosis sessions with a therapist and daily self-hypnosis, or to a control group involving daily relaxation and breathing exercises. Hypnosis was associated with an increase in forced expiratory volume in 1 s (FEV_1) of 4.3% ($p<0.05$). There was no significant difference between the groups in their incidence of wheezing or medication use [13]. In another randomized controlled study of 39 adults with mild to moderate asthma, patients who were naturally highly receptive to hypnotic suggestions demonstrated a significant reduction in reactivity to methacholine challenge testing, chronic bronchodilator use, and fewer asthma symptoms, as compared to patients who were less responsive to hypnotic suggestion or a control group that was not exposed to hypnosis [14]. The results of this study have yet to be replicated. In a 2-year randomized study of 28 children with asthma, those who were taught hypnosis had significantly reduced asthma severity and school absences [15]. Hypnosis also has been shown to help in the management of asthma in several anecdotal reports [16].

On the other hand, the literature has not consistently reported improvement of patients with asthma following use of hypnosis [16–18]. Possible reasons for this are that studies used insufficiently powered statistics or hypnosis techniques that provided suboptimal suggestions. Further, hypnosis might work best for patients with asthma whose presentation is complicated by anxiety since anxiety resolves easily with hypnosis [19–21]. As studies of hypnosis and asthma have not routinely prescreened for presence of anxiety, the potential effect of hypnosis for many patients with asthma may have been blunted as a result of inclusion of patients who did not have significant anxiety.

Hypnosis has been shown to be effective in randomized controlled trials for the treatment of other functional disorders, such as functional abdominal pain and irritable bowel syndrome [22]. For example, a 12-session hypnosis-standardized treatment protocol for adults with irritable bowel syndrome has been shown to reduce abdominal discomfort, increase quality of life scores, and decrease anxiety [23]. Similar results were reported in a study of children with functional abdominal pain or irritable bowel syndrome who were provided with six sessions of hypnosis [24]. Hypnosis also has been shown to be effective in randomized trials for the treatment of headaches, some of which may have been functional in nature [22].

Practical Application

When a patient is identified as having a physical or psychological symptom that might be addressed with hypnosis, the possibility of using this therapy can be introduced during a regular clinic visit [1]. In my experience, most patients are receptive to a mind/body therapeutic modality that can help them immediately. Demystifying hypnosis is essential with patients who have preconceived notions regarding its character, for example, "Are you going to make me quack like a duck?" Because of their relative lack of experience, children tend to have fewer misconceptions about hypnosis and also are more likely to embrace quickly a new way of using their imagination.

Clinicians who do not specialize in mental health should not offer to use hypnosis with patients who have severe psychological problems such as depression, bipolar disorder, or suicidal ideation. Further, sometimes, work with hypnosis uncovers significant psychological abnormalities. In such situations, patients should be given a referral to appropriate professionals who are experienced in the care of patients with mental health issues (Chap. 8). Depending on the clinical circumstances, the mental health professionals may choose to continue to use hypnosis to help patients cope or otherwise facilitate their ongoing therapy.

When a Patient Expresses Doubt

In practice, only a minority of patients express doubt that mind/body therapy can be applicable in their situation [1]. In such situations, I suggest that the mind can influence the perception of a symptom. For example, sometimes, athletes are unaware of an injury while they are participating in a competitive activity because they are so focused on the game that they pay little or no attention to their injury. Thus, even though a symptom might arise as a result of a physical problem, the way it is perceived is affected by a patient's state of mind. Further, most patients recognize that many symptoms are stress-related including headaches, stomach aches, chest pain, anxiety, and nervous habits. Thus, I wonder aloud whether the patient believes part of his or her symptoms might be stress-related, and if so, I explain that hypnosis can help patients modify their reactions to stress. In this way, hypnosis may be able to reduce the psychological impact in patients' presentations, which may in turn greatly simplify their medical management [8, 21, 22].

Following such an explanation, most patients are interested in a trial of hypnosis. Those who do not express an interest may not have established sufficient rapport with their health care provider [1]. Rapport should be established by the clinician's developing and maintaining an interest in the patient's feelings and thoughts. The clinician should be genuine and empathetic and seek to understand the patient's point of view, while keeping in mind that effective communication often includes nonverbal interactions [25]. Another possible reason for lack of interest in doing hypnosis is a conflict, such as having to give up a benefit (i.e., secondary gain) were hypnosis to be successful [25, 26]. For example, a child who has been taken out of an unpleasant gym class situation as a result of chest pain is less likely to be receptive to hypnosis that might resolve his pain because then he might be expected to return to that physical education class. Another type of conflict can arise when the patient's symptom serves as part of the basis for a lawsuit in which the patient stands to gain financially or otherwise as long as the symptom persists. In such circumstances, hypnosis is unlikely to be of benefit for a patient who at best is ambivalent about resolving the symptom (keeping in mind that all hypnosis is self-hypnosis). Notably, secondary gain issues also can interfere with a patient's receptiveness to other medical therapies.

Sometimes, it is patients' fears that preclude receptiveness to hypnosis, such as concerns raised as a result of religious beliefs. In such situations, when patients express ambivalence about hypnosis, I do not offer to teach them hypnosis immediately, because the patients are unlikely to use the skill, or may feel uncomfortable about a perceived pressure to use it. Instead, I counsel these patients to consider carefully the reasons they might not be receptive to hypnosis and offer to discuss these reasons with them. Further, as an alternative to hypnosis, I can suggest the possibility of the patient using biofeedback, breathing techniques, imagery, or relaxation [27].

Enhancing the Teaching Method for Hypnosis

Much of the effectiveness of hypnosis arises from the patients' expectations that it can help them. Thus, when the clinician has positive expectations about hypnosis and communicates these effectively as sufficient rapport has been established, the clinical results are more likely to be positive. For example, often as part of an introduction to hypnosis, I will tell patients, "I am very confident that I can help you to help yourself with hypnosis. I cannot promise that your symptom will resolve, but I am sure it will improve. How can I be so certain? Because every person has some mind/body control. Through the use of hypnosis you can achieve greater control over your mind and body and this is why you will improve" [1].

Once patients agree to learn hypnosis, the initial instruction time typically requires 10–30 min with adults, 5–10 min with older children, and even less time with younger children. Thus, hypnosis can be incorporated easily within a regular medical office appointment. There are many examples of successful hypnotic approaches in the literature [4, 28, 29]. Keys to successful hypnosis include establishment of rapport with the patients and their families (if applicable), facilitating the patients' ability to help themselves (i.e., self-mastery), and following patients' expectations, motivation, lead, and interests [4, 5]. For example, a child who enjoys playing football will tend to be much more responsive to hypnotic suggestions that involve his favorite sport (including how he might improve his athletic performance) rather than relaxation suggestions that involve thinking about a beach that may appeal to an adult, but which the child finds "boring."

An example of a simple hypnosis session that can be used successfully with most individuals who are preteen or older is shown in Table 12.1. The case studies illustrate other techniques for the treatment of functional respiratory disorders that can be used by appropriately trained clinicians who do not specialize in mental health.

Follow-up to the hypnosis intervention can be very brief, such as when patients report successful outcomes of self-hypnosis application. When patients state that their symptoms have not improved sufficiently but admit that they have not used hypnosis as recommended, a discussion regarding the reasons for their lack of "adherence" should take place. Solutions regarding how hypnosis might be utilized more reliably are developed with patients placed in the role of active consultants, for example, "I wonder how you could do this better to help yourself even more." When patients state that they have done hypnosis but it has not been helpful, modification of the hypnotic imagery can be recommended [1].

Clinical hypnosis can be billed as hypnotherapy or as counseling time under an evaluation and management code [6]. When time-based billing is used, the clinician should indicate in the medical record that "Over half of the encounter time was devoted to counseling."

The Benefits of Accredited Training in Hypnosis

Clinical hypnosis is best learned by health care providers through active participation in hypnosis workshops accredited by organizations specializing in medical hypnosis. It is unlikely that direct harm might be caused by clinicians who have not received sufficient training in hypnosis [1]. However, on infrequent occasions, patients may develop unanticipated distressing emotional reactions during hypnosis, which are termed "abreactions" [28, 30]. Training in hypnosis

Table 12.1 Hypnotic encounter for achievement of relaxation

"Before we get started, you need to understand that all hypnosis is self-hypnosis. Contrary to what you might see in cartoons or in shows, hypnosis is not sleep. When you are doing hypnosis you know what's going on and you can stop at anytime you want to because you are in control. I can teach you, if you like, how to use hypnosis to help you feel better. Would you like to know how to do that?"
"Good. One way that hypnosis works is through images in the mind. An image in the mind can affect the way your mind and body work. For example, what happens when you put two magnets a little apart from one another?"
"That's right. When the positive pole faces the negative pole the magnets attract. That's where the saying comes from: 'Opposites attract.' Now, hold your hands about 4 inches apart, and imagine, with your eyes open or closed, whichever is more comfortable, that your hands are giant magnets that can attract themselves all by themselves."
"That's right. Notice how the hands are coming together. Some people say that their hands tingle or feel warm as they come together, and others feel something else."
"That's right. Now that your hands are stuck together let me show you something else. Leave the magnets there. When I count to three, your job will be to leave the magnets there and try to separate the hands. I think you might be surprised by how that will feel. One… Two… Don't take the magnets away… Three!"
"How did that feel? [Pause]. How did it work? [Pause]. Was it something I did? Or did you do something? What did you do?"
"Now you begin to understand how an image in the mind can affect the body. Would you like another example?"
"Put both hands up in front of you. Now, imagine that in one hand you are holding a bucketful of wet sand, like you might have played with on the beach when you were younger. And in the other hand, imagine holding strings that are attached to many helium balloons of different colors. Now, notice how the hand holding the bucket can become heavier and heavier, while the hand holding the balloons can become lighter and lighter—all by itself."
"How did you do that?"
"Very good. Now, do you like relaxing?"
"Good. Then let me show you how you can relax with hypnosis. First I will tell you what you can do. Then you can do it. Afterwards we'll talk about the experience. In a few moments you can imagine going to a safe, relaxing place of your choice. It can be a place you've been to, a place you'd like to go to, or even an imaginary place. Now, once you are there, you can imagine what you might see, hear, smell, touch, and taste. Do you know why you want to imagine with all your senses?"
"The more you use your different senses the more real the experience can become, and the more relaxed you can be. Brain studies have shown that when you imagine a sense, you actually activate the same part of the brain that becomes active when you are literally experiencing that sense. Does that make sense to you?"
"In your relaxing place is there a place to sit or lay down comfortably?"
"Good. Then once you arrive in your relaxing place I will ask you to find a place to sit or lay down comfortably. Then, I will talk to you about relaxing from your head to your neck, to your arms, to your legs, down to your toes. How do you think you will feel then?"
"That's right. Now, here is an important part. You get to pick your own personal relaxation sign. This is a sign that you can use anytime you want to relax without using hypnosis. I suggest you pick a one-handed sign. Some people choose to touch their index finger to their thumb, while others cross their fingers, or make a fist. What would you like your sign to be?"

(continued)

Table 12.1 (continued)

"Very good. Once you make your sign in hypnosis, you can stay in your relaxing place for as long as you like. You can imagine being there for a minute, an hour, a year, or even forever. In hypnosis, time can mean whatever you want, so this will only take a few moments in real time. Once you are ready to return you can raise your hand and I will give you a few more instructions."

Once the patient indicates that he or she is ready to begin, the clinician provides instructions similar to those described above. Note that no further mention is made of eye closure, which is only necessary if the patient feels it would be helpful. Once the patient raises his or her hand during hypnosis, the instructions continue as follows:

"Very good. Now, before you come back you can tell yourself four things:

First, congratulate yourself for your excellent use of your imagination.

Second, remind yourself to practice your hypnosis every day for at least 2 weeks so that you can become very good with it. Hypnosis is a mind/body skill, so the more you use it, the better it becomes.

Third, remind yourself that whenever you want to relax without the use of hypnosis all you need to do is to make your relaxation sign.

Finally, now your mind is open to suggestions. You can offer good suggestions to yourself. The more you tell yourself these things the more they can come true. For example, you might tell yourself that you like how you feel right now and that you want to feel this way for the rest of the day. Or, you could tell yourself that you will become better and better at controlling discomforts that you may encounter. You might even imagine how good it will feel when you are better.

After you have told yourself all of the good things you need to hear—when the time is right, and you will know exactly when that time is—then come back."

Once the patient indicates he or she is back to usual awareness, the clinician may ask:

"Very good. How do you feel?"

"What has changed?"

"How did you do that?"

"What did you like about the experience?"

"Is there anything you didn't like, or wish was different?"

"Would you like to feel something neat?"

"Make your relaxation sign."

"What just happened?"

"Now you realize that you can control how you feel. The more you do hypnosis the more in control of yourself you can become. Isn't that great to know?"

"Good job."

Adapted from Anbar RD. Hypnosis for children with chronic disease. In: Wester WC, Sugarman LI, editors. Therapeutic Hypnosis with Children and Adolescents. Bethel, CT: Crown House Publishing; 2007. p. 357–85. With permission from Crown House Publishing.

is essential in learning how to deal with such situations. Further, indirect harm can be caused in a number of ways by insufficiently trained clinicians. First, as hypnosis is unlikely to work when used inexpertly, patients might conclude that hypnosis is not appropriate for their issues, or that the issues cannot be modified by a psychological approach. This can be a harmful incorrect conclusion that might unnecessarily prolong patients' discomfort or lead to additional ineffective treatments. Secondly, clinicians might conclude that hypnosis is unhelpful in particular clinical situations, which might be an erroneous assumption that will preclude other patients from benefiting from hypnosis [1].

Thus, clinicians who review the written material and view the hypnosis video links provided in this chapter as part of the case studies should not attempt to do hypnosis by copying what was done in the videos, without first receiving training in an appropriate workshop.

The use of language and nonverbal communication serve as the media through which hypnosis is applied [28]. Clinicians who are well trained in hypnosis learn to avoid communication difficulties that can inadvertently cause unintended harmful consequences [31]. For example, telling patients to "try" a treatment gives the negative suggestion that it may not be successful. Or, a clinician who checks the time frequently during a patient encounter is sending a nonverbal message that the clinician does not feel the patient is important, which can harm the therapeutic relationship. Patients respond well to clinician behavior that displays interest in them, such as remaining focused on the patient and displaying open body language [1].

Clinicians who have completed hypnosis training workshops usually find that their language and nonverbal interactions with patients improve, even when they are not employing formal hypnosis [4]. Please consult the appendix for information regarding the content and location of hypnosis training workshops.

Questions and Case Studies

The hypnosis instructions shown in Table 12.1 are sufficient to treat functional respiratory symptoms effectively approximately 70% of the time. The following series of questions and case studies will help to better understand better the nuances of hypnotic work. Choose the best answer.

Questions:

1. Why is it important for the patient to understand that all hypnosis is self-hypnosis?
   (a) In order to align the patient's expectations with those of the clinician
   (b) In order that the patient take charge of the experience
   (c) To help demystify hypnosis
   (d) So that the patient will become empowered
   (e) All of the above

2. What is the purpose of showing patients how to imagine their hands as magnets, or holding onto a sand pail and balloons?
   (a) Playing games helps improve rapport.
   (b) In order to help the patients realize that hypnosis is magical.
   (c) To allow patients to experience some effects of hypnotic imagery, which prepares them for further work with hypnosis.
   (d) As an essential ritual prior to every hypnosis encounter.
   (e) All of the above.
3. What is the benefit of the clinician telling the patient ahead of time what the instructions will be when the patient is asked to imagine a relaxation place?
   (a) This allows the clinician a chance to rehearse what is to be said.
   (b) The patient can let the clinician know verbally or nonverbally whether part of the proposed hypnotic experience might feel uncomfortable.
   (c) This is part of the informed consent process.
   (d) So that the patient will figure out in advance how to react to the hypnotic suggestions.
   (e) All of the above.
4. Why is the patient asked if he or she likes relaxing?
   (a) As a way of telling the patient what he or she must do to become healthier
   (b) To find out if the patient is paying attention
   (c) So that the patient will think of some relaxing situations
   (d) Some patients do not like to relax
   (e) All of the above
5. What is the purpose of teaching patients a relaxation sign?
   (a) This is a posthypnotic suggestion that patients can utilize later as needed.
   (b) The sign helps validate the hypnosis experience.
   (c) The sign can be used therapeutically instead of imagery when patients develop their symptoms.
   (d) The sign is another tool that empowers the patients.
   (e) All of the above.

Answers:

1. (e): Demystifying hypnosis, alignment of expectations, and allowing the patient to take charge enhance development of rapport and make hypnosis work much more likely to be successful [25]. Empowering the patient helps promote continued success with hypnosis.
2. (c): Demonstration of brief hypnosis induction techniques initially can help patients feel more comfortable with hypnosis. Unless the patient is young, playing games is unlikely to improve rapport. Implication of hypnosis as magical makes it seem

more mysterious, which can cause many patients to become wary of it. There is no one way to do hypnosis. Actually, a hypnotic ritual often is unnecessary.

3. (b): Allowing the patient to express their feelings about the proposed hypnotic experience helps the clinician individualize the hypnotic interaction, which makes it more likely to be relevant to the patient. (This is the reason that patients are prompted to identify their own relaxation imagery, rather than one of the clinician's choosing.) An informed consent usually is not necessary for hypnosis work. Responsiveness in hypnosis often is achieved without conscious intent, and thus, the patient should not attempt to plan responses in advance.
4. (d): Instructions to prompt relaxation given to patients who dislike relaxing will prompt patients to resist these hypnotic suggestions and interfere with the therapeutic work. Patients who say they dislike relaxation may be willing to use hypnosis in order to make themselves become more comfortable or happier. Hypnotic imagery should focus on achieving the patients' goals.
5. (e): When patients relax using their sign, which can seem automatic, it reinforces that something special has happened as a result of hypnosis. This helps raise the patients' expectations of success, which helps improve the efficacy of further hypnosis work.

Case 1: Chest Pain

A 30-year-old man with cystic fibrosis (CF) and moderate lung disease complained of recurrent sharp substernal chest pain for the past 2 years. The pain persisted for hours at a time and tended to occur when the patient was stressed, such as after a hard day at work. When the pain first occurred, it was associated with a burning quality and appeared related to eating of meals with a high-fat content. A 24-h pH probe study revealed mild gastroesophageal reflux, for which the patient was treated with omeprazole. The burning nature of the pain resolved following the anti-reflux therapy, but the sharp pain remained. The pain could not be elicited upon palpation of the chest. A chest CT scan revealed diffuse bronchiectasis that had not worsened over the last 2 years. An EKG was normal.

As the pain was thought to be functional in nature, the patient was instructed in self-hypnosis techniques to help improve his discomfort. He was taught how to imagine being in a relaxing place, using instructions similar to those in Table 12.1. He reported that when he was in his relaxing place, he could feel his discomfort, but it no longer bothered him.

As he was able to do hypnosis well, he also was taught two alternative imagery techniques for control of his discomfort.

House of control: The patient was instructed to imagine a house with his name on the door. Upon entering the house, the patient found various rooms, each labeled with a different part of his body. He was prompted to find the room that was labeled, "Chest." Upon entering the room, it was suggested that he would find panels that

controlled everything in his chest, including the frequency of his breathing, the rate of his heart, and control of sensation. He was asked whether the sensation in his chest was controlled on a panel with a lever or a dial. He replied, "a lever." The patient was instructed that he could lower the lever until the discomfort in his chest was improved sufficiently.
Glove anesthesia: With the patient's permission, while he was in a state of hypnosis, the clinician put an imaginary glove on the patient's right hand. The clinician acted as if the glove was a little small and therefore struggled some to put it on the patient's hand. The patient was instructed to imagine and describe the glove's color, texture, and temperature. Once the glove was firmly in place, the clinician demonstrated that when the gloved hand was pinched, there was a sensation of pressure but diminished pain, as compared to when the other hand was pinched. The patient responded that he perceived no pain in the gloved hand. He was told that the anesthesia induced by the imaginary glove could be moved anywhere in the body as he wished. For example, the patient was coached to place the gloved hand over his lower sternum and reported that his chest pain resolved.

The following videos of patients with CF are available:

(1) An 18-year-old describing how he utilized hypnosis for 7 years to help himself with his chronic illness (Video 12.1).
(2) A 19-year-old demonstrating use of relaxation imagery to control a headache (Video 12.2).
(3) A 19-year-old demonstrating use of house of control imagery to reduce discomfort associated with placement of an intravenous line (Video 12.3).
(4) A 9-year-old demonstrating use of glove anesthesia to control discomfort associated with phlebotomy (Video 12.4).
(5) An 18-year-old demonstrating how hypnosis can help change sensations (Video 12.5).

Questions:

1. Why is the patient's pain relabeled as discomfort by his clinician?

   (a) It is a matter of semantics. There is no particular reason.
   (b) When the word "pain" is used, it is a negative suggestion.
   (c) The clinician probably is personally uncomfortable with pain.
   (d) The patient might think that pain requires narcotic therapy.
   (e) None of the above.

2. Why was the patient taught about a house of control, rather than just about a room of chest control?

   (a) A room of control would not be believable to the patient.
   (b) A control room sounds too much like mission control.
   (c) A house of control implies the patient could control areas of the body other than the chest.

   (d) A house of control would help the patient feel as if he achieved the American dream.
   (e) All of the above.

3. Why did the clinician act as if it was a struggle to put on the patient's glove?
   (a) It helped focus the patient on the imagery technique.
   (b) The tactile stimulation is part of the hypnotic suggestion that this technique can change how the patient perceives discomfort.
   (c) It permitted more time for the patient to describe the experience and hence focus on it more deeply.
   (d) Rubbing of an area can diffuse the perceived signal from a sharp pain such as a pinch.
   (e) All of the above.

Answers:

1. (b): Even when hypnosis is not used formally, the language used by clinicians can have a profound hypnotic effect [4]. When a patient hears the word "pain," he needs to think about what this means and attend to such sensations from his body, which can magnify how these uncomfortable sensations are perceived. On the other hand, "discomfort" contains within it the positive suggestion that comfort is achievable, perhaps as simply as through elimination of "dis."
2. (c): The house of control imagery permits the patient to consider other ways he can help himself. Thus, it is yet another way of helping the patient become empowered. For example, some patients enjoy going into their brain rooms in order to gain more insight. Others choose to go into their leg rooms to help themselves run faster.
3. (e): The clinician's "struggle" was part of the hypnotic induction with this method. Clinicians using hypnosis often use physical responses, such as decreased sensation of pain as a result of rubbing, in order to reinforce the effectiveness of the hypnotic suggestion. For example, a clinician who suggests eye closure as part of a hypnotic experience can depend on eye fatigue setting in when a patient is asked to stare at a point above eye level for several moments.

Case 2: Dyspnea

A previously healthy 10-year-old boy complained of shortness of breath while watching TV when visiting his maternal grandmother's house 2 weeks after the sudden death of his maternal grandfather, as a result of a logging accident. The patient reported his dyspnea was unassociated with making a noise such as wheezing or stridor. The patient said it felt as if something was swelling in his throat and causing difficulty with his inhalation. Also, he had associated shakiness, but no dizziness, change in sensation (paresthesia), or nausea. The episode recurred once. His mother thought the symptoms might be attributable to anxiety or panic attacks, but his pediatrician said it might be from asthma. His mother also said she panicked when he developed his breathing problem because of what had happened to her father.

The patient described exercise-associated dyspnea with associated difficulty during inhalation, which started during the previous year when he began playing for a coach who loudly and aggressively encouraged his players. Also, the patient had noted that sometimes he caused himself to develop similar breathing problems when he thought about stressful issues.

The patient had seasonal allergies in spring and fall, for which he was started on oral montelukast. He said his breathing immediately felt better after beginning this therapy.

As part of the interview, he was asked what he would wish for if he was given one wish. He replied that he wished to be better at sports.

Hypnosis was explained to the patient in a fashion similar to that described in Table 12.1. Then, he was given a choice of whether to learn hypnosis and chose to do it by imagining that he went to Mexico as a place to relax.

Three weeks later, the patient reported that his dyspnea had improved greatly and that whenever it would occur he was able to resolve it with the aid of hypnosis, including his relaxation sign.

The following video is available:

This patient demonstrating how he was taught self-hypnosis for relief of dyspnea (Video 12.6)

Questions:

1. What is the significance of the mother's panic when the patient developed dyspnea?
   (a) The patient may have interpreted his symptoms as being more severe when he saw his mother becoming so anxious.
   (b) The mother caused the patient to develop anxiety.
   (c) This is consistent with a genetically based anxiety disorder.
   (d) This is suggestive of Munchausen's by proxy.
   (e) All of the above.
2. What is the most likely explanation for the patient's immediate improvement with montelukast therapy?
   (a) The patient's expectation of improvement with montelukast led to his relief.
   (b) Montelukast treated the patient's allergies effectively, which helped resolve his dyspnea.
   (c) Montelukast treated the patient's asthma effectively, which helped resolve his dyspnea.
   (d) The central nervous system effect of montelukast calmed the patient, which led to resolution of his dyspnea.
   (e) Any of the above might be true.

3. Why was the patient asked regarding what he might wish for?
   (a) As a way of making interesting conversation.
   (b) As an open-ended way to allow him to express what is important to him.
   (c) To check if the patient is imaginative.
   (d) To gauge how he would respond to an unexpected question.
   (e) All of the above.

Answers:

1. (a): Many factors impact how a symptom is perceived. For example, patients' intrinsic responsiveness can be affected by whether they are anxious, depressed, or excited [4]. Patients' behavior also is affected by extrinsic factors such as the expectations of their families and society. (Note this patient's apparent reaction to the pressure caused by his coach.)
2. (a): While montelukast can be of benefit in the treatment of exercise-induced asthma [32], in a patient whose dyspnea clearly is associated with stressful situations, it is more likely that the expectation of improvement (a component of the placebo effect) [33] was a more important factor for this patient. The effect of montelukast on allergy control is not immediate [32]. Calming is not a central nervous system effect of montelukast [32].
3. (b): By allowing the patient to express a wish, the clinician can use the answer to guide the hypnotic work for the patient. For example, with this patient, he could be offered an opportunity to learn how hypnosis could help his sports performance, which could help him become more enthusiastic about the use of hypnosis, and thus, it would be more likely to be effective for his medical condition. Conversely, another patient who appeared to be debilitated by a symptom might not even mention it as a possible wish, which would raise the question of whether the patient truly is interested in relief from his symptoms.

Case 3: Habit Cough

A 7-year-old boy presented with a 4-month history of recurrent harsh cough that began after *strep* throat. The cough had tended to occur more when the patient was upset, nervous, or stressed. The cough had been diagnosed as attributable to habit.

In a 3-min session, I offered to help the patient learn to do something else other than cough when he would become nervous or upset. In answer to my questions, the patient explained that he liked playing outdoors. We discussed how he could use each of his senses to imagine what it was like being outside. Then, I suggested that he pick a sign that would remind him how it feels to be outside. He said he liked playing basketball and made a loose fist with his right hand as a sign that would remind him of how it felt to play basketball. I instructed him that should he become nervous he could make his sign, which would calm him.

Two months later, the patient reported that he no longer was coughing, which he attributed to his decision to bounce a toy basketball to calm himself, as opposed to using his sign. I reminded him that he could use the sign to calm himself if a real toy basketball was unavailable.

The following videos involving patients with habit cough are available:

1. This 7-year-old patient learning how to use hypnosis (Video 12.7).
2. This 7-year-old describing his success with hypnosis (Video 12.8).
3. A 12-year-old first taught hypnosis in a fashion similar to that described in Table 12.1 and then turning down an imaginary cough lever (Video 12.9).

Questions:

1. Why did the hypnotic approach differ between the 7-year-old and the 12-year-old?
   (a) Hypnosis techniques should be matched to the developmental age of the patient.
   (b) A 7-year-old is unlikely to accept suggestions to relax, as he enjoys being active.
   (c) A 12-year-old is more likely to achieve and be impressed by hypnotic rituals (i.e., induction techniques) as described in Table 12.1.
   (d) The clinician should match the suggestions used to the interest of the patients.
   (e) All of the above.
2. Why did the 7-year-old choose to bounce a real toy basketball rather than use his loose fist sign?
   (a) He may have had oppositional-defiant disorder.
   (b) He wanted to show his independent thinking ability.
   (c) He is at a stage of development when the sign may be too abstract for him.
   (d) His parents gave him the idea.
   (e) All of the above.
3. Which of the following images/suggestions might be useful for the treatment of habit cough? [9]
   (a) If a cartoon character was causing the cough, what might it do instead?
   (b) Imagine a switch in the head that turns the cough on or off.
   (c) Imagine engaging in a pleasant activity in the absence of the cough.
   (d) Imagine colored air that brings in comfort with each breath.
   (e) All of the above.

Answers:

1. (e): For younger children, an introduction to hypnosis rarely is necessary. Hypnosis techniques for younger children should vary, depending on the developmental age of the child. For example, preschoolers tend to respond to storytelling, while school-age children often benefit from pretending they are favorite characters from books, movies, or television [4].

2. (c): Seven-year-olds tend to be concrete thinkers. Typically, children of this age do not vary hypnotic techniques on their own.
3. (e): Imagery specific for the habit cough or any other functional respiratory symptom can be as varied as the clinician and patients can imagine. The key is that the image used should be acceptable to the patient and ideally represent the patient's own ideas, which helps empower him.

Case 4: Vocal Cord Dysfunction

A 14-year-old girl presented with a 4-year history of activity-associated difficulty with inhalation. She reported feeling as if her throat closed up within a few seconds of exercise that prevented her from breathing, with an associated fluttering noise upon inhalation. When her symptoms occurred, the patient stopped her physical activity for 5–10 min, until the symptoms resolved, and she was able to restart her physical activity. Her pulmonary function was normal. Use of asthma medications did not help relieve her symptoms, nor did a tonsillectomy and adenoidectomy.

Based on her symptoms, at our center, she was diagnosed as having vocal cord dysfunction (Chap. 6). She was taught hypnosis for relaxation in a fashion similar to that shown in Table 12.1. When she imagined her hands were magnets, she could hardly separate them. As a place to relax, she picked a beach and a Go-Kart place at the same time, which is something she could not do in real life. Following hypnosis, the patient was asked to rate her level of relaxation before and after hypnosis on a scale of "0–10," wherein "0" meant she was as relaxed as she had ever been and "10" meant that the patient was as tense as she had ever been. She responded that her relaxation had improved from a "6" to a "1."

A month later, the patient reported that she no longer developed any activity-associated breathing difficulties.

Three videos involving this patient with vocal cord dysfunction are available:

1. Her history taking interview (Video 12.10).
2. Her hypnosis instruction (Video 12.11).
3. Her use of hypnosis to gain insight into the stressors that may have led to her breathing difficulty (Video 12.12). Notably, helping patients achieve such an understanding should be done only by practitioners of hypnosis who specialize in mental health [34].

Questions:

1. What does it mean when a patient cannot separate her hands when she imagines them to be magnets?

   (a) The patient has low self-esteem.
   (b) The patient is being noncooperative.
   (c) The patient does not understand the instructions given.

(d) The patient is a good hypnotic subject.
(e) None of the above.

2. Why did this patient imagine being in two places at once?

(a) She misunderstood the instructions.
(b) This is an example of trance logic.
(c) She was being noncooperative.
(d) The patient has attention deficit hyperactivity disorder.
(e) None of the above.

3. What was the purpose of asking the patient to rate her level of relaxation?

(a) This helps validate the experience for the patient.
(b) The patient's report of the relaxation ratings gives the clinician feedback regarding the effectiveness of the intervention.
(c) Asking for the rating shows respect for the patient's self-assessment, which empowers her.
(d) The patient can use the rating scale to gauge her progress over time.
(e) All of the above.

Answers:

1. (d): Good hypnotic subjects are able to experience hypnotic phenomena more easily and therefore frequently respond well to hypnotic suggestions. The keys to being a good subject include the patient's intrinsic hypnotic ability, rapport with the clinician, and the patient's level of motivation in using the hypnosis to help herself. Patients with high self-esteem tend to be more confident in their abilities and thus often can use hypnosis more easily.
2. (b): When patients are in hypnosis, they are able to visualize contradictory imagery comfortably. This situation arises as patients in hypnosis can focus intently on particular thoughts, which preclude their attending to other thoughts, such as "This cannot be." The ability to focus intently to the exclusion of other inputs is the reason patients in hypnosis can disregard physical stimuli that had led to perpetuation of their functional respiratory symptoms.
3. (e): When patients utilize a rating scale, they are more likely to recognize the degree to which hypnosis has been helpful to them, which enhances their belief in its utility, thus reinforcing their confidence in their ability to help themselves.

Case 5: Insomnia

A 24-year-old woman reported a 5-year history of difficulty falling asleep and awakening 2–3 times nightly because of recurrent nightmares. She explained that typically it took her approximately 2 h to fall asleep because she was worried about her lack of social life, inability to find a job, and also that she would be tired the next day, which would affect her academic performance in college. Her most common recurrent nightmare involved strangers being in her room who wanted to do something to her. She would awaken in fright before she would find out what they would do.

The patient already had worked on her sleep hygiene. She avoided caffeine, ate an early dinner, took 3 mg of melatonin 2 h before bedtime, dimmed the lights an hour before bedtime, got into bed consistently at around 11 pm, and did not watch television while in bed.

The patient was instructed about how to use hypnosis in order to relax, in a fashion similar to that described in Table 12.1. To help her fall asleep, she was given three options: (1) Imagine yourself in your relaxing place for as long as it takes to fall asleep. (2) Imagine seeing yourself fall asleep while you are in hypnosis, which will help you fall asleep in real life. (3) Imagine a "sleep dial" that you can manipulate. Turned one way, the dial will awaken you, while turned the other way, it can make you feel sleepy.

Helping patients achieve resolution of nightmares should be done only by practitioners of hypnosis who specialize in mental health [35]. In this case, the patient was coached to imagine herself in a movie theater, eating popcorn (which was suggested after she said she liked this food), and watching a movie of her nightmare. She was told that she could control the movie if she liked, by turning it off, turning down the volume, or removing its color. She was coached to watch the nightmare movie and to indicate the part at which point she would awaken. Then, she was coached to watch the remainder of the movie. She stated that at the conclusion of the movie, she found out that the strangers actually were there to protect her from harm.

Two weeks after the aforementioned interventions, the patient reported she was falling asleep within 20 min by imagining while in hypnosis that she was falling asleep and that her nightmare no longer recurred.

Questions:

1. How could a suggestion that the patient remain relaxed while in hypnosis "for as long as it takes" to fall asleep decrease the amount of time it would take for her to fall asleep?

   (a) By relaxing, the patient was preparing her body to fall asleep.
   (b) By focusing on her relaxing place, the patient could more easily stop thinking about her worrisome thoughts.
   (c) This suggestion takes advantage of time distortion that can occur with hypnosis [28]. She can imagine being in hypnosis for several hours or days, even as only a few moments pass in real time.
   (d) The suggestion implied that she would fall asleep.
   (e) All of the above.

2. Why was the patient told that she should imagine viewing her nightmare on a movie screen?
   (a) This gave her a feeling of control over the nightmare.
   (b) It made the nightmare seem unrealistic.
   (c) It helped her associate her nightmare with pleasant past movie experiences.
   (d) It made her nightmare seem bigger than life, so when she coped with it, she would feel more empowered.
   (e) All of the above.
3. Was it important for the patient to watch the nightmare until its conclusion?
   (a) Yes, because once it reached its end, it did not have to restart.
   (b) Yes, because once the patient realized its underlying message that she was protected, she felt safer.
   (c) No, because the nightmare likely would have resolved just by putting it on the movie screen.
   (d) No, because the conclusion may just have been made up by the patient during the hypnosis intervention and unrelated to what actually had occurred in her dream.
   (e) None of the above.

Answers:

1. (e): The success of many effective hypnotic suggestions is based on a number of factors, as shown in this instance. Clinicians who are just starting out with use of hypnosis sometimes inadvertently give contradictory suggestions. For example, with this patient, she was told about three options she could utilize to fall asleep, rather than three options she could "try" to use because "trying" suggests the possibility that none of the options might work.
2. (a): In addition to putting the nightmare on a movie screen, which distanced it from the patient and thus offered her some protection, she also was told she could control playing the movie as well as its sound and color. Prompting this patient to develop a sense of mastery over her frightening experience allowed her to explore more easily how it might be resolved. Implying that the nightmare was unrealistic does not honor how the patient has perceived it. Making a frightening experience bigger than life without safeguards can traumatize a patient.
3. (b): Helping patients understand the message behind their nightmares has been shown to help resolve them, often as patients end up gaining helpful insights from their dreams [35]. The type of suggestion used often is key to the success of hypnosis, although different patients require different types of suggestions. In terms of clinical outcome, it makes no difference whether the conclusion of a nightmare is "real" or made up on the spot by the patient. Either way, patients can improve.

Conclusions

Clinical hypnosis allows primary care physicians, pulmonologists, and other health care providers for patients with respiratory disorder to offer an efficient and effective tool for addressing patients with functional respiratory disorders, including those with chest pain, dyspnea, habit cough, and vocal cord dysfunction. The use of hypnosis in appropriate patients often can help preclude patients from undergoing unnecessary tests or receiving ineffective and possibly harmful treatment.

Index of Hypnosis Techniques in This Chapter

Table 12.1 and the case studies demonstrate several different hypnotic techniques that can be helpful for patients with functional respiratory disorders. These include:

Prehypnotic interview techniques:

Asking open-ended questions (Case 2, Video 12.10)

Induction techniques (helping a patient enter a hypnotic state):

Hands as magnets (Table 12.1, Video 12.11)
Sand pail and balloons (Table 12.1, Video 12.11)

Deepening techniques (helping a patient focus inwardly more intently):

Imagine what might be perceived with each of the senses (Table 12.1, Video 12.2)
Progressive relaxation (Table 12.1, Video 12.11)

Therapeutic hypnotic suggestions:

Cough lever (Video 12.8)
Ego-strengthening (helping the patient appreciate their own skills) (Table 12.1, Videos 12.1–12.7, Video 12.11):
House of control (Case 1, Video 12.3)
Glove anesthesia (Case 1, Video 12.4)
Relaxation/comfort sign (Table 12.1, Video 12.6)
Relaxation place (Table 12.1, Case 4, Case 5, Video 12.11)
Sleep dial (Case 5)
Time distortion (Case 5)

Validation techniques (helping a patient understand hypnosis has caused a change):

Relaxation scale (Case 4, Video 12.6, Video 12.11)
Relaxation sign (Table 12.1, Case 4, Video 12.6, Video 12.11)

Acknowledgements Portions of this chapter adapted from Anbar RD. Adding hypnosis to the therapeutic toolbox of pediatric respiratory care. Pediatr Asthma Allergy Immunol 2009; 22(4):209–14. With permission from Mary Ann Liebert, Inc.

References

1. Anbar RD. Adding hypnosis to the therapeutic toolbox of pediatric respiratory care. Pediatr Asthma All Immunol. 2009;22(4):209–14.
2. Anbar RD. Hypnosis in pediatrics: applications at a pediatric pulmonary center. BMC Pediatrics. 2002;2:11.
3. Wark DM, Kohen DP. A spiral curriculum for hypnosis training. Am J Clin Hypn. 2002;45(2):119–28.
4. Kohen DP, Olness K. Hypnosis and hypnotherapy with children. 4th ed. New York, NY: Routledge; 2011.
5. Wester WC, Sugarman LI, editors. Therapeutic hypnosis with children and adolescents. Bethel, CT: Crown House Publishing; 2007.
6. Anbar RD. Hypnosis: an important multifaceted therapy. J Pediatr. 2006;149(4):438–9.
7. Lahmann C, Nickel M, Schuster T, et al. Functional relaxation and guided imagery as complementary therapy in asthma: a randomized controlled clinical trial. Psychother Psychosom. 2009;78(4):233–9.
8. Anbar RD. Self-hypnosis for management of chronic dyspnea in pediatric patients. Pediatrics. 2001;107(2):395–6. e21.
9. Anbar RD, Hall HR. Childhood habit cough treated with self-hypnosis. J Pediatr. 2004;144(2):213–7.
10. Anbar RD, Hummell KE. Teamwork approach to clinical hypnosis at a pediatric pulmonary center. Am J Clin Hypn. 2005;48(1):45–9.
11. Anbar RD, Slothower MP. Hypnosis for treatment of insomnia in school-age children: a retrospective chart review. BMC Pediatrics. 2006;6:23.
12. Anbar RD, Geisler SC. Identification of children who may benefit from self-hypnosis at a pediatric pulmonary center. BMC Pediatrics. 2005;5(1):6.
13. Anon. Hypnosis for asthma: controlled trial. Br Med J. 1968;4(5623):71–6.
14. Ewer TC, Stewart DE. Improvement in bronchial hyper-responsiveness in patients with moderate asthma, after treatment with a hypnotic technique: a randomized controlled trial. BMJ. 1986;293(6555):1129–32.
15. Kohen DP. Relaxation/mental imagery (self-hypnosis) for childhood asthma: behavioral outcomes in a prospective, controlled study. Hypnos. 1995;22:132–44.
16. Brown D. Evidence-based hypnotherapy for asthma: a critical review. Int J Clin Exp Hypn. 2007;55(2):220–49.
17. Smith JM, Burns CLC. The treatment of asthmatic children by hypnotic suggestion. Br J Dis Chest. 1960;54:78–91.
18. Hackman RM, Stern JS, Gershwin ME. Hypnosis and asthma: a critical review. J Asthma. 2000;37(1):1–15.
19. Baron C. Role of panic attacks in the intractability of asthma in children. Pediatrics. 1994;94(1):108–10.
20. Ten Thoren C, Peterman F. Reviewing asthma and anxiety. Resp Med. 2000;94(5):409–15.
21. Anbar RD. Self-hypnosis for anxiety associated with severe asthma: a case report. BMC Pediatrics. 2003;3:7.
22. Hammond DC. Hypnosis in the treatment of anxiety- and stress-related disorders. Expert Rev Neurother. 2010;10(2):263–73.
23. Palsson OS. Standardized hypnosis treatment for irritable bowel syndrome: The North Carolina protocol. Int J Clin Exp Hypn. 2006;54(1):51–64.
24. Vlieger AM, Menko-Frankenhuis C, Wolfkamp SC, Tromp E, Benninga MA. Hypnotherapy for children with functional abdominal pain or irritable bowel syndrome: a randomized controlled trial. Gastroenterology. 2007;133(5):1430–6.
25. Anbar RD. User friendly hypnosis as an adjunct for treatment of habit cough: a case report. Am J Clin Hypn. 2007;50(2):171–6.

26. Schoen M. Resistance to health: when the mind interferes with the desire to become well. Am J Clin Hypn. 1993;36(1):47–54.
27. Anbar RD. Hypnosis for the pediatric respiratory care toolbox. Alter Complem Therapies. 2010;16(3):145–50.
28. Hammond DC, editor. Handbook of hypnotic suggestion and metaphors. New York, NY: WW Norton & Company; 1990.
29. Anbar RD. Hypnosis for children with chronic disease. In: Wester WC, Sugarman LI, editors. Therapeutic Hypnosis with Children and Adolescents. Bethel, CT: Crown House Publishing; 2007. p. 357–85.
30. Mott Jr T. Untoward effects associated with hypnosis. Psychiatr Med. 1992;10(4):119–28.
31. Lang EV, Hatsiopoulou O, Koch T, et al. Can words hurt? Patient-provider interactions during invasive procedures. Pain. 2005;114(1–2):303–9.
32. Diamant Z, Mantzouranis E, Bjermer L. Montelukast in the treatment of asthma and beyond. Expert Rev Clin Immunol. 2009;5(6):639–58.
33. Raz A, Raikhel E, Anbar RD. Placebos in medicine: knowledge, beliefs, and patterns of use. McGill J Med. 2008;11(2):206–11.
34. Anbar RD. Stressors associated with dyspnea in childhood: patients' insights and a case report. Am J Clin Hypn. 2004;47(2):93–101.
35. Linden JH, Bhardwaj A, Anbar RD. Hypnotically enhanced dreaming to achieve symptom reduction: a case study of 11 children and adolescents. Am J Clin Hypn. 2006;48(4):279–89.

Chapter 13
Speech Therapy for the Treatment of Functional Respiratory Disorders

Heather L. Hodges

This chapter contains videos, please download from
http://www.springerimages.com/videos/10.1007/978-1-61779-857-3_13

Abstract Speech therapy for the treatment of functional respiratory disorders serves as an efficient and effective means to resolving vocal cord dysfunction, chronic cough, and dysfunctional breathing patterns. Education regarding the laryngeal and respiratory mechanisms is an essential first step in treating such disorders. Various speech therapy techniques are tailored to the individual patient's needs and trigger situations. As the patient population is homogenous in diagnosis, but diverse in etiologies, triggers and contributing factors, specialized training in treatment techniques aids the clinician in recognizing treatment barriers, ways to desensitize hyper-functional respiratory responses, and ensures their ultimate resolution. This chapter offers an explanation and application of commonly used techniques, considerations for vocal hygiene and abuse/misuse, questions for comprehension, and case studies with video presentations.

Keywords Chronic cough • Dyspnea • Dysphonia • Paradoxical vocal fold motion • Speech therapy • Stridor • Throat clearing • Throat tightness • Vocal cord dysfunction

Background

The focus of speech therapy for the treatment of respiratory disorders centers on controlling vocal cord dysfunction (VCD), eliminating chronic cough, and/or reversing dysfunctional, airflow limiting breathing patterns. Each disorder is discussed individually below with accompanying background regarding various appropriate treatment techniques. Potential causes, triggers, and comorbidities lead to

H.L. Hodges (✉)
Department of Rehabilitation Services, National Jewish Health,
1400 Jackson Street, Denver, CO 80206, USA
e-mail: hodgesh@njhealth.org

R.D. Anbar (ed.), *Functional Respiratory Disorders: When Respiratory Symptoms Do Not Respond to Pulmonary Treatment*, Respiratory Medicine,
DOI 10.1007/978-1-61779-857-3_13, © Springer Science+Business Media, LLC 2012

heterogeneity within the patient population, and thus the described techniques should be individualized to each patient's needs [1]. While the elements of education, instruction, and retraining can be provided by a primary care physician, the time invested in the tailoring of techniques, desensitization of triggers, and attending to the vocal pathology of these patients is most often referred to the care of a speech-language pathologist (SLP).

Vocal Cord Dysfunction

During the breathing cycle, the vocal folds should remain in an open, or abducted state. It is important to note that they should be at their greatest abduction during inhalation and may slightly adduct upon exhalation. As their primary biological function is airway maintenance, they provide protective functions by means of coughing, throat clearing, and complete adduction during swallowing and/or breath holding. When provoked by an irritant, which may commonly include postnasal drainage (PND), gastroesophageal reflux (GER)/laryngopharyngeal reflux (LPR), allergens, or environmental exposures such as chemical fumes, they can develop an overprotective response leading to VCD. VCD, also commonly known as paradoxical vocal fold motion (particularly among SLPs), is the paradoxical adduction of the vocal folds during inspiration, expiration, or both (see Chap. 6). This adduction leads to breathing restriction that can cause feelings of dyspnea, tightness, or symptoms of stridor or tension. Moreover, dyspnea-evoked anxiety or stress may also increase muscle tension within the larynx and create an environment of hypervigilance. Pairing a laryngeal irritant and/or laryngeal tension with the protective nature of the larynx, the system essentially becomes conditioned or trained to protect in this manner of hyperadduction behavior. While speech therapy can be a cornerstone of treatment for VCD [2, 3], the etiology of the dysfunction will include medical, functional, or a combination of comorbidities. Addressing these etiological comorbidities is vital to the successful *complete* resolution of VCD. Because of this, the treatment of VCD often requires a team approach and, along with the SLP, may include a primary care physician, otolaryngologist, allergist, pulmonologist, gastroenterologist, psychologist/psychiatrist, athletic coach/trainer, recreation therapist, or neurologist [4–7]. However, given the vocal folds muscular makeup, the (re) training of the laryngeal mechanism out of the overprotective adduction behaviors via speech therapy or other techniques, such as hypnotherapy (Chap. 12), often is necessary, even when the airway irritant or threat is eliminated.

While identified in medical writings as long as 28 years ago, speech therapy as a treatment for VCD can historically be attributed to Dr. Florence Blager [8, 9]. Her treatment focus is on making speech sounds during exhalation, often referred to as "s breathing", "f breathing", or "s-h breathing" [2]. Diaphragm engagement for speech differs from its engagement for breathing. This change in engagement takes some of the load off the respiratory mechanism, including the larynx, thereby relaxing the respiratory system out of a VCD attack. It also provides respiration-affirming auditory feedback, which takes attention away from inhalation. This is especially helpful in patients whose VCD manifests as a feeling they "cannot get enough air in" [2, 10].

Other speech treatments for VCD have included panting [2] and maneuvers to open the posterior oropharynx such as yawning, feigning a yawn, or attempting to lower the base of the tongue. In a case study presented by Pitchenik [11], an individual with severe dyspnea and inspiratory stridor presented with flow volume loops demonstrating significant upper airway obstruction. An organic cause was ruled out following a thorough workup, and during the plethysmography, airway resistance measures were observed to be within normal limits. This finding led to engaging the subject to pant during times of an attack. This panting was described as breathing as rapidly and shallowly as possible, i.e., "pant like a dog." The subject was noted to reverse out of his attacks successfully and repeatedly. He further reported that his attacks diminished over several weeks' time. Additionally, patients have reported successful reversal of attacks when instructed to lower the base of their tongue, yawn, feign yawning, or perform "wide open throat breathing" [2, 9, 12]. These maneuvers widen the laryngopharynx, [2, 11, 13–15] thereby increasing the available supra- and subglottal space for air to flow. Moreover, the vocal folds tend to abduct during a yawn, allowing for ease of airflow.

Both panting and widening the upper airway can aid in the reversal of an acute VCD episode. In the expansive patient population treated at National Jewish Health in Denver, CO, neither method appears to completely abate VCD and, for many patients, can be difficult to implement during moderate to severe episodes of vocal fold adduction. It seems that reverting to a rapid, shallow breathing pattern or attempting posturing consistent with a yawn (i.e., relaxing) is uncomfortable or difficult to execute in times of dyspnea, tightness, or stridor.

Practical Application

The following treatment techniques are directly extracted from the approaches employed by the current speech-language pathology team at National Jewish Health, the preeminent institution in the discovery, diagnosis, and treatment of VCD. Fran Lowry, voice pathologist and colleague of this author, is credited with the development of these techniques [16]. A breakdown of the following techniques, each falling under the classification, *pursed lip breathing*, is found in Fig. 13.1.

Education Regarding the Laryngeal Mechanism

Initially, a thorough intake is obtained and includes the patient's symptoms, onset, triggers, vocal hygiene, and the co-occurring medical issues potentially causing the VCD (most often PND or GER/LPR but including exercise, an irritant exposure, or psychological condition such as anxiety). Subsequently, education is provided as a

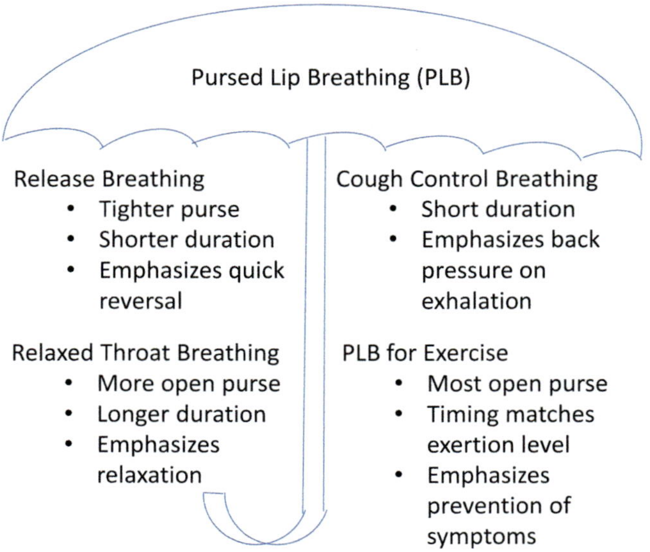

Fig. 13.1 Potential variations on pursed lip breathing techniques and their various terms

part of the treatment process [17]. As most patients do not fully understand the function of the larynx, and only consider the vocal folds during times of voice change, voice loss, or vocal performance, education regarding the protective mechanism of the larynx is the key to understanding the upper airway's involvement in breathing difficulties and/or chronic cough [18]. We find that even our patients as young as age 5 years are intrigued by the functions of the larynx as they pertain to their VCD symptoms. Further, the public's notion of speech therapy typically involves aiding those with difficulty speaking, rather than difficulty breathing. It is explained to the patient that their vocal folds are the mechanism for airway maintenance by means of coughing, throat clearing, adduction during swallowing, and in breath holding. This information alone is often empowering and will frequently cause the misconceptions of speech therapy to melt away, thereby creating an increased sense of trust and understanding of the treating clinician.

Following the explanation regarding the normal protective mechanisms of the larynx, the abnormal hypervigilant response of vocal fold closure (VCD) during breathing is explained and demonstrated [16] using visual aids including anatomical drawings and models. Within the overprotective response of the vocal folds, a chronic dry cough may also exist and is addressed in education and treatment. It should be noted that a patient with VCD may or may not have a chronic dry cough, just as someone with an unproductive cough may or may not have VCD. Regardless of an unproductive cough standing alone or along with the symptom complex of VCD, it is treated with the same techniques explained below. Special considerations will be highlighted when dealing with cough. With the patient holding an increased

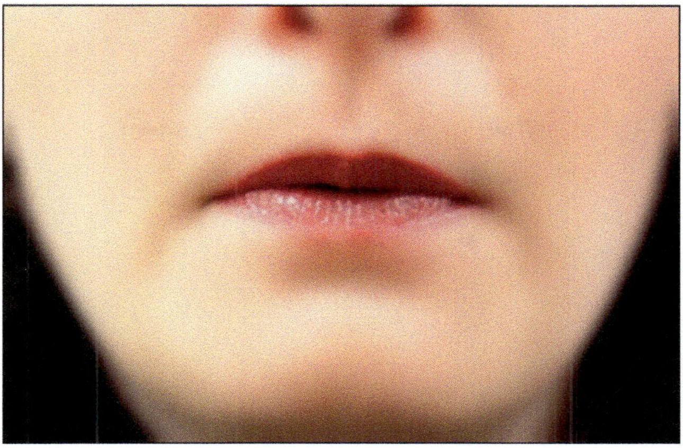

Fig. 13.2 Lip posture during exhalation for release breathing technique

understanding of the laryngeal mechanism, education then serves as a bridge to the treatment portion of therapy. The clinician frequently will first demonstrate and explain the technique(s) utilized for the patient's individual case. The rationale, or physics, behind the breathing is also explained to further empower the patient.

One of two main techniques will be most commonly used as the treatment base. For both techniques, based on Lowry [16], the patient is instructed to lower his or her shoulders and employ a diaphragmatic breathing pattern. We observe many patients to have a thoracic, or shallow, breathing pattern. To optimize more filling and relaxed breathing, the breath should come from diaphragmatic excursion upon inhalation. The two actions of lowering the shoulders and optimizing diaphragmatic breathing will eliminate extrinsic laryngeal tension that perpetuates throat tightness and vocal fold adduction, by instead encouraging relaxation. In the first potential technique employed, here forth referred to as *release breathing,* a quick yet relaxed inhalation through the nose or mouth occurs, within less than 1 second. As many people associate a quick breath with extrathoracic movement, upper body relaxation is emphasized. The same amount of air then is immediately exhaled through slightly tight pursed lips for 2–3 s. Patients may benefit from the visualization of "as if you are holding a grain of rice between your lips" (see Fig. 13.2). This pursed lip exhalation allows for back pressure, consistent with the Bernoulli principle, to build behind the lips and within the airway, yielding a strong stream of air to build subglottally. This increased air pressure abducts the vocal folds into an open and relaxed position. Over successive repetitions, the larynx relaxes, the vocal folds remain open, and the patient has effectively reversed a VCD episode.

The other main technique that can be implemented is *relaxed throat breathing*. While it is also a pursed lip exhalation technique based on subglottic air pressure encouraging upper airway abduction, it differs in that it is a longer and more relaxed breathing cycle. Additionally, upon exhalation, the lips are more open, with the visualization of "as if you are making a candle flicker" (see Fig. 13.3). As it involves

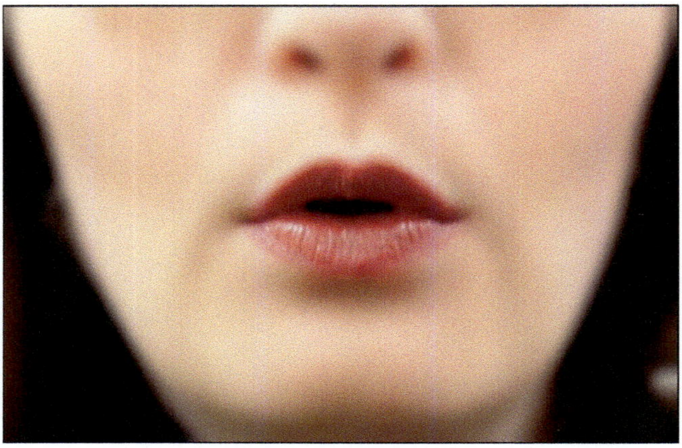

Fig. 13.3 Lip posture during exhalation for relaxed throat breathing technique

a deeper inhalation, it tends to be more relaxing and therefore more comforting for those patients with significant anxiety or hyperventilation syndrome that may trigger or are caused by a VCD attack. For some patients, practice with both techniques and determination of which is more comfortable and easier to implement acutely is beneficial. They can then focus their treatment using one of the two techniques. Others may find that each works in different circumstances. For example, a patient may report the release breathing is preferred when exercising, while the relaxed throat breathing is better at controlling symptoms during times of stress.

In contrast to acute treatment of VCD via panting, maneuvers to widen the laryngopharynx, or heliox [2], patients do not just complete their breathing technique(s) during an episode of VCD but also implement them as a retraining and a pretreatment tool. Consistent with the motor learning and skill acquisition principles of frequent, distributed, daily practice (i.e., intense practice) [19, 20], the patient is instructed to complete these exercises when asymptomatic [21–24]. By practicing these techniques intensively, even when asymptomatic, patients affect a change in behavior (i.e., vocal fold adduction as in VCD). As VCD occurs in pediatric, adult, and geriatric populations, the daily dose of release breathing practice is tailored to the age of the patient. For instance, we find clinically most pediatric patients require less daily practice than adult populations for effective results. This daily training encourages frequent open and relaxed vocal fold configuration, thereby working to retrain the muscle response of overprotection by means of muscle tightness (i.e., vocal fold adduction). Frequent practice also ensures this breathing becomes an automatic response, such that at the onset of dyspnea, tightness, stridor, etc. the patient is confident and capable of quickly implementing the release or relaxed throat breathing for symptom reversal. In times of symptom exacerbation, the patient is encouraged to complete as many pursed lip breathing cycles as necessary for episode reversal.

Additionally, treatment with the above techniques includes use of the release or relaxed throat breathing in trigger situations. Some patients may have identified no specific triggers for their VCD, while others will have an extensive list. Triggers for a VCD episode can range from stress or tension, hot or cold temperatures, temperature changes, and strong odors [25], fumes from paint or car exhaust, smoke, and exercise [26], to talking or laughing. Oftentimes, these triggers are not harmful to breathe [27], despite the dramatic respiratory symptoms they can induce. Achieving VCD control around such triggers is vital. For example, a patient triggered by strong fragrances may go so far as avoiding grocery stores because passing the cleaning and laundry aisles will trigger a VCD attack. By using one or both of the above techniques before, during, and after exposure to a patient's triggers, VCD control is achieved, as is long-term desensitization of the laryngeal VCD response to such irritants. An example of desensitization is provided later in this chapter. In some patients with co-occurring asthma [28, 29] for whom rescue inhalers provide limited relief of dyspnea or even "make breathing worse" (i.e., act as a trigger), use of pursed lip breathing before, between, and after doses of their asthma medication serves to keep the vocal folds relaxed and ensures full delivery of their inhaled medication to the lower airways.

Prior to education and treatment, a patient with identifiable triggers frequently will hold his or her breath to avoid inhaling the offending agent. Similarly, a high-performing athlete may employ breath holding during times of thoracic stabilization (e.g., a basketball player stabilizes his "core" when making a lay-up, a track athlete controls her body to jump a hurdle, or a soccer player exerting force when making a shot on goal). All patients should be reminded that vocal fold adduction occurs when holding one's breath and can therefore trigger or perpetuate a VCD attack. By instead utilizing the patient's preferred pursed lip breathing technique, they will relax the vocal folds open before trigger exposure, maintain control during the exposure, and leave the situation controlled and calm by implementing several breaths post exposure.

Many patients are not aware of breath holding behavior or how to recognize the onset of the subtle first signs and symptoms of VCD, thus specific irritant challenges with the SLP as a means toward desensitization can be an empowering and compelling means toward treatment buy-in, adherence, VCD control, and ultimately, VCD resolution. There are many considerations when challenging a patient to an irritant.

First, patient consent should be obtained. Next, and most importantly, the irritant should not be noxious to inhale, such as bathroom or oven cleaner, as this can cause or trigger lower respiratory disorders such as asthma. Appropriate irritants for a challenge may include, but are not limited to, perfume, lit scented candles, walking into cold air, or exertion.

Second, the challenge should target a trigger specific to that patient. Someone sensitive to perfume should be challenged with perfume and not cold air, just as a soccer player should be challenged with running/sprinting and not isometric exercises.

Third, patients should be allowed to trigger their symptoms to a mild degree. We have them rate their symptoms throughout the challenge on a scale from 0 to 10.

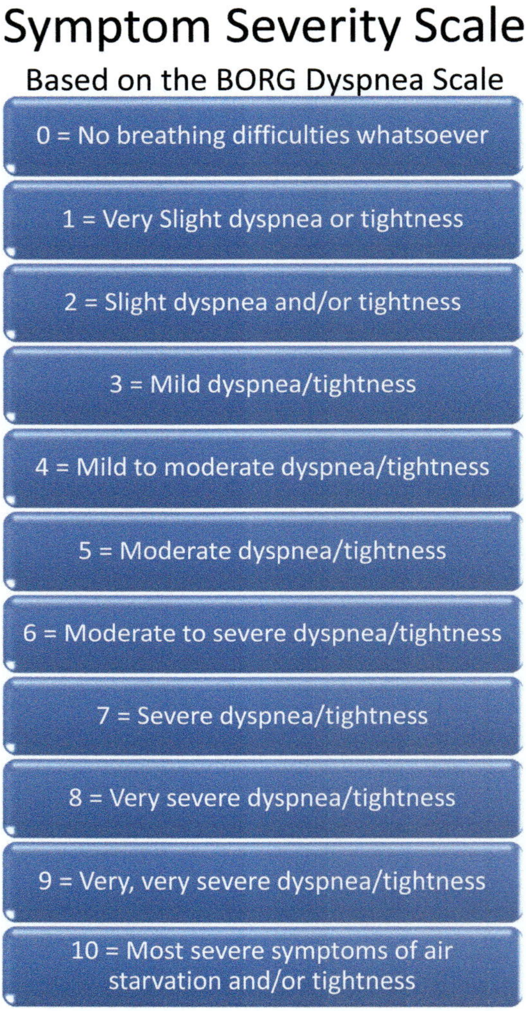

Fig. 13.4 An adaptation of the BORG scale which is used in multiple disciplines to obtain patient self-ratings of dyspnea

with 0 being no symptoms and 10 equal to most severe symptoms (similar to the BORG scale of dyspnea; see Fig. 13.4). Depending on anxiety levels and severity of the individual's VCD, most patients will be removed from the trigger situation once symptoms reach a subjectively measured "2 or 3." They will complete their preferred pursed lip breathing technique until symptoms reverse ideally back to a perceived "0," although a level of "1" may be acceptable. At this point, the patient is reintroduced into the trigger situation, always using their pursed lip breathing, until symptoms return. Even in the first session of desensitization work, the patient will tolerate longer and longer trigger exposures before eliciting their VCD. Moreover, when the patient is removed from the situation with continued use of their pursed lip

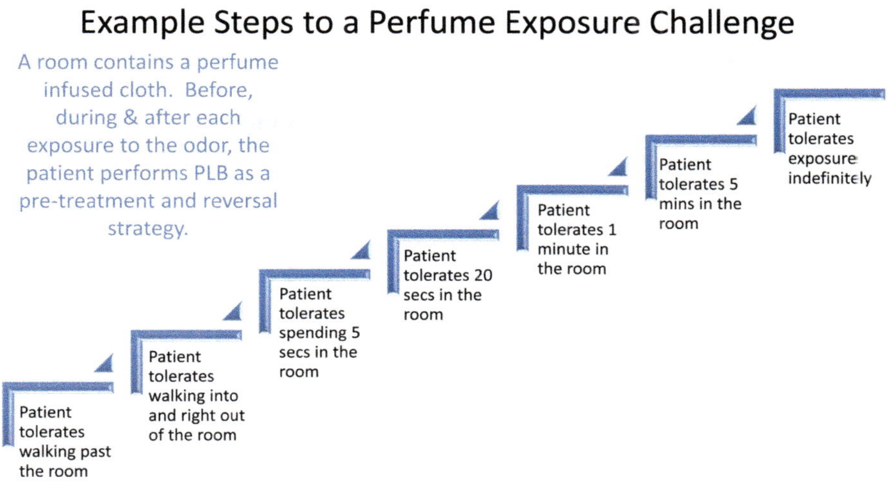

Fig. 13.5 Schematic of the stepwise progression of a patient-tailored irritant challenge

breathing, the time to reverse out of a VCD episode becomes shorter and shorter. Not only is the patient desensitizing their VCD response but also is empowered over breathing difficulties that otherwise can leave a VCD patient feeling debilitated, anxious, avoidant, and at the mercy of their breathing difficulties.

Finally, the challenges should be taken in "baby steps." This is particularly true for patients with VCD subsequent to exposure to an airborne irritant of a dangerous nature. Such exposures include home/workplace mold, chemical fires, chemical spills, and fine particulate construction dust [3] as in the case of the first responders to the World Trade Center on 9/11. Such irritants can cause an immediate irritation of the mucous membranes of the upper airway [30]. In these cases, the heightened protective response to an agent potentially threatening to the lungs is so great and so acute that it is almost like a protection switch was turned "on" and is stuck in that position. These patients typically have more identifiable triggers, a greater sense of anxiety, and take longer to treat. While most glaringly evident in patients postnoxious exposure, *consideration of a heightened protective response should be undertaken with all patients no matter what triggers or etiological factors exist.*

With the patient performing the release or relaxed throat breathing technique before, during, and after each exposure, an example of a "baby steps" approach during a perfume irritant challenge is found in Fig. 13.5. Please note the subtle exposure progression. It is important to state that before stepping up, mastery of VCD at the prior step should occur. Both points are in accordance with systematic desensitization (Chap. 9) [27]. As patients will be highly encouraged by these developments, they should be left at the end of the session with the reminder that trigger exposures should remain in the spirit of "baby steps." Success in controlling VCD is a powerful motivator; left unwarned, a patient may push too far too fast, hindering their recovery and increasing their frustration.

Considerations for Exercise-Induced VCD or Cough

The range of exertion triggering a VCD attack is as varied as the patient population itself [1]. From the patient unable to walk more than 2 min without onset of dyspnea, to one with difficulty climbing stairs, to the high school soccer player, and to the Olympic track hopeful, VCD occurs across the board of athletic prowess. With this knowledge, it is key to find out what activity triggers one's VCD (e.g., a triathlete is only triggered during swimming events and not running or cycling), how long it takes to trigger an attack (this can also be helpful in differentiating between when symptoms are attributable to VCD versus asthma or both), and what are their first symptoms of an episode. Beginning the exercise challenge with a warm-up will allow the muscles to loosen up, while the patient begins the challenge with a relaxed upper airway via implementation of pursed lip breathing at the onset of exertion.

Breathing during physical exertion, especially high-level cardio exercise, requires a heavier, harder, and faster breathing pattern than at rest. Thus, execution of a tight pursed lip exhale or slow relaxed breathing pattern highlighted as the main two techniques above may not be possible. Therefore, the technique is adjusted and simplified for exercise. The patient is encouraged to inhale through the nose or mouth as is comfortable, and on the exhale, a more open "blowing out a candle" cue is given. The time spent during inhalation and exhalation is not emphasized, as the level of cardio exertion will dictate the rate of the breathing cycle. Someone walking will have a slower, longer breathing cycle, with capability to purse his or her lips tighter than someone sprinting. Conversely, an athlete in a sprint will have a rapid breathing cycle with perhaps minimal pursing of the lips (refer to Fig. 13.6). The exhale will remain somewhat longer than inhalation since the air is passing through a space partially restricted by the pursing of the lips.

Several parallels exist between an airborne irritant challenge and an exercise challenge. As many athletes are accustomed to pushing themselves to maximal performance levels despite discomfort, pain, or dyspnea, they often push beyond mild symptoms before acknowledging VCD onset. Therefore, it is often more imperative to remind these patients to alert when their first symptoms appear, "at a level 2 or 3" (refer to Fig. 13.4). Also similar to an irritant challenge, once the patient reports mild symptoms, he or she should be removed from the trigger situation. In this case, employing pacing strategies and their reversal breathing technique effectively takes them out of the trigger environment without taking them "out of the game." The pacing strategy involves slowing the rate of physical activity and allows a patient's work of breathing to decrease such that rescue breathing can be executed. In the exertion VCD population, the most commonly preferred rescue technique is release breathing. Once they have reversed their symptoms to a "0 or 1" on the symptom severity scale, their faster rate of exercise and the open "candle blow" exhalation technique are then resumed. Also, parallel to a patient triggered by an airborne irritant, an athlete patient gaining control of

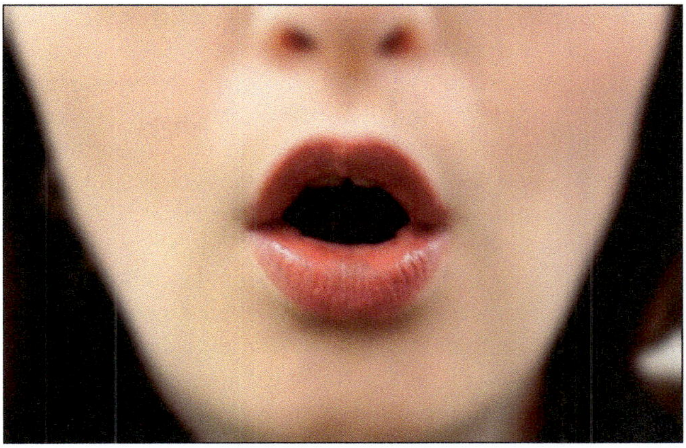

Fig. 13.6 Lip posture during exhalation for pursed lip breathing for exercise

his or her VCD will notice an increasing duration of exercise before VCD is triggered. Similarly, when VCD is triggered, use of pacing and rescue breathing resolves their symptoms more quickly.

Application of Techniques to Dry Chronic Cough

Various strategies for cough control are found in the literature. These include modified swallowing techniques, sucking ice chips, pursed lip breathing, relaxed throat breathing, substituting a laugh for coughing, and abdominal breathing [9, 13, 18, 31, 32]. Current practices at National Jewish Health are similar to the above programs for VCD resolution. As with VCD, the use of pursed lip breathing (Fig. 13.1) is applied to the treatment of dry chronic cough and includes daily, frequent, distributed practice when asymptomatic, as well as using it before, during, and after exposure to a known cough trigger; however, use for symptom control is modified slightly. The patient is first encouraged to use the pursed lip breathing at the onset of impending cough. Tuning the patient into the first signs or symptoms of impending cough may be warranted [18, 31, 32]. The first signs and symptoms at which to implement pursed lip breathing for prevention of cough may include a "tickle" sensation in the throat, increased thoracic or clavicular tension, breath holding as means to stifle a cough, or even one's hand moving toward the mouth in order to cover it before a cough begins. Clueing the patient into these signs and symptoms allows them to immediately begin pursed lip breathing for cough prevention purposes. These patients are also instructed to complete as many breathing cycles as needed to resolve their cough symptoms.

Often, the onset of a cough can be too quick or too intense to successfully implement cough control breathing for prevention purposes, and thus the patient is instructed regarding cough interruption. When a dry cough is occurring the patient is encouraged to purse his or her lips and cough through the restricted oral space. It is pointed out that they are not to try to stifle the cough, as the increase in subglottic pressure and extrinsic muscle tension of a stifle often leads to an exacerbated cough response. Instead, they are to move the air coming out during the cough through tight lips, creating a controlled increase in air pressure used to open the glottis, which relaxes the vocal folds out of the cough response.

Depending on the individual's cough severity and sensitivity of their laryngopharynx, the breathing cycle is usually quick, as in release breathing, but the force of the exhale is a little greater to allow for optimal back pressure within the glottis as it forces abduction of the folds. If a patient's laryngopharynx is particularly irritated from significant PND, LPR, or the laryngeal abuse of the cough act itself, the patient is instructed to reduce the force of the exhale, and/or increased focus on relaxation breathing may be needed. Tailoring the technique to an individual's tolerance, while optimizing the level of back pressure upon exhalation, is the balance to strike when applying these techniques to dry cough.

Use of an Inspiratory Muscle Trainer for Athletes with VCD

Exercise-induced VCD and inspiratory muscle weakness have similar sign and symptom presentations including tachypnea and effortful breathing during intense exercise [33–36]. Moreover, studies have shown an inverse relationship between inspiratory muscle strength and perceived dyspnea and work of breathing in various populations, including healthy and highly trained athletic populations [33, 36–38]. Given this backdrop, Mathers-Schmidt and Brilla [39] applied the use of an inspiratory muscle trainer (IMT, described below) to a teenage soccer player with known VCD that was triggered during intense exercise. While she was provided education on the laryngeal mechanism and information on relaxed throat breathing prior to beginning IMT work, the investigators found during treatment periods focused on IMT the patient's maximum inspiratory pressure (MIP) and maximal exercise measures increased over time, while exertional dyspnea ratings and VCD symptom occurrences decreased. Use of an IMT as an adjunct to traditional VCD treatment at National Jewish Health has thus been adopted in certain cases where VCD exists in intensely competitive athletes.

First, the patient's baseline MIP is taken via use of a manometer (see Fig. 13.7): The nares are occluded via nose clips, while the patient breathes through a mouthpiece connected to the valve of the manometer. After several quiet breathing cycles, the patient is instructed to exhale maximally. Upon maximum forceful inhalation, the valve is closed and the MIP in cm H_2O is measured. The best measurement over 3–4 trials is used as the starting point.

Consisting of a mouthpiece and adjustable valve as described by Sapienza et al. [40], the IMT has adjustable threshold levels set as a percentage against the individual's MIP. Once the set threshold level is met during inhalation, the IMT's

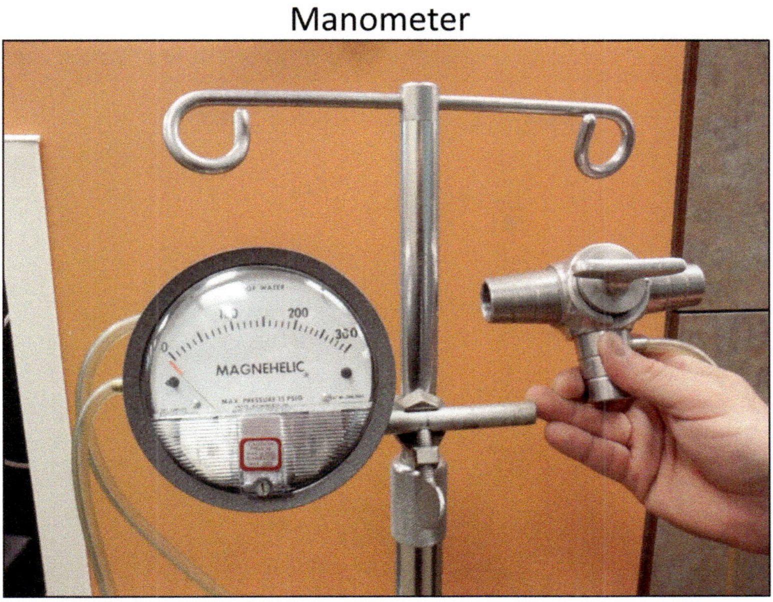

Fig. 13.7 An example of a manometer used to take a patient's maximum inspiratory pressure (MIP)

intake valve closes, allowing the patient to inhale against resistance. This resistance challenges the inspiratory muscles, thereby strengthening them over time. The IMT threshold is increased each week and is set as a percentage against the patient's weekly MIP (see Fig. 13.8). Following the protocol of Mathers-Schmidt and Brilla, 5 sets of 12 breaths into the IMT are completed with 1 min of rest between sets. This protocol occurs within treatment sessions with the speech-language pathologist, as well as during independent home practice occurring five days a week.

During times of IMT, the patient is also implementing daily release/relaxed throat breathing practice as above, as well as implementing pursed lip breathing and pacing for exercise. Easily incorporated into the IMT consult and follow-up sessions, the supplementation of pursed lip breathing maximizes the treatment outcomes for athletes with VCD.

Dysfunctional Breathing Patterns

Individuals experiencing dyspnea may benefit from therapy solely focused on maximizing breath support via diaphragmatic breathing. These individuals may not have VCD or upper airway involvement whatsoever. Instead, this population may present with general complaints of running out of air, increased work of breathing, or decreased breath support for speech secondary to a thoracic or clavicular breathing pattern. Such paradoxical breathing patterns are associated with increased breathlessness

Inspiratory Muscle Trainer Protocol

Week #	% of MIP (in cm H20) for IMT Resistance
1	25%
2	25%
3	50%
4	50%
5	75%
Additional Weeks (as needed)	75%

Fig. 13.8 The weekly progression of settings on an inspiratory muscle trainer as a percentage of a patient's MIP

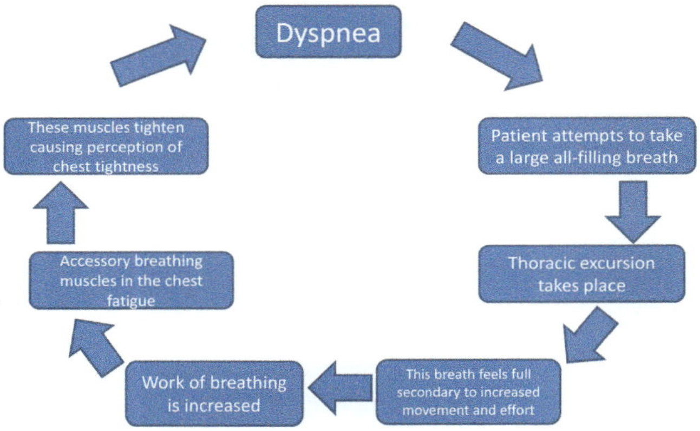

Fig. 13.9 This figure represents the perpetuating cycle of dyspnea and a thoracic breathing pattern on the interplay between work of breathing and chest tightness

[32] and respiratory load [41, 42] and have been observed in VCD and non-VCD patients. These patterns may have become habitual as a result of obesity or pregnancy that limit diaphragmatic excursion for inhalation or may be a maladaptive response to a respiratory or pulmonary compromise (e.g., asthma, COPD, acute bronchitis, etc.). Given clinical observations and patient interviews, it is the sense of this author that a thoracic breathing pattern can develop as a poor compensation to "get a deep breath." The upper body movement during a thoracic or "chest" breath feels large and effortful. This sense of working for a deep breath provides sensory misinformation that one has taken "as big a breath as possible," when in fact, diaphragmatic breathing, being most efficient, feels small or diminished as a result of its own efficiency. This creates a vicious cycle of sensory misinformation (see Fig. 13.9).

In a society concerned with a fit and trim physique, diaphragmatic excursion may be limited by "sucking the stomach in," thus putting the load of breathing on the chest muscles instead of allowing them to be the *accessory* breathing muscles that augment rather than drive the breathing pattern. Putting the breathing load on accessory muscles is not only inefficient and limiting but taxes them to the point of exhaustion, creating a feeling of discomfort or extrinsic chest tightness. This chest tightness may thereby increase work of breathing, cause feelings of dyspnea, and perpetuate the chest breathing pattern.

Treatment aimed at increasing diaphragmatic excursion should begin with education. Amazingly, many, especially adults, have an opposite notion of the breathing cycle, thinking the abdomen should move inward during inhalation and relax outwardly during exhalation. Providing demonstration or illustration of outward abdominal movement on inhalation is often eye opening. Tactile feedback by placing the hand or something with bulk, such as a book, on the abdomen of a patient in a reclined position may help him/her better appreciate appropriate activation of the diaphragm. Some patients benefit from increasing the pressure of the hand, pushing it inward during exhalation, allowing for an increase in the elastic bounce back of the diaphragm during the next inhalation. Pairing this increased breath support with phonation activities (i.e., speech and singing) may be indicated. These means are beneficial for individuals with or without VCD associated dyspnea.

Considerations for Vocal Abuse and Misuse

Optimizing the health of the laryngeal tissues ensures healing and release of laryngeal muscle tension and expedites resolution of VCD, cough, or dyspnea. During initial intake, information regarding vocal hygiene is obtained, including smoking habits, how much water and other beverages contributing to hydration are consumed daily, and how much daily caffeine and alcohol are consumed. If the laryngeal tissues are dry, they are more irritable, less likely to heal if damaged from throat clearing and/or coughing and more likely to continue behaviors of coughing, throat clearing, and dysphonia. Optimizing hydration [18], while controlling for the drying effects of tobacco smoke, caffeine, and alcohol, will expedite the efficacy of the treatment techniques.

Elimination of chronic throat clearing [43, 44] is another factor in breaking the overprotective behavior(s) of the vocal folds as well as managing vocal abuse. Oftentimes, the sensation of a tickle precedes the urge to clear one's throat. This tickle may result from PND or other secretions on or near the glottis. The act of throat clearing will move the offending element away from the glottis but is typically unproductive in fully expectorating it. Eventually, inhalation, gravity, or both allow the secretions to reenter the hypopharynx, and the need to clear one's throat recurs. This inefficient action can trigger a perpetual cycle of forceful vocal fold adduction. However, simply instructing a patient to "not clear your throat anymore" is insufficient. The secretions or PND need to be managed. In addition to nasal irrigation or use of nasal steroid sprays, swallowing techniques are useful in moving secretions from the hypopharynx into the digestive tract where they can be passed from the body. Swallowing sips of water may help, but adding force to the swallow is often required due to the sticky nature of the body's secretions. Therefore, the patient is instructed to implement a chin-tuck posture to swallow, or to swallow effortfully. Both techniques allow for increased muscle contraction of the upper swallow mechanism, thereby clearing the laryngopharynx most effectively. The patient is instructed to use the swallowing technique of their preference, optimally prior to but also following throat clearing.

Laryngeal muscle tension, especially that of muscle tension dysphonia (MTD), also may require treatment by the SLP for successful resolution of VCD or chronic dry cough [43, 44]. Muscle tension existing in the larynx of such a patient typically has multifactorial origins. First, intermittent dysphonia often is a symptom of VCD [45], during which many patients feel compelled to push their voice production since adequate breath support for speech is often lacking. Pushing the voice occurs when the patient, usually unintentionally, forces vocal production through means of hyperfunction. Signs of hyperfunction during a laryngeal exam may include false-fold hyperfunction or anterior-posterior hyperfunction, or a visible "squeeze" of the supraglottic structures. This causes strain on the vocal folds. Such misuse also is seen in patients with a chronic cough or throat clearing, wherein the lamina propria (layers of collagen elastin fibers existing within the vocal folds) is damaged by the forceful repeated slamming of the vocal folds during these behaviors. This damage will inhibit the natural vibration of the vocal folds, which results from air moving through the glottis during speech, also leading one to potentially strain for phonation. Finally, muscle tension during speech may be a long-standing behavior stemming from personality ("I am just a soft spoken person"), preference ("I don't like how high pitched my voice sounds"), or psychological influences ("When I spoke too loudly as a child, I was punished"). This misuse of one's voice may not have been previously terribly impactful on an individual, but once VCD or a chronic cough comes into play, this underlying tension will encourage a tight, tense laryngeal environment, exacerbating VCD/cough or providing a hurdle to successful treatment outcomes.

For some patients, introducing pursed lip breathing that abducts the vocal folds will de-bundle their laryngeal tension and be sufficient to actually resolve MTD caused during a VCD episode. Other patients may require more extensive voice therapy in addition to VCD/cough treatment. This therapy may focus on appropriate air flow during phonation, improved vocal resonance, and/or optimizing one's pitch or loudness when speaking.

Questions and Case Studies

To help enhance comprehension regarding speech therapy for functional respiratory disorders, please answer the following questions.

Questions:

1. Treatment techniques for VCD may include:
   (a) Making speech sounds such as a prolonged "fffff" on exhalation
   (b) Pursed lip breathing exercises
   (c) Yawning
   (d) Panting
   (e) All of the above

2. Why is education regarding the laryngeal mechanism as it relates to breathing, phonating, coughing, throat clearing, breath holding, and VCD a prominent component to a patient's initial consult with the SLP?
   (a) Patients may not be familiar with the vocal folds role in breathing difficulties or cough.
   (b) The idea of a speech therapy referral for treatment of dyspnea may seem to come out of "left field."
   (c) It builds the patient's trust and confidence level that the SLP understands their condition.
   (d) Increasing understanding of the upper airway mechanism empowers the patient over their VCD/cough.
   (e) All of the above.

3. What is the rationale for using pursed lip breathing techniques to treat VCD/cough?
   (a) The diaphragm engages differently, lessening the work of breathing.
   (b) Exhaling through pursed lips creates back pressure subglottally, forcing vocal fold abduction.
   (c) Breathing in such a silly way makes the patient laugh at themselves, thereby relaxing the laryngeal mechanism.
   (d) All of the above.
   (e) Pursed lip breathing is not a frequently implemented means to treat VCD/cough.

4. Why should an abdominal breathing pattern be encouraged over a thoracic/clavicular (e.g., "chest") breathing pattern?
   (a) Because all people with VCD and cough will have chronically poor diaphragmatic excursion; eliminating chest breathing will cure VCD and cough on its own.
   (b) It should not be encouraged. Breathing from the chest will relax the larynx.
   (c) Putting the load of breathing on the diaphragm will decrease work of breathing, relax the upper body, and improve breath support for phonation.
   (d) In the time it takes to achieve an abdominal breathing pattern, someone in a VCD attack will be sufficiently distracted from their dyspnea to allow for relaxation to reverse their symptoms.
   (e) (a), (c), and (d).

5. In addition to breathing retraining for VCD, cough, and dyspnea, the SLP may also address what during treatment?
   (a) The patient's hydration habits
   (b) Chronic throat clearing
   (c) Muscle tension
   (d) Dysphonia
   (e) All of the above

Answers:

1. (e): Each of these techniques has been used in the successful treatment of those with VCD. Pursed lip breathing techniques are the treatments most often implemented by the speech pathology team at National Jewish Health where an average of 32 new VCD cases are received weekly. Compared to "f" breathing, yawning-type maneuvers, and panting, it is observed to have the quickest treatment effect and is used to prevent, interrupt, and eliminate a VCD response.
2. (e): Even when provided initial education by the referring physician, many people do not fully comprehend the intricacies of the vocal tract. This education also serves as opportunity to clear up any questions or misunderstandings the patient may have about the vocal folds. Additionally, most people perceive speech therapy as helping those who have difficulty communicating. This interaction helps the patient see how speech therapy can help their specific non-communication-related symptoms. Finally, education empowers patients that something can be done to resolve their cough or breathing difficulties. Oftentimes, patients have been previously diagnosed with asthma that may not exist or may be suboptimally treated due to vocal fold adduction, limiting intake of their inhaled medication. Such patients can be frustrated or feel hopeless that their symptoms will not resolve.
3. (b): By pursing the lips on exhalation, a bottleneck is created behind the lips. This creates back pressure through the respiratory system, thereby creating a strong stream of air that will push the vocal folds open. Employing an abdominal breathing pattern will further relax the larynx but may require focus to achieve. Laughing can actually be a trigger for VCD and cough and is not part of the treatment focus.
4. (c): Breathing from the abdomen not only helps to decrease extrinsic laryngeal tension by taking the load of breathing off the upper body but also benefits those with dyspnea from inefficient chest breathing and/or difficulty with breath support for speech. Many people with VCD or cough revert to chest breathing during times of symptoms. While panting may help reverse an acute VCD attack, breathing from the chest tends to exacerbate VCD and dyspnea. Achieving a relaxed state often will improve dyspnea, VCD, and/or cough, but distraction is not an ideal means for treating such conditions, particularly for long-term benefit.
5. (e): Dehydrated laryngeal tissues, vocal abuse of throat clearing, and vocal misuse occurring from or resultant to muscle tension or dysphonia will impede the resolution of VCD, cough, and dyspnea and may exacerbate their presentations.

Case 1: Dyspnea (Occurring Without VCD)

A 42-year-old male with a history of chronic cough and moderate intermittent GER/LPR complained of difficulty getting enough air when singing. He has completed speech treatment for his cough, which has been resolved for 4 weeks. He began over-the-counter PPI treatment and reported that his GER/LPR symptoms had resolved. Based on a pulmonary functional test (PFT) and methacholine challenge, asthma and obstructive or restrictive pulmonary disorders have been ruled out. Laryngoscopy revealed no laryngeal masses, tissues without edema or erythema, and the vocal folds vibrated normally during phonation with no inappropriate adduction during the breathing cycle. He noted a recent 20-pound weight increase due to poor eating habits as a result of an erratic performance schedule, leading him to eat at all hours of the day and frequently at restaurants.

At rest, he exerts an appropriate diaphragmatic breathing pattern. When asked to perform a song, he is observed to exert a thoracic breathing pattern. After less than 1 min of singing, a visible tension of the shoulders and neck is observed. The patient is not holding out notes as he should; instead, he is taking replenishing breaths at an increasing frequency.

Education: The patient acknowledges an excellent understanding of the pattern of diaphragmatic engagement during the respiratory cycle. Reminding him of abdominal excursion upon inhalation and abdominal retraction on exhalation is not enough to revert his breathing out of the thoracic pattern.

External cueing: The patient is placed in front of a mirror. Modeling of chest versus abdominal breathing is provided by the clinician. The patient acknowledges seeing his backward pattern but improves it minimally. Next, the patient is encouraged to place his hand on the abdomen and asked to tune into making his hand move outwardly on inhalation. This improves his diaphragmatic breathing pattern. Finally, he is encouraged to use his hand to press his abdomen inwardly on exhalation. This produced an optimal elastic response of the diaphragm upon the inhalation immediately following, as observed by the abdomen moving outward while the chest moves minimally. This pattern is solidified via successive repetitions. Visual, external, and kinesthetic cues are systematically dropped as soon as the patient achieves independence. Cues are revisited at times when thoracic breathing returns, typically occurring during times of increased load from songs with difficult pitch and tempo profiles or need for prolonged continual phonation as in "holding a note out." Practice across singing situations and song difficulty during three follow-up appointments occurs to ensure optimal carryover. The patient reports progressive increased control of his breathing during singing and use of cues when he feels his "breathing slip up." By the end of treatment, he reports resolution of dyspnea with singing and improved vocal performance as a result.

Questions:

1. Despite having excellent pretreatment understanding of diaphragmatic breathing, why may have this gentleman slipped into a thoracic breathing pattern?
   (a) His recent weight gain provided increased abdominal pressure, making diaphragmatic excursion more difficult.

   (b) He began breathing from his chest as it subconsciously felt larger, and the effort involved made him feel as though he was breathing at his deepest.
   (c) His dyspnea during singing led him to increase his work of breathing, calling on his accessory breathing muscles in the chest to engage more than they are intended to.
   (d) All of the above.
   (e) None of the above.

2. What steps helped this patient to achieve an appropriate breathing pattern maximizing diaphragmatic involvement?

   (a) Education alone
   (b) Education, visualization, tactile cueing, and kinesthetic cueing
   (c) Education and clinician instruction to belly breathe
   (d) Education, visualization, and the patient enrolling in yoga classes
   (e) All of the above

3. Without specific work on diaphragmatic breathing the patient likely:

   (a) Would have been fine. His breathing pattern would work itself out eventually.
   (b) Would have gone on a diet. Losing weight around his abdomen would have regulated his breathing pattern.
   (c) Would have had continued difficulty with his breath support during singing, perhaps with worsening of symptoms.
   (d) All of the above.
   (e) None of the above.

Answers:

1. (d): All of the above are potential reasons for recent onset of a chest breathing pattern. This also represents a progression of how chest breathing not only began but became a pattern. His weight gain may have prohibited diaphragmatic excursion happening easily, breathing from the chest required more upper body movement making it feel large and filling, and chest tightness with feelings of dyspnea were perpetuated by exhausting the accessory breathing muscles of the chest.
2. (b): Education occurred first but was not sufficient in breaking the chest breathing pattern. Adding visualization in front of the mirror and the tactile feedback of his hand moving in and out furthered his progression, and the pushing of the hand solidified the diaphragmatic breathing pattern. The term "belly breathing" is used frequently in diaphragmatic work, often highlighted in yoga classes.
3. (c): Leaving his complaints of dyspnea alone likely would not result in spontaneous recovery. Catching a bad motor habit early allows for the most immediate and complete resolution of his inefficient breathing pattern. Left alone, the tension created with an ever-increasing chest breathing pattern may lead to difficulties with breath support for speech or even MTD. Weight loss would lead to ease in

diaphragmatic excursion but, on its own, may not resolve his dyspnea or inefficient breathing pattern.

The following video clips of abdominal breathing remedying dyspnea are available:

1. Use of education and cueing to achieve abdominal breathing in this 42-year-old patient (Video 13.1)

Case Study 2: Vocal Cord Dysfunction with Exercise

A 31-year-old female has experienced shortness of breath and occasional stridor with exercise since high school. She was initially treated with albuterol used as a pretreatment prior to exercise and for emergent use when symptomatic. Her symptoms did not improve with use of the inhaler, and occasionally, when using it for rescue purposes, her symptoms worsened. Methacholine challenge, exercise-induced bronchospasm (EIB) challenge, and PFT revealed no pulmonary involvement. She was then told to discontinue inhaler use. Laryngoscopy following EIB revealed moderate VCD characterized by almost full adduction of the vocal folds upon inhalation. Otherwise, her laryngeal structures were normal with no masses or signs of laryngeal irritation and normal vibratory pattern during phonation. She has a history of LPR and PND secondary to environmental allergies. She takes oral lansoprazole twice daily to control her reflux, completes nasal saline irrigation for PND control, and takes cetirizine for her allergies.

She notes her symptoms do not occur when using an elliptical trainer nor when playing softball. Instead, her symptoms are most significant when playing basketball and soccer. During the initial consultation, education on VCD is provided, as well as an introduction of release breathing. She implements the release breathing to practice, 5 reps, 20 times daily, and at times of symptom exacerbation. While she reports good symptom reversal, she does not have initial success in preventing her symptoms from occurring during soccer or basketball games.

An exercise challenge is performed with basketball as the patient was in the midst of an adult basketball league season. During a warm-up consisting of stretching and light jogging, the patient demonstrates the pursed lip breathing for exercise appropriately. No symptoms are reported during warm-up. Basketball-related activities including taking lay-ups and completing "suicide sprints" drills (see Fig. 13.10) take place. During the lay-up portion of the challenge, the patient implements PLB appropriately except for a brief observable breath hold upon jumping and releasing the ball toward the backboard. Within 1 min of this drill, she has triggered mild symptoms of tightness, rated as a "2 or 3" on a scale from 0–10. When asked, she notes not realizing the breath holding had occurred. When instructed to exhale via pursed lips upon her jump, she implements this appropriately and completes 5 min of lay-up drills with no symptoms reoccurring. She notes that typically, she would have significant symptoms at this point in a basketball practice.

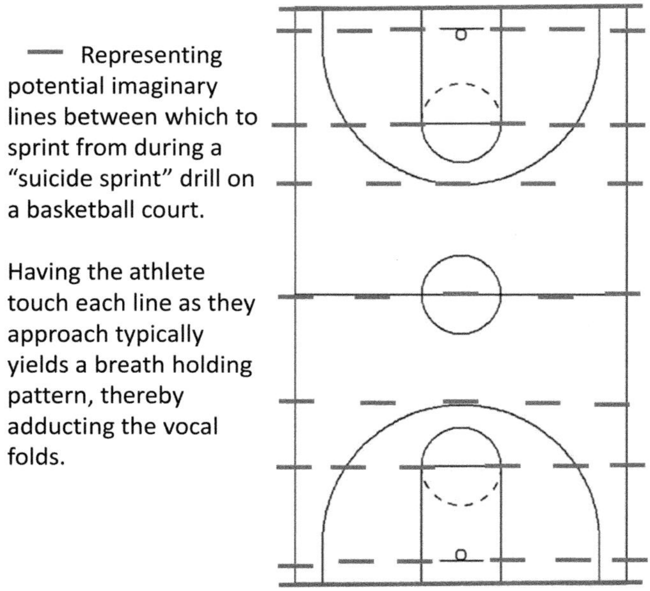

Fig. 13.10 Representing potential imaginary lines between which to sprint from during a "suicide sprint" drill on a basketball court

During suicide sprints (see Fig. 13.10), the patient is noted to have increased shoulder tension when poised at the starting line waiting for the call to "go." Although with increased awareness for breath holding during thoracic stabilization, she is observed to briefly hold her breath when stopping to touch each line. Additionally, as the drill progresses, increasing upper body tension is observed. She complains of VCD-associated symptoms within 30 s prior to completing one full cycle of the drill. Her symptoms trigger quickly to a "5" on the 0–10 severity scale. She is instructed to slow her pace and begin a tighter pursed lip breathing pattern consistent with the release breathing. She does so appropriately, and her symptoms reverse to a "1" after implementing these strategies for 45 s. Given clinician cueing to lower her shoulders before and during sprinting, and to breathe through the line-touch portion of the drill, she successfully controls her symptoms on the next trial of suicide sprints. Following this single follow-up appointment, the patient notes rare, minimal VCD occurring with basketball. Her symptoms briefly increase during springtime soccer, but after increasing her allergy control regimen per her allergist, her episodes of VCD again resolve.

Questions:

1. Why might this patient's VCD symptoms vary between sports/activities?
   (a) She is not invested in playing softball competitively, so her VCD is not triggered during this sport.

(b) The continuous running and need to quickly change direction during play that occurs in basketball and soccer make her symptoms harder to control.
(c) Her basketball and soccer coaches in high school must have been meaner than her softball coach, thereby evoking a psychological response during these sports.
(d) All of the above.
(e) None of the above.

2. Why did her symptoms worsen during soccer?

   (a) Her allergies likely worsened during the spring, and running outside on grass increased PND which irritated her VCD.
   (b) By the time her spring season started, she had forgotten how to do her breathing exercises for VCD control.
   (c) As a midfielder in soccer, she was running more than she had been in basketball.
   (d) All of the above.
   (e) None of the above.

3. Why may have the patient had increased shoulder tension during the suicide sprints but not on lay-ups?

   (a) The anticipation of the signal "Go" to start the sprints caused her increased tension.
   (b) Sprinting exacerbated her competitive nature which in turn made her more tense.
   (c) Bending down to touch each line created upper body tension.
   (d) All of the above.
   (e) None of the above.

Answers:

1. (b): Softball requires brief periods of running followed by periods of relative rest, allowing for recovery breathing between plays. The work of breathing is greater in basketball and soccer, and thoracic stabilization during plays is more likely. These factors make VCD harder to control and may encourage breath holding that exacerbates VCD. While increased outside pressure may lead to stress-induced VCD, assuming option C is a stretch in this case given the patient's control over VCD during subsequent basketball and soccer play.
2. (a): Increased irritation to the vocal folds occurs from PND or reflux, which can exacerbate her VCD. Resolution occurred via controlling her allergy-related PND. Patients are instructed to maintain daily practice of pursed lip breathing techniques and their implementation during exercise, so she should not have forgotten her techniques. Varying exertional levels can lead to some sports being more likely to trigger VCD than others. Repeat exercise challenges may be indicated when new sports are attempted. Based on her resolution of symptoms following increased allergy control, the VCD was not worsened by soccer alone.

3. (d): Given the observation of increased shoulder tension before the drill began indicates choice (a) while sprinting does appear to trigger highly competitive patients more so than other drills. Additionally, body movement requiring shoulder or arm flexion can induce upper body tension.

The following video clips of pursed lip breathing techniques for VCD are available:

1. This 31-year-old patient demonstrating release breathing (Video 13.2)
2. This 31-year-old patient learning pursed lip breathing for exercise (Video 13.3)
3. This 31-year-old patient implementing pursed lip breathing during a running warm-up (Video 13.4)
4. This 31-year-old patient using prevention and reversal while running on a treadmill (Video 13.5)
5. A 10-year-old female learning the release breathing (Video 13.6)
6. A 10-year-old female learning the relaxed throat breathing techniques (Video 13.7)

Case Study 3: Chronic Cough

A 34-year-old male has a history of chronic dry cough lasting 6 months. He believes his cough started as productive as a result of an upper respiratory infection. Following resolution of his URI, his cough has not resolved. In fact, he finds it to be progressively worsening. Chest CT and PFT testing rule out lung disease or infection. Sinus CT reveals pansinusitis, while laryngoscopy reveals signs of LPR including moderate laryngeal edema and hypertrophy of the posterior arytenoid process. Additionally, a small varix on the left vocal folds is noted (which is a prehemorrhagic sign of laryngeal trauma). Vocal fold motion during phonation and respiration is within normal limits. Given the sinus CT and laryngoscopy findings, he is started on twice daily nasal saline irrigation, nasal steroid spray, and oral omeprazole.

He reports no dyspnea but did endorse dysphonia ("My voice is deeper than usual and gets gravely") and chronic throat clearing. His cough does not awaken him and, while mostly occurring without a pattern, does appear to worsen upon exposure to cold air. He reports good daily liquid intake, mostly of caffeinated coffee (six cups per day), a glass of water, and one beer nightly. He was never a smoker.

Following thorough intake, the patient is encouraged to increase daily consumption of clear, decaffeinated, nonalcoholic beverages and to minimize caffeine and alcohol consumption. Also, he is instructed on cough control breathing exercise to be used:

1. To practice 5 reps, 20 times daily
2. To prevent an impending dry cough
3. To interrupt breakthrough dry cough
4. Before, during, and after exposure to cold air

Additionally, throat-clearing techniques are implemented, with the patient preferring the chin-tuck posture to swallow small sips of water prior to, and after, throat clearing.

He returns for follow-up two weeks later and reports a decrease in cough by 50% overall, with some success in interrupting breakthrough cough as well. He notes a decrease in his throat-clearing behavior and adds that his awareness for throat clearing has increased greatly. He further reports fewer occurrences of his raspy voice. After 6 weeks, he notes complete resolution of cough, throat clearing, and dysphonia.

Questions:

1. If his significant PND and reflux were being addressed, why pursue speech therapy?
   (a) It should not have been pursued. Treating these irritants is enough to stop a cough.
   (b) Because of the patient's voice complaints. Voice therapy should have occurred to remedy his raspy voice while PND and LPR treatment addressed his cough.
   (c) PND and LPR are never causes for a cough, so he must need speech therapy.
   (d) Due to the muscular makeup of the vocal folds, they can be trained or can learn to cough. This learned behavior will need addressing in addition to medically eliminating the laryngeal irritants.
   (e) All of the above.
2. Why was throat-clearing elimination added to the treatment?
   (a) The vocal folds are showing signs of trauma from forceful repeated adduction.
   (b) Throat clearing is vocally abusive and may be worsening his dysphonia.
   (c) Adding in swallowing techniques to prevent or minimize throat clearing also helps manage PND in the laryngopharynx.
   (d) Throat clearing will serve to perpetuate the adduction pattern of coughing.
   (e) All of the above.
3. Why was the patient told to improve his hydration habits?
   (a) Dehydrated laryngeal tissues will be less responsive to treatment.
   (b) Hydrated tissues will heal more easily.
   (c) Dry laryngeal tissues are more susceptible to further damage.
   (d) Increasing hydration will improve his vocal quality.
   (e) All of the above.

Answers:

1. (d): Once a cough has become chronic, solely treating the underlying causes may not resolve it. While the patient's voice complaints—and varix—would be a stand-alone reason for a speech therapy referral, completing voice therapy alone would not likely resolve his cough. That being said, if his voice complaints continued or worsened, he may have required voice therapy as an adjunct to treatment. By breaking the slamming adduction patterns of the vocal folds, they are retrained and allowed to heal.

2. (e): Controlling for throat clearing will decrease the damage to the vocal folds, improve the rapidity of healing, expedite the effects of the cough control breathing, and indirectly manage mucus irritating the larynx.
3. (e): Even without the patient exhibiting a prehemorrhagic sign of laryngeal trauma (i.e., the varix), chronic throat clearing is damaging to the vocal folds, will limit the retraining designed to encourage open relaxed vocal folds, and will keep his vocal quality compromised.

The following video clips of cough control breathing are available:

1. This 34-year-old patient discussing cough control breathing (Video 13.8)
2. This 34-year-old patient demonstrating cough control breathing to interrupt his cough (Video 13.9)

Conclusions

Speech therapy for the treatment of functional respiratory disorders serves as an efficient and effective means to resolving VCD, chronic cough, and dysfunctional breathing patterns. Education regarding the laryngeal and respiratory mechanisms is an essential first step in treating such disorders. Various speech therapy techniques are tailored to the individual patient's needs and trigger situations.

Acknowledgments Many of the ideas and literature included in this chapter have been discussed over the years with other members of the speech-language pathology team at National Jewish Health. I want to expressly thank Julie Bergquist, MA, CCC-SLP and Fiona Briggs, MA, CCC-SLP for these thoughtful discussions, collaboration in all educational endeavors, and for their editing eyes as this chapter was written.

References

1. Mathers-Schmidt BA. Paradoxical vocal fold motion: a tutorial on a complex disorder and the speech-language pathologist's role. Am J Speech Lang Pathol. 2001;10:111–25.
2. Brugman SM, Simons SM. Vocal cord dysfunction: don't mistake it for asthma. Phys Sports Med. 1995;26(5):63–85.
3. Perkner JJ, Fennelly KP, Balkissoon R, et al. Irritant-associated vocal cord dysfunction. J Occup Environ Med. 1998;40(2):136–43.
4. Murry T, Tabaee A, Aviv JE. Respiratory retraining of refractory cough and laryngopharyngeal reflux in patients with paradoxical vocal fold movement disorder. Laryngoscope. 2004;114(1):341–5.
5. Altman KW, Simpson CB, Amin MR, Abaza M, Balkissoon R, Casiano RR. Cough and paradoxical vocal fold motion. Otolaryngol Head Neck Surg. 2002;127(6):501–11.
6. Sandage MJ, Zelanzy SK. Paradoxical vocal fold motion in children and adolescents. Lang Speech Hear Serv Sch. 2004;35(4):353–62.
7. Vertigan AE, Theodoros DG, Gibson PG, Winkworth AL. Voice and upper airway symptoms in people with chronic cough and paradoxical vocal fold movement. J Voice. 2007;21(3):361–83.

8. Christopher KL, Wood 2nd RP, Eckert RC, Blager FB, Raney RA, Souhrada JF. Vocal-cord dysfunction presenting as asthma. N Engl J Med. 1983;308(26):1566–70.
9. Martin RJ, Blager FB, Gay ML, Wood 2nd RP. Paradoxic vocal cord motion in presumed asthmatics. Semin Respir Med. 1987;8:332–7.
10. Patterson DL, O'Connell EJ. Vocal dysfunction: what have we learned in 150 years? Insight Allergy. 1994;9(6):6–12.
11. Pitchenik AE. Functional laryngeal obstruction relieved by panting. Chest. 1991;100(5):1465–7.
12. Gallivan GJ, Hoffman L, Gallivan KH. Episodic paroxysmal laryngospasm: voice and pulmonary assessment and management. J Voice. 1996;10(1):93–105.
13. Adrianopoulos MV, Galliva GJ, Gallivan KH. PVCM, PVCD, EPL, and irritable larynx syndrome: what are we talking about and how do we treat it? J Voice. 2000;14(4):607–18.
14. Bahrainwala AH, Simon MR, Harrison DD, Toder D, Secord EA. Atypical expiratory flow volume curve in an asthmatic patient with vocal cord dysfunction. Ann Allergy Asthma Immunol. 2001;86(4):279–84.
15. Blager FB. Paradoxical vocal fold movement: diagnosis and management. Curr Opin Otolaryngol Head Neck Surg. 2000;8:180–3.
16. Hicks M, Brugman SM, Katial R. Vocal cord dysfunction/paradoxical vocal fold motion. Prim Care. 2008;35(1):81–103.
17. Goldman J, Muers M. Vocal cord dysfunction and wheezing. Thorax. 1991;46(6):401–4.
18. Vertigan AE, Theodoros DG, Gibson PG, Winkworth AL. Efficacy of speech pathology management for chronic cough: a randomised placebo controlled trial of treatment efficacy. Thorax. 2006;61(12):165–9.
19. Brown AB, McCartney N, Sale DG. Motor control and learning: a behavioral emphasis. Champaign, IL: Human Kinetic Publishers; 1990.
20. Verdolini K. Principles of skill aquisition applied to voice training. In: Acker M, Hampton B, editors. The vocal vision: views on voice. New York: Applause; 1997.
21. Stelmach GE, Requin J, editors. Frequent augmented feedback can degrade learning; evidence and interpretations. Tutorials in motor neuroscience. Boston, MA: Kluwer; 1991
22. Schmidt RA, Bjork RA. New conceptualizations practice: common principles and three paradigms suggest new concepts in training. Psychol Sci. 1992;3(4):207–17.
23. Rosenbaum DA, editor. Human motor control. San Diego, CA: Academic Press; 1991.
24. Singer RN. Motor learning and human performance; an application to motor skills and movement behaviors. New York: Macmillan; 1980.
25. Bahrainwala AH, Simon MR. Wheezing and vocal cord dysfunction mimicking asthma. Curr Opin Pulm Med. 2001;7(1):8–13.
26. Levin M. Vocal cord dysfunction complicating asthma. Curr Allergy Clin Immunol. 2003;16(1):12–4.
27. Van den Bergh O, Stegen K, Van Diest I, et al. Acquisition and extinction of somatic symptoms in response to odours: a pavlovian paradigm relevant to multiple chemical sensitivity. Occup Environ Med. 1999;56(5):295–301.
28. Murray DM, Lawler PG. All that wheezes is not asthma. Anaesthesia. 1998;53(10):1002–11.
29. Borer H, Hanni P, Schoenenberger RA. Vocal cord dysfunction: an important differential diagnosis of brittle asthma. Respiration. 2001;68(3):318.
30. Weiss SM, Lakshminarayan S. Acute inhalation injury. Clin Chest Med. 1994;15(1):103–16.
31. Blager FB, Gay ML, Wood RP. Voice therapy techniques adapted to treatment of habit cough: a pilot study. J Commun Disord. 1988;21(5):393–400.
32. Sandage M. Sniffs, gasps, and coughs; irritable larynx syndrome across the lifespan. The ASHA Leader. July 11, 2006;16–21
33. Volianitis S, McConnell AK, Koutedakis Y, McNaughton L, Backx K, Jones DA. Inspiratory muscle training improves rowing performance. Med Sci Sports Exerc. 2001;33(5):803–9.
34. Romer LM, McConnell AK, Jones DA. Inspiratory muscle fatigue in trained cyclists: effects of inspiratory muscle training. Med Sci Sports Exerc. 2002;34(5):785–92.
35. Mador MJ, Acevado FA. Effect of respiratory muscle fatigue on subsequent exercise performance. J Appl Physiol. 1991;70(5):2059–65.

36. Boutellier U. Respiratory muscle fitness and exercise endurance in healthy humans. Med Sci Sports Exerc. 1998;30(7):1169–72.
37. Kellerman BA, Martin AD, Davenport PW. Inspiratory strengthening effects on resistive load detection and magnitude estimation. Med Sci Sports Exerc. 2000;32(11):1859–67.
38. Williams JS, Wongsathikun J, Boon SM, Acevedo EO. Inspiratory muscle training fails to improve endurance capacity in athletes. Med Sci Sports Exerc. 2002;34(7):1194–8.
39. Mathers-Schmidt BA, Brilla LR. Inspiratory muscle training in exercise-induced paradoxical vocal fold motion. J Voice. 2005;19(4):635–44.
40. Sapienza CM, Brown J, Martin D, Davenport P. Inspiratory pressure threshold training for glottal airway limitation in laryngeal papilloma. J Voice. 1999;13(3):382–8.
41. Mador MJ. Respiratory muscle fatigue and breathing pattern. Chest. 1991;100(5):1430–5.
42. Lim TK. Vocal cord dysfunction presenting as bronchial asthma: the association with abnormal thoraco-abdominal wall motion. Singapore Med J. 1991;32(4):208–10.
43. Broaddus-Lawrence P, Treole K, McCabe RB, Allen RL, Toppin L. The effects of preventive vocal hygiene education on the habits and perceptual vocal characteristics of training singers. J Voice. 2000;14(1):68–71.
44. Roy N, Gray SD, Simon M, Dove H, Corbin-Lewis K, Stemple JC. An evaluation of the effects of two treatment approaches for teachers with voice disorders: a prospective randomised clinical trial. J Speech Hear Res. 2001;44(2):286–96.
45. Vertigan AE, Theodoros DG, Winkworth AL. Perceptual voice characteristics in chronic cough and paradoxical vocal fold movement. Folia Phoniatr Logop. 2007;59(5):256–67.

Chapter 14
Pharmacologic Therapy in Patients with Functional Respiratory Disorders

Charles R. Harris, Joseph F. Zastrow, and Ran D. Anbar

Abstract When a patient with a functional respiratory disorder does not improve in response to non-pharmacological interventions, the addition of pharmacological treatments may be considered. These treatments should be based on the patient's symptom severity, precipitating factors (such as exercise-induced vocal cord dysfunction), type of functional respiratory dysfunction, or presence of a concurrent additional psychological disorder(s). Treatments such as anticholinergic therapy, psychiatric medications, and heliox are appropriate in limited circumstances. This chapter also describes medications that frequently have been used in patients with functional respiratory disorders who have been misdiagnosed or who have concurrent organic respiratory disease. Important side effects of these medications are described that can overlap symptoms of functional respiratory disorders and thus complicate making the diagnosis. Case studies are presented that will challenge the reader to decide whether and which pharmacologic therapy should be utilized in the treatment of patients with functional respiratory disorders.

Keywords Botulinum toxin • Habit cough • Ipratropium bromide • Heliox • Lidocaine • Psychiatric medications • Vocal cord dysfunction

C.R. Harris
Department of Psychiatry, SUNY Upstate University Hospital, Syracuse, NY, USA

J.F. Zastrow
Primary Care Associates, Lake Norman, Mooresville, NC, USA

R.D. Anbar (✉)
Department of Pediatrics, SUNY Upstate Medical University, 750 East Adams St., 13210-1834, Syracuse, NY, USA
e-mail: anbarr@upstate.edu

R.D. Anbar (ed.), *Functional Respiratory Disorders: When Respiratory Symptoms Do Not Respond to Pulmonary Treatment*, Respiratory Medicine,
DOI 10.1007/978-1-61779-857-3_14, © Springer Science+Business Media, LLC 2012

Introduction

When a physician or clinical practitioner first evaluates a patient with wheezing, dyspnea, or other respiratory symptoms common in a functional respiratory disorder (FRD), typically, FRD is low in the differential diagnosis. Commonly, the symptoms may not even have been thought of as possibly stemming from an FRD. Ideally, a clinician should take a thorough history and develop a differential diagnosis ranging from most to least likely; however, in patients with symptoms resulting from an FRD, this typically is not the case. The low ranking of FRDs in the differential diagnosis reflects their apparent lesser importance to clinicians who are very concerned about misdiagnosing an "organic" etiology leading to harm as a result of an incorrect treatment plan.

Clinicians also consider the impact of a trial of medication therapy when treating a disease that is high in their differential diagnosis. For example, a patient may present as a result of sudden onset of dyspnea and wheezing after perfume exposure. A clinician might consider the possibility that the wheezing is a result of the chemical exposure as more important than psychologically induced wheezing that has been triggered by a recalled memory of a reaction to perfume exposure. The risk of not treating an allergic reaction appears *moderate*, and treatment with an inhaler is a simple solution. Conversely, failure to diagnose an FRD is associated with apparent *low* risk. Therefore, in this setting, the clinician is likely to prescribe a medication. A complicating result of this scenario is that often, patients with FRDs exhibit an improvement as a result of a placebo response to medication [1,2]. This apparent response to medicine reinforces the clinician's belief in the differential diagnosis; e.g., the patient becomes temporarily better, and both the clinician and patient attribute the improvement to the medication. Thus, the possibility of an FRD may not even be entertained. Unfortunately, this leads to a misdiagnosis resulting in application of an "incorrect treatment plan" that the clinician was attempting to avoid!

If the cause of wheezing in response to perfume exposure has in fact been created by the remembrance of the perfume coupled with a past repressed traumatic event, it brings up an interesting problem in the paradigm through which clinicians approach this symptom. Since psychological exploration is a relatively benign therapy that could result in a permanent resolution of symptoms, this would seem optimal to employ first. However, because of the clinician's time constraints and limited psychosocial training, fully engaging in this process usually is challenging [3]. Thus, non-pharmacologic alternatives are rarely considered first.

Our cultural reliance on external therapies and substances in particular and the expectation that doctors will prescribe them as primary therapy is another driving force resulting in inappropriate prescription of medications [4]. When such expectations are met, any side effects of the therapy render a medication, at least in part, an "active placebo" [5,6]. In this situation, the patient can interpret the side effect as demonstrating the efficacy of a medication, and this belief can help promote an improvement in the clinical condition, especially in the case of a patient with an FRD. This reinforces the reliance on external therapies rather than non-pharmacologic interventions that often depend on employment of internal resources.

Common clinical aphorisms are:

"When all else fails, take a history."
"If you can name it, you can treat it."

Both of these adages are important in assessing the interface of medicine use for organic disease and FRD. Often, a patient will have been through a number of medication trials before a detailed psychological history finally is obtained. Clinicians then will obtain an environmental, family, and social histories in an attempt to identify the cause of functional pulmonary problems. Insurance companies often pay only if a diagnosis can be coded. Hence, clinicians are pressed to label a patient with a diagnosis as soon as possible in order to apply a known treatment.

Patients with FRD issues who are seen in a primary care clinic almost invariably begin with a misdiagnosis and a trial of medication. These medications often help symptom control and can lead to a diagnosis; but many times, the results of a medication trial can hamper the diagnosis of an FRD. A common medical school axiom is, "Not all asthma wheezes, and not all that wheezes is asthma." A corollary should be, "Not all that responds to an inhaler is asthma." Many patients with FRD may find temporary relief in medications; virtually, all will have tried some medication, and some will be unwilling to discontinue medications even after identification of an FRD as the likely sole cause of their symptoms.

Although there are symptom codes such as "wheezing" (786.07), payment is structured to disease and not symptoms. Thus, a diagnosis such as "asthma" (393.90) is commonly applied. Now, the patient carries a label: He/she is "an asthmatic." If the patient improves with medication and later deteriorates as a result of a psychological process, it will be interpreted as a worsening of their asthma. A clinician may conclude that the treatment is ineffective and in reaction add more medications. These medicines can further cloud the true diagnosis with temporary symptom control. A polypharmacy regimen may result in significant side effects or worsened symptoms. For example, if anxiety is the reason for underlying FRD symptoms, using a beta agonist may worsen anxiety symptoms [7]. These increased anxiety-related symptoms could lead to the prescription of even more medications such as prednisone, which could lead to the development of further side effects, including even psychosis.

Pharmacotherapy in the treatment of FRDs is indicated only in particular situations. These will be discussed in Sect. I of this chapter. We will discuss the benefits and drawbacks of utilizing medications in this setting and provide guidance regarding their appropriate use. Section II describes medications that frequently have been used in patients with FRDs who have been misdiagnosed or who have concurrent organic respiratory disease. This will be especially helpful to practitioners who may not be familiar with commonly used respiratory medications. This section describes important side effects of these medications that can overlap symptoms of FRDs and thus complicate making the diagnosis. More detailed information regarding the use of these medications, particularly for the diagnosis of asthma, can be found in a variety of comprehensive texts and guidelines [8–10]. Section III presents case studies that will challenge the reader to decide whether and which pharmacologic therapy should be utilized in the treatment of patients with FRDs.

Section I: Pharmacologic Therapy for Functional Respiratory Disorders

The primary forms of treatment for FRDs are non-pharmacologic, including cognitive behavioral therapy (CBT, see Chap. 9), biofeedback (Chap. 10), breathing relaxation techniques (Chap. 11), hypnosis (Chap. 12), and speech therapy (Chap. 13). If the patient does not improve in response to non-pharmacological interventions, the addition of pharmacological treatments may be considered. These treatments should be based on the patient's symptom severity, precipitating factors (such as exercise-induced vocal cord dysfunction [VCD]), type of functional respiratory dysfunction, or presence of a concurrent additional psychological disorder(s). Although published data are limited to case reports and small clinical trials mostly involving VCD, some specific patients with FRDs may respond well to pharmacological treatments.

Pharmacological treatments that have been reported as useful for FRDs can be divided into five main subgroups:

Recommended for use in specific circumstances:

1. Anticholinergic therapy
2. Psychiatric medications
3. Heliox therapy

Not recommended for use:

1. Botulinum toxin
2. Lidocaine

Anticholinergic Therapy

Rationale

VCD (Chap. 6) has been described as presenting as two subtypes: (1) Spontaneous VCD (SVCD) occurs in the absence of any known triggers. (2) Exercise-induced VCD (EIVCD) occurs solely in the presence of strenuous activity. EIVCD has been reported to respond to anticholinergic therapy, while SVCD does not [11].

Mechanism of Action

EIVCD is thought to arise through stimulation of the vagal nerve [11]. As vagal nerve activity is driven by acetylcholine, application of an anticholinergic drug decreases this effect, with an associated improvement or resolution of VCD. Anticholinergic therapy may not be as efficacious in the treatment of SVCD because this condition might be triggered by central nervous system involvement that is mediated through other mechanisms, e.g., in a patient who develops VCD following a psychologically traumatic event [1].

Literature Review

Doshi [11] reported six patients with EIVCD that resolved after their use of ipratropium bromide before exercise. Of these six patients, two also had concomitant SVCD that was controlled following speech therapy. In our experience, use of once daily tiotropium bromide also was efficacious in the prevention of EIVCD in four patients.

Potential Side Effects

The side effects of inhaled anticholinergic drugs are mild, with dry mouth being the only commonly reported side effect [12].

Recommendation

We recommend that anticholinergics be considered as first-line therapy for EIVCD since their use before physical activity prevents onset of the symptom. This therapy does not necessitate disruption of the activity in order to employ interventions such as specialized breathing techniques. Relaxation techniques, such as achievable with hypnosis (Chap. 12) or speech therapy (Chap. 13), also can be applied prior to physical activity to prevent EIVCD. One disadvantage of anticholinergic therapy for EIVCD is creation of dependence on a medication that may not be necessary with the application of a non-pharmacologic approach. As EIVCD primarily is a disorder of youth, side effects of anticholinergic therapy are rarely a significant problem.

Psychiatric Medications

Rationale

The relationship between FRDs and psychological issues is complex. FRDs often have a psychological basis and present with psychological comorbidity. It has been estimated that up to 73% of patients with FRDs have a comorbid psychiatric condition [13,14]. Psychiatric disorders such as mood, anxiety, psychosomatic, and personality disorders can make the treatment of FRDs very difficult. For instance, patients with anxiety disorders may be resistant to first-line treatments such as behavioral therapy, speech therapy, biofeedback, or hypnosis because they feel too anxious to accept the absence of identifiable organic causes for their symptoms. For such patients, it may prove useful to temporarily treat coexisting psychiatric disorders using psychiatric medications.

Mechanism of Action

The psychiatric medications that have been reported to be useful in the treatment of FRDs fall into four classes:

- Antidepressants used to treat depression and anxiety
- Anxiolytics used to treat anxiety
- Antipsychotics for symptoms such as associated hallucinations and delusions
- Mood stabilizers for bipolar disorder involving both depression and mania

Typical antidepressants that have been used for FRDs include citalopram and venlafaxine, extended release. It should be emphasized that neither drug has been approved by the food and drug administration (FDA) for use in the treatment of FRDs [15]. Citalopram is a selective serotonin reuptake inhibitor (SSRI), while venlafaxine is a serotonin and norepinephrine reuptake inhibitor (SNRI). SSRIs increase availability of serotonin in the brain, and SNRIs also increase norepinephrine [15]. Both of these neurotransmitters are thought to ameliorate the symptoms of depression and anxiety gradually over time. It should be noted that recent studies regarding the treatment of mild or moderate depression have proposed that the effect of antidepressants is only marginally more effective than placebo [16].

Benzodiazepines are a commonly reported class of anxiolytic drugs that have been used in the treatment of FRDs [17]. These drugs are thought to decrease anxiety through decreasing neuronal activity, especially in the more emotionally reactive parts of the brain such as the amygdala [17]. This, in turn, decreases anxiety [15]. Benzodiazepines also have been postulated to attenuate the Kratschmer reflex, which is a protective laryngeal reflex that results in temporary closure of the vocal cords [18].

Haloperidol, an antipsychotic that has been reported to have been used in the treatment of FRDs, works by decreasing the activity of dopamine in the limbic structures of the brain, which decreases psychotic symptoms and is associated with a calming effect [15,19].

Lithium, the oldest mood stabilizer that remains in common use today, has an unknown mechanism of action, but likely stabilizes neuronal membranes via calcium-mediated mechanisms and promotes better neuronal plasticity [15].

Literature Review

There have been several case reports of patients with VCD who were treated successfully with psychiatric medications. In one case study, a woman who had been diagnosed with VCD via laryngoscopy also carried the diagnosis of asthma, chronic rhinosinusitis, gastroesophageal reflux disease, fructose intolerance, and obesity [14]. This patient had a history of major depressive disorder and anxiety that were treated with venlafaxine for 5 years, but not at the time of her development of VCD. She was followed by an allergist, pulmonologist, otolaryngologist, primary care, and speech therapist. The allergist referred her to a psychiatrist because the patient showed no improvement after instruction to avoid irritants and fumes that were believed to be the precipitating trigger for her VCD. She had been to the emergency room monthly and had been intubated twice prior to the psychiatric referral.

The patient was treated with combined psychotherapy and medication. She was treated with citalopram and showed no response. She then was switched to venlafaxine XR with only a partial response. Lithium was then added as an adjunct for depression [20]. The combination of psychotherapy, lithium, and venlafaxine was sufficient to provide remission of the anxiety, depression, and VCD. It appeared that the medication enabled the patient to gather insight and implement the suggested behavioral therapy such as relaxation techniques [14].

Another case report describes an 18-year-old man with a 10-day history of stridor, dyspnea, and hoarseness that disappeared when he spoke [21]. The patient also had a history of asthma. Upon initial presentation, the patient was treated for an exacerbation of asthma. However, he did not respond to inhaled bronchodilators, oxygen, and corticosteroids. The patient then was administered diazepam IV for anxiety because it was observed that his dyspnea subsided during sleep. Despite these treatments, his condition did not improve. A trial of continuous positive airway pressure (CPAP) was not tolerated due to neck pain and headache. A psychiatric consultation did not uncover underlying depression or anxiety, and it was suggested that the patient had a conversion disorder for which he was given haloperidol IV. The patient's symptoms resolved. However, haloperidol side effects of akathisia, restlessness, dizziness, and dystonic reactions prevented its long-term use. After the haloperidol was discontinued, the symptoms recurred [21].

In the anesthesiology literature, there have been a few case reports of individuals who were treated successfully with various benzodiazepines for VCD [18,22,23].

Potential Side Effects

Side effects are the main problem with use of psychiatric drugs in the treatment of FRDs. Most psychiatric drugs have an extensive list of possible side effects ranging from mild GI discomfort to lethal cardiac arrhythmias [24,25]. However, some psychiatric drugs are considered safer than others.

For instance, SSRI and SNRI generally are considered to have a safe side-effect profile, which includes development of gastrointestinal discomfort, dry mouth, ejaculatory dysfunction, increased anxiety, headaches, tremor, and sweating. However, these drugs also are associated with rare but serious side effects including serotonin syndrome, neuroleptic malignant syndrome, akathisia-like movements, and seizures [24]. The risk of suicide is yet another rare side effect of antidepressant therapy, which is increased in teenagers [26].

Benzodiazepines have a relatively safe side-effect profile, which can include drowsiness, ataxia, amnesia, dizziness, and confusion [17]. However, this class of drug is notorious for its abuse and overdose potential, dependence, paradoxical agitation, respiratory suppression, and withdrawal symptoms [26].

Lithium has a very complex side-effect profile affecting many different organ systems. Lithium can cause nausea, thyroid damage, diarrhea, weight gain, tremors, kidney damage, polyuria, polydipsia, seizures, ataxia, coma, and death can occur [25]. This is a class D drug, as it is associated with severe teratogenic effects during pregnancy. Lithium has a narrow therapeutic window, and an overdose can be fatal. Therefore, lithium therapy requires frequent monitoring of lithium levels in addition to monitoring of thyroid, cardiac, and kidney function.

Haloperidol and other antipsychotic drugs also have a very extensive side-effect profile consisting of metabolic syndrome, arrhythmias, neuroleptic malignant syndrome, dystonia, parkinsonism, akathisia, severe extrapyramidal symptoms, tardive dyskinesia, galactorrhea, drowsiness, and sudden death [25].

Recommendation

Psychiatric drugs can be beneficial for some patients with FRDs who are refractory to first-line non-pharmacological treatments, but the severity of their associated side-effect profiles limits their use. We believe that in the absence of a primary psychiatric disorder for which psychotropic medication is indicated, the long-term use of such medications in order to treat FRDs should be reserved as a treatment of last resort.

Heliox Therapy

Rationale

Heliox gas has been described as a safe and effective means of alleviating stridor associated with acute upper airway obstruction including VCD. In severe cases, it can help decrease patients' anxiety that had developed as a result of their associated respiratory distress.

Mechanism of Action

Heliox is a gaseous mixture of 20–40% oxygen and helium [27]. During an episode of VCD, the reduced gas viscosity of the oxygen/helium mixture causes reduced airflow turbulence as compared to ambient air or oxygen. This is associated with reduced resistance to gas flow leading to a reduction in the airway obstruction during an episode of VCD [27,28].

Literature Review

Five cases have been published regarding use of heliox in the treatment of VCD [27]. In four of the cases, the VCD symptoms improved. In the fifth, a patient with concomitant asthma and VCD did not improve until he was taught laryngeal relaxation techniques.

Side Effects

There are no dangerous side effects reported with the use of heliox [29].

Recommendation

The use of heliox generally should be limited to one-time "reliever" therapy to alleviate acute symptoms of VCD. Recurrent use of heliox may be counterproductive in that it might discourage patients from seeking non-pharmacologic therapy for VCD, such as hypnosis or speech therapy. In addition, heliox is difficult to administer outside of the medical setting and is costly. Also, it should be noted that if heliox is used in cases of stridor due to causes other than VCD (e.g., an organic upper airway pathology such as glottic or subglottic narrowing), the symptoms could be masked by the effects of heliox [27], which could delay the diagnosis and application of definitive therapy, and potentially put the patient at risk.

Botulinum Toxin

Rationale

Botulinum toxin injected into the vocal cords causes paralysis of the cords, which resolves the vocal cord adduction that causes symptoms in VCD [30]. It can also reduce irritation of the vocal cords that otherwise can perpetuate habit cough [31].

Mechanism of Action

Botulinum toxin inhibits the release of acetylcholine by neurons. This causes a flaccid paralysis of the affected muscles [32]. Typically, the effect of injected botulinum toxin wears off after 3–4 months [33].

Literature Review

There has been only one case report of permanent resolution of VCD following treatment with use of botulinum injection. In this case, the patient was injected once and had full recovery with the aid of psychotherapy and speech therapy [34]. In two other cases, botulinum injection for VCD yielded relief of symptoms for only 1 week and for 4 months [35,36]. In one instance, use of botulinum injection in the treatment of VCD was followed by the development of severe stridor for which the patient was administered IV midazolam that resulted in instantaneous resolution of the symptoms [23]. One report cites three cases of children with habit cough whose vocal cords were injected with botulinum toxin without achievement of permanent relief [31].

Potential Side Effects

Side effects associated with administration of botulinum toxin into the vocal cords include development of dyspnea, dysphagia, and severe stridor [23,37].

Recommendation

Given that botulinum toxin does not appear to reliably resolve FRDs, the likely need to readminister it every few months, its potential morbidity, its associated administration costs, and availability of other effective therapies for FRDs, we recommend against its use.

Lidocaine

Rationale

Inhaled lidocaine has been used in the treatment of habit cough in conjunction with other non-pharmacologic techniques. Application of nebulized lidocaine to the trachea may decrease the sensation that triggers the cough, thus allowing the patient time to master the non-pharmacologic techniques that can provide definitive treatment.

Mechanism of Action

Lidocaine decreases neuronal discharge by decreasing sodium movement into the nerve, thus leading to localized anesthesia [38].

Literature Review

Lokshin et al. [39] described nine patients with habit cough who were treated with a combination of lidocaine and suggestion therapy. The patients were administered nebulized lidocaine as a distractor during 15-min suggestion therapy sessions during which the cough ceased. In long-term follow-up (up to 9 years), six of seven patients reported complete resolution of their symptoms; one reported sporadic cough that was controlled through use of self-suggestion. Sherman [40] describes a case of an eight-year-old boy who after one treatment with nebulized lidocaine experienced complete remission of his habit cough.

Potential Side Effects

Side effects of nebulized lidocaine include dyspnea, chest tightness, and bronchoconstriction [41].

Recommendation

As non-pharmacologic therapy alone usually is effective in the treatment of habit cough, use of lidocaine probably is not of additional benefit. Therefore, we recommend against its routine use.

Section II: Medications Used with Misdiagnosed FRDs or Concurrent Organic Disease

Pulmonary medications are commonly used to treat patients prior to their diagnosis with an FRD, or to treat an organic respiratory disease that occurs concurrently with an FRD. These medications fall into six classes:

1. Beta-2 agonists
2. Corticosteroid inhalers
3. Leukotriene modifiers
4. Methylxanthines
5. Oral corticosteroids
6. Cough suppressants: narcotic and non-narcotic

It should be emphasized that none of these medications are effective in the treatment of an FRD. However, organic respiratory disease often improves with some of these medications, which can delay or prevent recognition of a concurrent FRD. Further, clinicians should be alert to the possibility that the side-effect profiles of some of these medications can overlap and thus be confused with symptoms that can be associated with an FRD.

Beta-2 Agonists

The bronchial tree has small smooth muscles that surround the airway tubes, which regulate their closure, termed "bronchoconstriction," or opening, termed "bronchodilation" [42].

Beta-2 agonists relax the muscles around the airways. This is useful therapeutically to open tightened airways that can occur as a result of asthma attack or chronic obstructive pulmonary disease. Beta-2 agonists are most commonly inhaled, but may be administered orally or rarely intravenously or intramuscularly.

The side effects of beta-2 agonists include stimulation of other beta receptors commonly found throughout the body. Thus, agitation, anxiety, restlessness, tremor, and tachycardia are common side effects, which can be confused with symptoms arising as a result of psychological issues associated with an FRD. Inhaled beta-2 agonists at recommended doses have few side effects [42].

Examples of short-acting beta-2 agonists (yielding 4–6 h of bronchodilation) include albuterol (with brand names such as ProAir, Proventil, Ventolin), levalbuterol (Xopenex), pirbuterol (Maxair), and terbutaline (Brethaire). Examples of long-acting beta-2 agonists (12 h) include formoterol (Foradil) and salmeterol (Serevent).

Corticosteroids Inhalers

Corticosteroid inhalers are medications that when used regularly suppress and control the underlying inflammation that is the principle driving force in persistent asthma.

At the recommended doses, there are few side effects with these medicines [43].

Examples of corticosteroid inhalers include beclomethasone (Qvar), budesonide (Pulmicort), ciclesonide (Alvesco), flunisolide (AeroBid), fluticasone (Flovent), and mometasone (Asmanex).

Corticosteroid inhalers also are available in combination with long-acting beta-2 agonists. Examples of these include budesonide/formoterol (Symbicort), fluticasone/salmeterol (Advair), and mometasone/formoterol (Dulera).

Leukotriene Modifiers

Medications in the leukotriene modifier category help prevent asthma or allergy symptoms by blocking the action of leukotrienes. When stimulated, leukotriene receptors cause bronchial muscle closure and airway mucous formation.

Side effects with leukotriene modifiers are few [10].

Examples of leukotriene modifiers include montelukast (Singulair), zafirlukast (Accolate), and zileuton (Zyflo).

Methylxanthines

Three important classes of methylxanthines are caffeine, theobromine, and theophylline (including its synthetic analog aminophylline). Their mechanism of action is unknown [10].

These medicines are similar to caffeine, and therefore, side effects include nausea, vomiting, jitteriness/tremulousness, insomnia, anxiety, palpitations, and heart irregularities [10]. These side effects can mimic many symptoms associated with

FRDs. Because of the advent of improved therapies for obstructive pulmonary disease, this class of medicine is not used with great regularity any longer.

Examples of theophylline oral tablet/capsule brands include Quibron, Slo-Bid, Theo-24, Theo-Dur Sprinkles, Theo-Dur, and Uniphyl.

Oral Corticosteroids

Oral corticosteroids are potent anti-inflammatory agents that are used in the acute setting for moderate-to-severe flare-ups of obstructive lung disease that are poorly responsive to bronchodilators.

Long-term use of oral corticosteroids can contribute to hyperglycemia (high blood sugars), especially in patients with a predisposition to diabetes mellitus, mood disturbances, psychosis, high blood pressure, cataracts, loss of bone density, and increased susceptibility to infections [43].

Examples of oral corticosteroid tablets include methylprednisolone (Medrol) and prednisone. Oral corticosteroids in liquid form include prednisolone (Orapred, Pediapred, Prelone) and prednisone (Deltasone).

Cough Suppressants: Narcotic and Non-narcotic

Cough suppressants can be divided into two major classes: central acting (in the brain) and peripheral acting medications. Central acting medications consist primarily of narcotics (such as codeine) and dextromethorphan. Peripheral acting medications include guaifenesin and benzonatate [44,45].

The side-effect profile of narcotic central acting cough suppressants includes dependency, respiratory depression, sedation, nausea, and constipation [44,45]. Side effects associated with peripheral acting cough suppressants include nausea, vomiting, hives, and abdominal pain [46].

Examples of cough suppressant brands include benzonatate (Tessalon Perles, Zonatuss) and guaifenesin (Mucinex, Tussin, a component of DayQuil mucus control and Robitussin chest congestion).

Section III: Case Studies

Case 1: Cough

A 13-year-old girl presents with a persistent nonproductive "honking" cough. The cough started in association with an upper respiratory infection 6 months ago, changed in character from "quiet" to "honking" 2 weeks after its onset, and has persisted despite resolution of the other URI symptoms. The patient reports that a “tickling” in the throat causes her to cough. She denies other associated symptoms such as fever, rhinorrhea, wheezing, or heartburn. The mother reports that the cough is not present at night. The patient was prescribed three different antibiotics that she took as directed, without relief. The family has tried throat lozenges, diphenhydramine, guaifenesin, and speech therapy (Chap. 13), which have not helped. There are no new house pets, or changes in the patient’s diet. Notably, the patient’s mother remarried around the time of the cough onset. The patient’s physical examination is normal.

Questions:

1. The most likely diagnosis for this girl is:
   (a) Chronic bronchitis
   (b) Habit cough
   (c) Laryngeal carcinoma
   (d) Influenza
   (e) Allergic rhinitis
2. All of the following would be appropriate for evaluating this patient *except*:
   (a) Laryngoscopy
   (b) CBC with differential
   (c) Allergy evaluation
   (d) Chest X-ray
   (e) Lung biopsy
3. Which of the following therapies is most likely to be effective in this case?
   (a) Guaifenesin and codeine cough suppressant
   (b) Another trial of speech therapy
   (c) Hypnotherapy
   (d) An empiric trial of medications for gastroesophageal reflux
   (e) No therapy, as cough should improve without treatment

Answers:

1. (b): The characteristic “honking” cough, throat “tickle,” absence of the cough during sleep, and recent change in family dynamics (the mother’s remarriage) are consistent with a diagnosis of habit cough (Chap. 5). Although the child presents with a chronic cough after experiencing an upper respiratory infection, the diagnosis of chronic bronchitis can be excluded by the facts that the patient’s cough subsides with sleep and absence of sputum production. Influenza is unlikely to persist for half a year. Laryngeal carcinoma is unlikely to occur in a 13-year-old. Allergic rhinitis presents with sneezing, nasal congestion, and/or rhinorrhea [47], which are not present in this case.

2. (e): A laryngoscopy would be reasonable to evaluate for an upper airway mass or foreign body that might be triggering the cough. A CBC with differential would be useful in evaluating for infectious causes of cough. An allergy evaluation would be useful to evaluate for a possible allergic trigger. A chest X-ray would be helpful for excluding pulmonary abnormalities that could be associated with persistent cough such as peribronchial cuffing related to asthma, or findings consistent with tuberculosis or interstitial lung disease. A lung biopsy would be inappropriate without radiographic demonstration of lung pathology that would warrant such an intervention, e.g., an interstitial lung disease pattern.
3. (c): Hypnotherapy has been shown as very effective in the treatment of habit cough. Guaifenesin and codeine are ineffective in its treatment. Speech therapy is not a usual therapy for habit cough and already failed in this patient. The patient reports no symptoms suggestive of gastroesophageal reflux. Without therapy, habit cough can persist for years [39].

Case 2: Shortness of Breath

A 17-year-old girl presents with a history of shortness of breath when she engages in competitive cross-country meets. Her respiratory symptoms typically begin after she has run for 5 min and are associated with difficulty with inhalation and an associated soft inspiratory "squeak." The patient reports no associated cyanosis, headaches, tremors, chest pain, palpitations, paresthesia (tingling or numbness in extremities), nausea, or shakiness. When her dyspnea occurs, the girl first tries to fight through the sensation, slows her running, and often has to stop for 5–10 min until her symptoms resolve. When she starts running again, she again often develops her symptoms.

The girl initially was diagnosed with asthma by her primary care provider, but has failed trials of pre-exercise-inhaled albuterol, budesonide/formoterol inhalation therapy, and montelukast. The girl has no history of prolonged coughing or wheezing in association with upper respiratory infections. She recalls that at the beginning of the school year, she was tossing popcorn in the air and tried to catch it in her mouth when she choked on one kernel and then coughed it up. She has a strong family history of asthma and anxiety.

She is an elite athlete who has been recruited for colleges as a result of her success with running during her high school sophomore and junior years.

Questions:

1. The diagnosis for this girl most likely is:

   (a) Congenital tracheomalacia (floppy airway)
   (b) Exercise-induced asthma

(c) Foreign body aspiration
(d) Panic and hyperventilation
(e) VCD

2. All of the following would be appropriate for evaluating this patient *except*:

   (a) Laryngoscopy during exercise
   (b) Laryngoscopy at rest
   (c) Pulmonary function testing during exercise
   (d) Pulmonary function testing at rest
   (e) Chest X-ray

3. Appropriate interventions for this girl include all of the following *except*:

   (a) Hypnotherapy
   (b) Inhalation of heliox before track meets
   (c) Speech therapy
   (d) Use of ipratropium bromide by inhalation before competitive races
   (e) (b) and (d)

Answers:

1. (e): In the setting of a high-achieving female athlete, VCD is the most common cause of exercise-associated dyspnea, especially given her difficulties during inhalation (Chap. 6). A congenital laryngeal lesion would likely have caused symptoms from early childhood. An inhaled foreign body and asthma would not cause symptoms only during competitive meets. Further, asthma does not cause difficulty during inhalation. This girl does not report symptoms consistent with hyperventilation such as tremors, palpitations, or paresthesia.
2. (e): Even though the patient has no symptoms at rest, she may be found to have an abnormal laryngoscopic examination or pulmonary function that could guide therapy. However, patients with VCD typically demonstrate adduction of the vocal cords with inhalation and flattening of their inspiratory loop during pulmonary function testing only when they are symptomatic. Thus, this patient may benefit from evaluation during and immediately after exercise that triggers her symptoms. A chest X-ray is not indicated as the patient's symptoms are suggestive of an upper airway process, and thus an X-ray of the chest is unlikely to demonstrate an abnormality.
3. (b): EIVCD responds to hypnotherapy, speech therapy, and pretreatment with ipratropium bromide. An advantage of learning self-hypnosis is that the patient can generalize its use for some other issues, if necessary (e.g., improving test anxiety or enhancement of her athletic performance). Use of heliox has not been demonstrated to prevent VCD, and its administration in the non-urgent care setting is impractical because of logistical and financial considerations.

Case 3: Chest Pain

A 50-year-old obese man is rushed to the emergency department for the fourth time in half a year with complaints of severe chest pain, palpitations, sweating, and tremor. On each occasion, he has feared for his life because he has believed he was suffering from a heart attack. Each time, his medical work-up revealed no acute physical cause of his symptoms. His electrocardiograms and chest X-rays were normal. He was diagnosed with anxiety.

The patient smoked two packs of cigarettes a day for 30 years, until quitting after his first trip to the emergency department this year. He is known to have high serum cholesterol, but has not been able to tolerate long-term use of a statin drug because he had developed a neuropathy as a side effect. He has been told that he has prediabetes, borderline hypertension, and a fatty liver. He reports that usually, it takes him 1–2 h to fall asleep, and typically, he awakens multiple times at night and has difficulty falling back asleep. The patient has no intrusive thoughts or compulsive behaviors. A sleep study did not demonstrate obstructive apnea.

The patient's paternal grandfather and father both died of myocardial infarctions between the ages of 40 and 50.

The patient lost his job 9 months ago and since then has stayed mostly at home, where he watches many hours of television every day. He has not spoken much with his wife for the past half year. He has not looked for a new job because he has stated that no one wants to hire someone his age. He refuses to see a counselor.

Questions:

1. In addition to anxiety, this patient also demonstrates symptoms of:
   (a) Depression
   (b) Malingering
   (c) Obsessive compulsive disorder
   (d) Selective mutism as a result of his neuropathy
   (e) Transient ischemic attacks
2. All of these patient's symptoms might be considered functional *except*:
   (a) Anxiety
   (b) Chest pain
   (c) Diaphoresis
   (d) Tremor
   (e) None of the above (all of his symptoms could be considered functional)
3. Appropriate therapy for this patient includes all of the following *except*:
   (a) Ativan, nightly
   (b) CBT, weekly
   (c) Exercise program

(d) Selective norepinephrine reuptake inhibitor (SNRI), daily
(e) SSRI, daily

Answers:

1. (a): The patient has sleeping difficulties, has become socially withdrawn, and also demonstrates hopelessness and worthlessness concerning his work prospects. All of these symptoms are associated with depression [48]. The patient also has a significant life event, i.e., loss of job, which is a risk factor for the development of depression [48]. The patient has no intrusive thoughts or compulsive behavior indicative of obsessive-compulsive disorder. The patient has no external incentives to suggest malingering (Chap. 1). The patient's decreased verbal interaction with wife likely is a manifestation of decreased interest in his relationship with his wife, which is a symptom of depression rather than of selective mutism. The patient's symptoms and exam findings do not suggest transient ischemic attack.
2. (a): Anxiety is a psychiatric diagnosis. Functional symptoms can be defined as physical complaints that do not have an identifiable physiologic cause.
3. (a): Nightly use of Ativan would cause dependence and not be helpful in the treatment of this patient's depression. All of the other options may be appropriate. Further, concurrent use of CBT, exercise, and pharmacotherapy likely would be more effective in the treatment of this patient than any of these therapies used alone.

Case 4: Asthma

A 12-year-old with severe asthma has required chronic use of systemic steroids for nearly 10 years in order to control her asthma symptoms [49]. She was diagnosed with asthma at a year of age when she presented with recurrent coughing, wheezing, and rapid breathing associated with upper respiratory tract infections. She responded to use of bronchodilator therapy during her acute illnesses. However, because of her frequent exacerbations, she was started on inhaled steroids by the time she was 2 years old. Despite this, she continued to develop severe exacerbations of her asthma for which she required multiple visits to emergency departments and frequent hospitalizations including intensive care.

As a result of the severity of her asthma, the patient was given frequent courses of oral prednisone that controlled her symptoms, but within a few days to weeks, her symptoms recurred. Therefore, she was started on therapy with chronic oral steroids that kept her symptoms under control.

By the time she was 10 years old, the patient already had been hospitalized 14 times because of her asthma, including five times in intensive care. During her one hospitalization, it was noted that the patient was anxious, and she was referred for evaluation by a psychiatrist who recommended family therapy. The patient and her parents participated in ten therapy sessions but did not feel this was of benefit and therefore stopped.

At 12 years of age, the patient reported that she was short of breath frequently, despite her chronic use of oral and inhaled steroids. She reported that she needed to use her inhaled bronchodilator at least four times daily for her shortness of breath. She said that she always was worried that her asthma could flare severely enough that she would require yet another hospitalization, or even place her life in danger. As a result of side effects of her steroid therapy, she was short and obese.

The patient was an only child, whose parents were very concerned about her health.

Questions:

1. Evidence that this patient's asthma may have been complicated by anxiety includes:
   (a) Her frequent need for bronchodilator therapy
   (b) Her need for use of chronic oral prednisone
   (c) Her multiple hospitalizations
   (d) Her expressed fear that she might develop a severe asthma exacerbation
   (e) Her complaint of frequent shortness of breath
2. The patient's development of anxiety in this setting likely was the result of:
   (a) A common response in the setting of a chronic illness
   (b) Steroid psychosis
   (c) Participation in family therapy
   (d) Attention-seeking behavior
   (e) A psychiatric disorder related to her parents' excessive concern about her health
3. Appropriate first-line interventions for this patient include all of the following *except*:
   (a) Biofeedback
   (b) CBT
   (c) Hypnotherapy
   (d) Relaxation techniques
   (e) Treatment with an SSRI

Answers:

1. (d): All of the other options could arise as a result of severe asthma without associated anxiety.
2. (a): Anxiety frequently develops in patients with asthma as a result of their learning to associate asthma exacerbations with unpleasant outcomes. Anxiety does not typically occur as a side effect of corticosteroid therapy. It can occur as a result of bronchodilator therapy, especially if the medication is administered systemically. Parental anxiety often influences their children's psychological reactions, but this does not mean that the children are suffering from a psychiatric disorder. The

patient's anxiety led to the recommendation for family therapy. Thus, family therapy was not its cause.

3. (e): An SSRI should be used in this setting as a last resort, as all of the other options are likely to yield a significant improvement in the patient's anxiety and be associated with decreased dependence on pharmacotherapy.

Conclusions

The initial and most important action in the management of patients with FRDs is obtaining a good patient history and physical exam that helps identify the disorder and exclude other possible causes. Once the diagnosis has been made, definitive treatment with non-pharmacological interventions should begin. As the patient improves, medications that had been initiated to treat other suspected respiratory conditions may be decreased if there is a concomitant organic respiratory disorder, or discontinued if the FRD has occurred in isolation.

If the patient with an FRD presents in acute distress or is unresponsive to non-pharmacological interventions, certain drugs such as psychiatric medications or heliox can be used temporarily to augment treatment. In the case of EIVCD, treatment with an anticholinergic agent prior to exercise often is useful.

References

1. Leo RJ, Konakanchi R. Psychogenic respiratory distress: a case of paradoxical vocal cord dysfunction and literature review. Prim Care Comp J Clin Psychiatry. 1999;1(2):39–46.
2. Kellman RM, Leopold DA. Paradoxical vocal cord motion: an important cause of stridor. Laryngoscope. 1982;92(1):58–60.
3. Committee on Psychosocial Aspects of Child and Family Health. American Academy of Pediatrics. The new morbidity revisited: a renewed commitment to the psychosocial aspects of pediatric care. Pediatrics. 2001;108(5):1227–30.
4. Watson RL, Dowell SF, Jayaraman M, Keyserling H, Kolczak M, Schwartz B. Antimicrobial use for pediatric upper respiratory infections: reported practice, actual practice, and parent beliefs. Pediatrics. 1999;104(6):1251–7.
5. Rubin LC. Merchandising madness: pills, promises, and better living through chemistry. J Pop Cult. 2004;38(2):369–83.
6. Thomson R. Side effects and placebo amplification. Br J Psychiatry. 1982;140:64–8.
7. Coffman KL, Levenson JL. Lung Disease. In: Levenson JL, editor. Textbook of psychosomatic medicine, Chapter 20. Washington, DC: American Psychiatric Publishing Inc.; 2005.
8. Kaminsky DA. Asthma. In: Hanley ME, Welsh CH, editors. Current diagnosis & treatment in pulmonary medicine, Chapter 6. New York: McGraw-Hill; 2003.
9. Expert panel report 3: Guidelines for the diagnosis and management of asthma (EPR–3 2007). NIH Publication No. 08-5846. Bethesda, MD: U.S. Department of Health and Human Services; National Institutes of Health; National Heart, Lung, and Blood Institute; National Asthma Education and Prevention Program, 2007.
10. Barnes PJ. Pulmonary pharmacology. In: Bruton LL, Chabner BA, Knollmann BC, editors. Goodman & Gilman's The pharmacological basis of therapeutics, Chapter 36. 12th ed. New York, NY: McGraw-Hill; 2011.

11. Doshi DR, Weinberger MM. Long-term outcome of vocal cord dysfunction. Ann Allergy Asthma Immunol. 2006;96(6):794–9.
12. Brown JH, Laiken N. Muscarinic receptor agonist and antagonists. In: Bruton LL, Chabner BA, Knollmann BC, editors. Goodman & Gilman's The pharmacological basis of therapeutics, Chapter 9. 12th ed. New York, NY: McGraw-Hill; 2011.
13. Newman KB, Mason UG, Schmaling KB. Clinical features of vocal cord dysfunction. Am J Respir Crit Care Med. 1995;152(4 Pt 1):1382–6.
14. Thurston NL, Fiedorowicz JG. Improvement of paradoxical vocal cord dysfunction with integrated psychiatric care. Psychosomatics. 2009;50(3):282–4.
15. Stahl SM. Stahl's essential psychopharmacology. 3rd ed. New York, NY: Cambridge University Press; 2008.
16. Kirsch I. Antidepressants and the placebo response. Epidemiol Psichiatr Soc. 2009;18(4): 318–22.
17. Mihic SJ, Harris RA. Hypnotics and sedatives. In: Bruton LL, Chabner BA, Knollmann BC, editors. Goodman & Gilman's The pharmacological basis of therapeutics, Chapter 17. 12th ed. New York, NY: McGraw-Hill; 2011.
18. Roberts KW, Crnkovic A, Steiniger JR. Post-anesthesia paradoxical vocal cord motion successfully treated with midazolam. Anesthesiology. 1998;89(2):517–9.
19. Bo P, Ongini E, Giorgetti A, Savoldi F. Synchronization of the EEG and sedation induced by neuroleptics depend upon blockade of both D1 and D2 dopamine receptors. Neuropharmacology. 1988;27(8):799–805.
20. Bauer M, Adli M, Bschor T, et al. Lithium's emerging role in the treatment of refractory major depressive episodes: augmentation of antidepressants. Neuropsychobiology. 2010;62(1):36–42.
21. Karaman E, Duman C, Alimoqlu Y, Islidak H, Oz F. Paradoxical vocal cord motion—haloperidol usage in acute attack treatment. J Craniofac Surg. 2009;20(5):1602–4.
22. Tousignant G, Kleiman SJ. Functional stridor diagnosed by the anaesthetist. Can J Anaesth. 1992;39(3):286–9.
23. Baldwin MK, Benumof JL. Paradoxical vocal cord movement: a unique case of occurrence and treatment. Anesthesiology. 2007;107(2):359.
24. O'Donnell JM, Shelton RC. Drug therapy of depression and anxiety disorders. In: Bruton LL, Chabner BA, Knollmann BC, editors. Goodman & Gilman's The pharmacological basis of therapeutics, Chapter 15. 12th ed. New York, NY: McGraw-Hill; 2011.
25. Meyer JM. Pharmacotherapy of psychosis and mania. In: Bruton LL, Chabner BA, Knollmann BC, editors. Goodman & Gilman's The pharmacological basis of therapeutics, Chapter 16. 12th ed. New York, NY: McGraw-Hill; 2011.
26. Strahl NR. Clinical study guide for the oral boards in Psychiatry. 3rd ed. Washington DC: American Psychiatric Publishing, Inc; 2009.
27. Weir M. Vocal cord dysfunction mimics asthma and may respond to heliox. Clin Pediatr. 2002;41(1):37–41.
28. Patel PM, Patel HH, Roth DM. General anesthetics and therapeutic gases. In: Bruton LL, Chabner BA, Knollmann BC, editors. Goodman & Gilman's The pharmacological basis of therapeutics, Chapter 19. 12th ed. New York, NY: McGraw-Hill; 2011.
29. Gupta VK, Cheifetz IM. Heliox administration in the pediatric intensive care units: an evidence-based review. Pediatr Crit Care Med. 2005;6(2):204–11.
30. Tilles SA. Vocal cord dysfunction in children and adolescents. Curr Allergy Asthma Rep. 2003;3(6):467–72.
31. Sipp AJ, Haver KE, Masek BJ, Hartnick CJ. Botulinum toxin A: a novel adjunct treatment for debilitating habit cough in children. Ear Nose Throat J. 2007;86(9):570–2.
32. Hibbs RE, Zambon AC. Agents acting at the neuromuscular junction and autonomic ganglia. In: Bruton LL, Chabner BA, Knollmann BC, editors. Goodman & Gilman's The pharmacological basis of therapeutics, Chapter 11. 12th ed. New York, NY: McGraw-Hill; 2011.
33. Scheinberg A. Clinical use of botulinum toxin. Austral Prescr. 2009;32(2):39–42.
34. Maillard I, Schweizer V, Broccard A, Duscher A, Liaudet L, Schaller MD. Use of botulinum toxin type A to avoid tracheal intubation or tracheostomy in severe paradoxical vocal cord movement. Chest. 2000;118(3):874–7.

35. Vlahakis NE, Patel AM, Maragos NE, Beck KC. Diagnosis of vocal cord dysfunction: the utility of spirometry and plethysmography. Chest. 2002;122(6):2246–9.
36. Goldstein R, Bright J, Jones SM, Niven RM. Severe vocal cord dysfunction resistant to all current therapeutic interventions. Respir Med. 2007;101(4):857–8.
37. Novakovic D, Waters HH, D'Elia JB, Blitzer A. Botulinum toxin treatment of adductor spasmodic dysphonia: longitudinal functional outcomes. Laryngoscope. 2011;121(3):606–12.
38. Catterall WA, Mackie K. Local Anesthetics. In: Bruton LL, Chabner BA, Knollmann BC, editors. Goodman & Gilman's The pharmacological basis of therapeutics, Chapter 20. 12th ed. New York, NY: McGraw-Hill; 2011.
39. Lokshin B, Lindgren S, Weinberger M, Koviach J. Outcome of habit cough in children treated with a brief session of suggestion therapy. Ann Allergy. 1991;67(6):579–82.
40. Sherman JM. Breaking the cycle: lidocaine therapy for habit cough. J Fla Med Assoc. 1997;84(5):308–9.
41. Cullen L, Taylor D, Taylor S, Chu K. Nebulized lidocaine decreases the of nasogastric tube insertion: a randomized, double-blind trial. Ann Emerg Med. 2004;44(2):131–7.
42. Westfall TC, Westfall DP. Adrenergic agonists and antagonists. In: Bruton LL, Chabner BA, Knollmann BC, editors. Goodman & Gilman's The pharmacological basis of therapeutics, Chapter 12. 12th ed. New York, NY: McGraw-Hill; 2011.
43. Schimmer BP, Funder JW. ACTH, Adrenal steroids, and pharmacology of the adrenal cortex. In: Bruton LL, Chabner BA, Knollmann BC, editors. Goodman & Gilman's The pharmacological basis of therapeutics, Chapter 42. 12th ed. New York, NY: McGraw-Hill; 2011.
44. Chung KF. Currently available cough suppressants for chronic cough. Lung. 2008;186 suppl 1:S82–7.
45. Dicpinigaitis PV. Current and future peripherally-acting antitussives. Respir Physiol Neurobiol. 2006;152(3):356–62.
46. Smith SM, Schroeder K, Fahey T. Over-the-counter (OTC) medications for acute cough in children and adults in ambulatory settings. Cochrane Database Syst Rev. 2008;1:CD001831. doi:10.1002/14651858.CD001831.pub3.
47. Hayes BF, Soderberg KA, Fauci AS. Introduction to the immune system. In: Fauci AS, Braunwald E, Kasper DL, Hauser SL, Longo DL, Jameson JL, Loscalzo J, editors. Harrison's principles of internal medicine, Chapter 308. 17th ed. New York, NY: McGraw Hill; 2008.
48. Loosen PT, Shelton RC. Mood disorders. In: Ebert MH, Loosen PT, Nurcombe B, Leckman JF, editors. Current diagnosis & treatment psychiatry, Chapter 18. 2nd ed. New York, NY: McGraw-Hill; 2008.
49. Anbar RD. Self-hypnosis for anxiety associated with severe asthma: a case report. BMC Pediatr. 2003;3:7.

Chapter 15
The Healing Energy of Breath in Traditional Chinese Medicine and Other Eastern Traditions

Reinhild Draeger-Muenke and Maximilian Muenke

"The breath is the intersection of the body and mind."

–Thich Nhat Hanh

Abstract The first breath and the last breath traditionally determine the span of a life from birth to death. Many different traditions have understood the importance of breath for the well-being of mind, body, and spirit. The importance of breath as a part of healing from physical disease and emotional suffering is based on ancient Eastern traditions as well as more recent Western approaches. Here, we explore the power of breath and its contribution to maintaining and restoring health in Traditional Chinese Medicine (TCM) and other Eastern modalities, and its incorporation into complementary medicine approaches in the twenty-first century.

Keywords Acupressure • Traditional Chinese Medicine • Acupuncture • Breath • Hypnosis • Integrative medicine • Eastern medicine • Energy flow • Self-regulation • Mind-body medicine

Background

Few health-care practitioners following a Western model of physical treatment of disease will know to wonder how, for example, asthma, eczema, and experiences of loss and grief may be connected. Thousands of years ago, Traditional Chinese

R. Draeger-Muenke (✉)
Independent Private Practice, 329 Bryn Mawr Avenue, Bala Cynwyd, PA 19004, USA
e-mail: rmuenke@aol.com

M. Muenke (✉)
Medical Acupuncture and Complementary Medicine, 329 Bryn Mawr Avenue, Bala Cynwyd, PA, USA
e-mail: maxmuenke@aol.com

R.D. Anbar (ed.), *Functional Respiratory Disorders: When Respiratory Symptoms Do Not Respond to Pulmonary Treatment*, Respiratory Medicine,
DOI 10.1007/978-1-61779-857-3_15,

Medicine (TCM) developed a complex concept of such diseases and formulated answers to health-care questions that are rarely, if ever, asked in Western medicine. TCM provides perspective regarding the complex connections between the physical, emotional, and spiritual dimensions of human beings, their health and disease. For a Western practitioner, it can be an intriguing journey to discover that there is more to the adequate intake of air than pulmonary functioning. TCM's more comprehensive approach to the understanding of health and disease has the capacity to broaden the Western paradigm with its primarily physical and symptom amelioration orientation. TCM can enable Western health-care providers to respond more knowledgably to the ever-increasing patient demand for care that makes sense of symptoms with multiple causes and gives overarching meaning to what ails them.

Through a TCM paradigm, patients—together with their care providers—understand that their physical, emotional, and spiritual life determines health or disease and that they can influence their health status by tending to all three dimensions knowledgably. For example, in the case of pulmonary disease, a patient can be offered Western standard treatment in conjunction with acupressure stimulation of specific energy points and a practice of mindful moving and breathing to ameliorate secondary symptoms such as physical and emotional stress and its sequelae. Similarly empowered, patients' motivation to participate in the care for their health increases, as they move from being passive victims of a random illness to actively pursuing quality of life and health management that supports mind, body, and spirit.

Breathing can be considered the most important function of the body. Without breath, life and all other bodily activities will cease within minutes. Therefore, breath has been associated with life itself, and from the beginning of humankind, breath has been appreciated in its physical and spiritual dimensions. In many creation myths, the giver of the original breath gives life and creates order out of chaos. Breath in many cultures and spiritual traditions therefore is considered to be a direct manifestation of spirit, the carrier of the soul, or breathed into humans by a higher being. In Hebrew, the words for breath (*neshem*) and soul (*neshama*) are closely related, indicating that breath may connect humans to a higher plane. *Ruach*, the Hebrew word for wind, breath, mind, or spirit given to a living creature by the Creator, denotes both the power and the creative ability to give such life (Genesis 1:2). The Latin *spiritus* provides the foundation for the words "spirit" as well as for "breath," as in "inspiration/expiration." The Greek *pneuma* signifies both "god inspired wind," spirit, and breath. Sanskrit's *Prana* and the Tibetan *Lung*, as well as the Chinese *Qi*, signify breath as life's energy and vitality together.

The English language makes many references to the act of breathing, such as taking, holding, regaining, saving, catching, or losing one's breath, and being out of breath. Other references connect breath with an emotional state: to say something under one's breath; to have one's breath taken away; to waste one's breath; in the same breath; one breath at a time; with bated breath; breathing a sigh of relief; breathing freely; taking a breather; a breath of fresh air, and many others. Such frequent referencing to the act of breathing in everyday language may well signify the importance of breath itself and its many nuances in daily living.

It is well understood that one can learn to control emotions through breathing. As fear affects breathing via the activation of the sympathetic nervous system, breathing mindfully can be utilized to reconnect with the parasympathetic system to slow the body down and restore itself. Unintegrated emotions find their physical manifestation in restricted movement and muscle tensions that negatively impact the available physical and emotional energy for daily living. Learning to control one's breathing is a powerful means to regenerate energy flow and "dynamic harmony," allowing for a flexible and appropriate response to the actual needs and possibilities of the present moment.

Many healing approaches in the East and in the West focus on breath, with the understanding that breath, beyond its mechanical qualities, connects the physical, emotional, and spiritual realms. Here, we will provide an introduction into the concept of breath as healing life energy in both Eastern and Western traditions.

Breath in Traditional Chinese Medicine and Other Eastern Traditions

TCM has long made the connection between correct breathing and health, as opposed to impeded breathing and disease. Breathing can be considered the most essential physical activity a body can perform, aiding in maintaining and obtaining Qi, life's energy. Quite simply, without breath, all physical activity eventually ceases, and ultimately life itself ends.

The connection between breath and Qi is complex. Basic tenets hold that a person's original Qi is inherited from his/her ancestors and, from the moment of conception, is also influenced by the environment [1]. Therefore, the amount of Qi available to the individual differs from person to person. Qi is thought to flow through channels (meridians) that comprise an energy network connecting every organ and every cell in the body. Twelve main meridians are connected to specific internal organs, after which they are named. The Lung meridian (see Fig. 15.1) is of special interest here, as it is closely connected with the physical breathing apparatus and a person's vital Lung Qi. A person's life span, according to TCM, is determined by the amount of available Qi. To put it simply, when all available Qi is used up, death occurs.

Every person's original Qi decreases over the course of a lifetime. The rate of decline is determined by the inherited Qi and the net gains and losses of living one's life. Thus, "external pathogens" such as environmental factors leading to physical illness, (e.g., respiratory distress), and/or "internal pathogens" such as unbalanced emotions (e.g., prolonged sadness leading to depression or other mental illness), may combine and interact to deplete available Qi. To minimize the loss of Qi, a life in both physical and emotional balance and moderation can help maintain available Qi.

According to TCM, Qi can be regained or rebalanced through four different means: (1) acupuncture, i.e., the insertion of fine needles into acupuncture points on the surface meridians of the body (e.g., Lung meridian; see Fig. 15.1), or acupressure, i.e., using pressure at acupuncture points [2, 3]. The application of heat at acupuncture points, called moxibustion, has a similar effect; (2) Qi also can be balanced through movement such as Qigong or T'aichi, (3) utilizing Chinese herbs and consuming healthy food in moderation; and (4) last, but not least, breathing properly is an additional means to restore and replenish Qi.

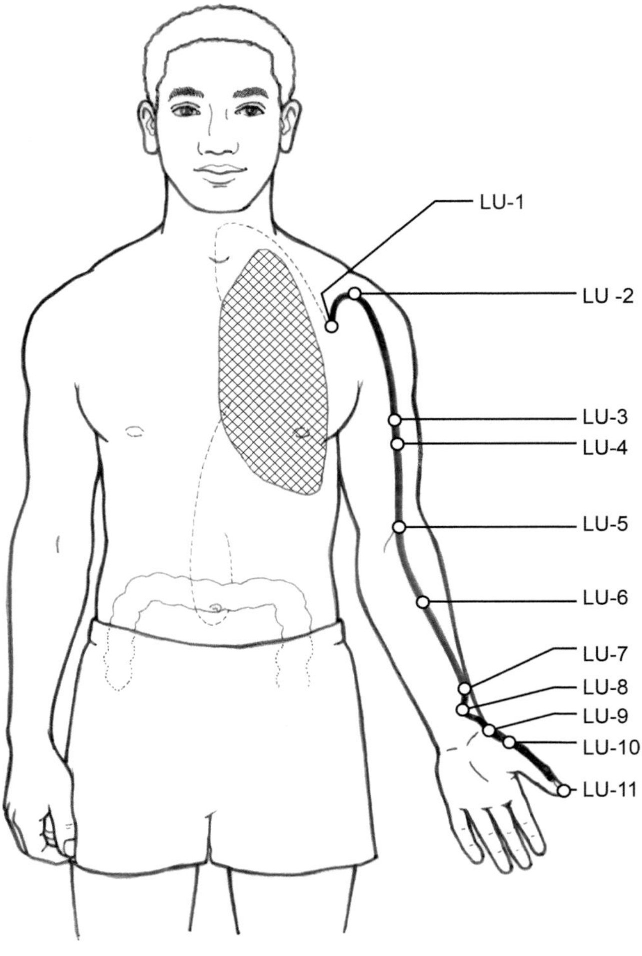

Fig. 15.1 *Lung meridian*: Acupressure points LU-1 through LU-11 along the lung meridian (*bold line*) and their connection to the associated organs, lungs and large intestine (*dotted lines*)

As in Western understanding, TCM considers the lungs to be the vehicle for breathing. In addition, TCM understands that the organ "Lung" is important for the formation and movement of Qi. Not only does the TCM organ "Lungs" govern the lungs, but the "Lungs rule the exterior of the body" [1], influencing the nose, sweat glands, body hair, and skin. It is important to note that TCM understands skin to function as the third lung, as skin with its pores combines with the two lobes of the lung to form the "Foundation of Qi"—generating specific Lung Qi through inhaling "Natural Air Qi" [1]. Defective Lung Qi then leads to the co-occurrence of skin and lung diseases, such as the combination of eczema and asthma, a presentation well known in Western medicine.

TCM teaches that in order for the Natural Air Qi to penetrate deeply into the body, to be "grasped," and for the inhalation process to be completed and well utilized, proper breathing and the generation of Lung Qi require the help of the Kidneys, which are therefore considered the "root of the Qi." Kidneys thus assist the Lungs in their generation of "Defensive" Qi and provide resistance to fight "internal" and "external" pathogens that threaten life's energy. It follows that TCM considers Kidney difficulties a root cause for respiratory problems such as chronic asthma.

TCM considers the Lungs "tender organs," easily affected by what Kaptchuk calls "fleeting" events [1], such as breathing itself, an acute respiratory illness, or emotional reactivity. Not surprisingly, TCM has long understood the physical underpinnings of human emotions and has developed an intricate system (Five-Element theory [4]) to make sense of, and give meaning to, the mind-body connections established by living one's life.

In focusing on the Lungs, it is important to note that TCM considers the Lungs the storage place for our "Animal Soul" ("Poo")—the part of our energy that is best described as untamed, erratic, and reacting emotionally to all the pressing demands of human life. When the "Animal Soul" is healthy, it reacts with flexibility to the emotional demands of living and quickly rebalances by being able to evaluate the "bigger picture." When the Animal Soul is not able to react flexibly, a person may find himself or herself either emotionless or overly emotional. The great challenges to our "Animal Soul" are the experiences of mourning, loss and grief, and the inability to find completion. Therefore, the Lungs are quickly affected by loss, longing, and unresolved grief—and, vice versa, when the Lung Qi is disturbed by chronic respiratory illness, a sense of unresolved grief, loss, and longing can develop [1].

Focusing on the mechanics of breathing means focusing on the short-term aspects of Lung Qi: Inhalation as the means of bringing outside Qi (in the form of natural air) in contact with the Qi inside the body via the Lungs, which propel Qi downward and help disseminate it, and exhalation to expel "impure" air. The nose is considered the "thoroughfare for respiration," the functioning of which is closely connected to the Lungs. The throat, including the vocal cords, functions as the "door" of the Lungs. Therefore, TCM will treat nose and throat disorders through treating the Lungs [1]. When breathing is healthy and unobstructed, the rhythm of exchange is smooth and even. An imbalance or obstruction interfering with Lung functioning will lead to symptoms such as asthma, cough, or dyspnea—not the other way around! Since the Lungs and their Qi are connected to the Qi of the chest and with that to the movement of all Qi in the body, Lung disharmony, especially in the case of a chronic lung disorder, leads to deficient Qi everywhere in the body affecting other organs and their energy systems as well.

As mentioned above, the Lungs affect the exterior of the body through the skin, sweat glands, and hair, regulating body temperature and offering protection from external pathogens. The Lungs' ability to disseminate Qi influences the capacity of the Protective Qi to protect the body. If the Lung Qi is weak, the sweat glands may produce too little or too much sweat, which in turn will affect the Protective Qi's ability to resist harmful influences. In that case, for example, a person may contract recurrent "colds," as they will be unable to resist "what is going around."

By now, it has become evident that in TCM, the cause, the process, and the outcome of illness merge. Instead of simple causality, there are circles of constant feedback loops involving Qi. Different parts of a person's energy system resonate with each other either in an overall pattern of environmental, internal, physical, emotional, and spiritual harmony or disharmony, supporting a person's health or being unable to prevent disease [1].

Acupressure as an Aid in Functional Respiratory Disease

Acupressure, or Tuina, exerting concentrated pressure at specific acupuncture points to activate the flow of energy along meridians, has been described in numerous works of TCM [5]. Over the past several decades, acupressure has been presented to the Western world mostly through descriptions in self-help books [2, 6–9]. While identification of pressure points can be learned from written instructions, it is advisable to also experience the precise activation of such points by a health-care professional trained in the broader healing context of TCM. Thus, the following description of points and their applications, as well as examples of accompanying interventions, serve the purpose of elucidating our approach but are not intended as instruction for unsupervised self-practice.

Following TCM's principle that the prevention of disease is preferable to treating it [10, 11], several point combinations have been chosen for their use in health maintenance and well-being. We will introduce here the most commonly utilized points: the "Four Gates" (Fig. 15.2) [1, 3, 12] and their expanded version, the "Five Golden Points" (Fig. 15.3) [2, 3], and several points related to lung functioning and breathing. According to TCM, activating the points of the Four Gates, one on each foot and each hand (see Fig. 15.2), results in a better flow of energy not only in the associated meridians but throughout the entire body. The Five Golden Points consist of the Four Gates and additional points on the knees, elbows, and the crown of head (see Fig. 15.3) [12, 13]. Those additional points stimulate the immune system as well as invite general calm and well-being. Even though the location of the acupuncture points along the meridians is (mostly) identical regardless of the source or textbook used, individual names may vary. Here, we use the standard Western nomenclature for the points along the meridian that derives their name from the associated internal organs, and we will give the points' Chinese names with English translation.

Description of the points of the *Four Gates* and the *Five Golden Points* (Fig. 15.2): **LI-4**, Large Intestine 4, *He Gu* ("Joining Valley") is located in the middle of the webbing between the thumb and index finger of each hand. Grab the webbing from both sides with the tip of your thumb on one side of the webbing and your index finger on the other side to press the muscle in the webbing. **LR-3**, Liver 3, *Tai Chong* ("Great Rushing") is the corresponding point located between the first and second toes on both feet. Use your index finger to find the point. Move from the toes

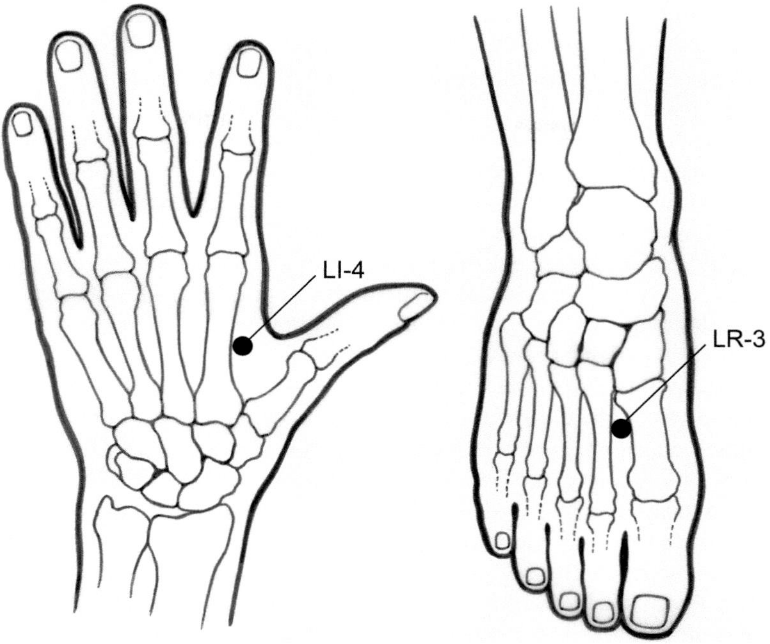

Fig. 15.2 The acupressure points of the Four Gates

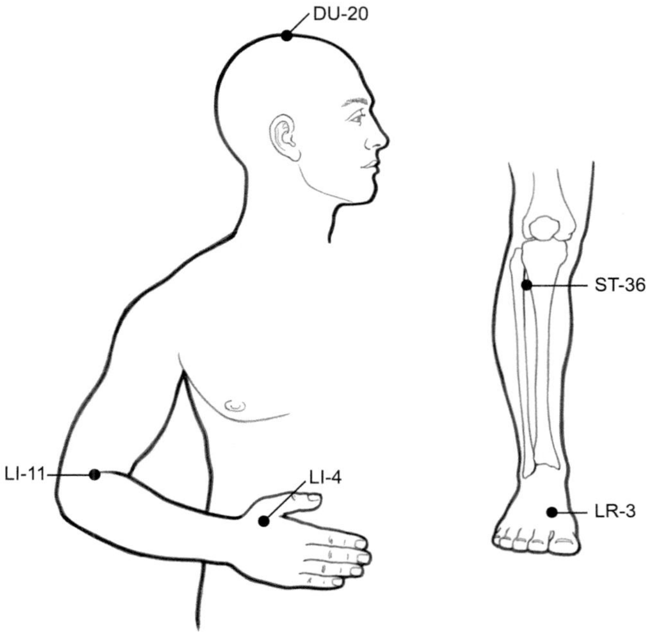

Fig. 15.3 The acupressure points of the Five Golden Points

toward the foot and come to a stop where the metatarsal bones join, and exert gentle pressure downward. **DU-20**, DU meridian with pressure points along the body's midline, is also called Governing Vessel (GV). *Bai Hui* ("Hundred Meetings"), the highest point of the head ("Crown Chakra" in Indian tradition), is located at the midpoint of an imaginary line between the tips of the ears and a line between the tip of the nose and the middle of the head. **LI-11**, Large Intestine 11, *Qu Chi* ("Pool at the Crook"), with the elbow bent at a right angle, the point is at the outside end of the elbow crease. **ST-36**, Stomach 36, *Zu San Li* ("Leg Three Miles") is situated on the outside of the lower leg below the knee. With the upper and lower leg bent at a right angle, the point is located the width of four fingers below the kneecap and one fingerbreadth to the outside of the crest of the shinbone.

At specific surface points along the meridians, so-called acupuncture or acupressure points Qi can be manipulated to increase the flow of energy along these meridians. Activation of energy on these specific points can be experienced as a tingling sensation, electricity, or a feeling of warmth, and is called the "DeQi" sensation. Traditionally, pressure at acupuncture points has been applied by the pads of the thumb and index finger, with slowly increasing pressure in a circular or back-and-forth motion for approximately a minute each, until DeQi sensation has been experienced, confirming that contact has been made with the energy at that pressure point. It is understood that open sores, bruises, swelling, or other points of acute discomfort should be avoided, and acupressure at points in the vicinity of the injury should be applied only after medical consultation (for details of contraindications see [2, 6, 7]).

In an acupuncturist's office, acupressure is considered part to be part of the overall treatment. In contrast, in a mental health-care setting, touch is not part of most treatments offered. Therefore, with careful consideration being given to specific patient-therapist variables, acupressure may be offered or simply demonstrated by the mental health-care provider, who identifies acupressure points of the head, upper body, and extremities on a chart or on the therapist's hands, feet, and crown of head and invites the patients to identify and experience those points on themselves. When the activation of acupressure points becomes part of treatment, it can serve as an additional tool for grounding, calming, and providing positive sensory feedback, especially when negative energy in the form of anxiety or posttraumatic disturbance is present. Once incorporated into self-care, acupressure is a portable self-regulatory tool, extending treatment between office visits and allowing the patient to take charge of maintaining and solidifying treatment gains.

It cannot be emphasized enough that successful treatment of mind-body and spirit depends on the creation of an overall tension and distraction-free inner and outer atmosphere of calm and focused healing. Just as electronic devices need to be silenced, so do inner chatter and errant thoughts need to quiet in order to allow the mind to focus on the acupressure points that are being stimulated, as well as on the sensations at those points as Qi is generated and begins to move.

Specific Energy Centers and Acupressure Points Related to Lung and Breathing

TCM refers to three major centers of energy, the Upper, Middle, and Lower Dantien, corresponding, respectively, to the space between the eyebrows, the solar plexus, and the lower abdominal region. Each of these energy centers is believed to harbor Shen energy, which in Chinese philosophy denotes the concept of spirit, god-given energy, awareness, and consciousness. Three different centers of energy are referred to as Triple Heater: The Upper Heater is located in the chest above the diaphragm, the Middle is in the upper abdomen between the umbilicus and the diaphragm, and the Lower heater is in the lower abdomen below the umbilicus. They are associated with the overall movement of Qi between the organs located within the Upper, Middle, and Lower Heater. Their energy is activated via acupuncture, acupressure, and/or focused breathing [14] in order to regulate and harmonize the energy exchange between the major internal organ networks.

Shen energy residing in the Upper Dantien is thought to be responsible for controlling the basic energy of the mind, clear thinking, and awareness. It generates consciousness that is communicated through a person's eyes. When the Upper Dantien is open and energized, a person is able to experience strong intuition and a sense of real purpose. When it is closed, the attention is weak and scattered, and a person may be distracted and indecisive [15]. Thus, it is logical to stimulate this central acupressure point between the eyebrows for mental clarity and focus and to pair it with conscious, deep abdominal breathing.

In order to support the flow of Shen energy in the Middle Dantien, a body midline acupressure point (Conception Vessel (CV)-16) right at the end of the breastbone where the lowest right and left ribs meet and where the abdominal cavity begins, can be gently massaged. Again, pairing this massage with focused breathing will enhance the distribution of energy throughout the body.

Deep abdominal breathing is considered an effective way to maintain the proper flow of Shen energy in the Lower Dantien as well, effectively quieting a person's brain and mind. A pressure point a hand width below the navel (CV-4) can be stimulated in conjunction with focused abdominal breathing to affect Lower Dantien energy flow. TCM postulates that keeping the Lower Dantien open and active results in increased Qi in all cells and tissues of the body and the brain. Overall, Shen energy supports healing and well-being and is considered to be a foundation for psychospiritual growth [15].

Special emphasis needs to be given to the acupressure points located on the body's midline that are part of the GV and CV meridians. These two meridians can be considered as reservoirs for extra energy which when stimulated can enhance the effects of the overall acupressure treatment by helping to balance energies [2]. When stimulated and paired with focused slow and deep breathing, acupressure points on these two meridians invite deep centering and tapping into what may best be called one's own wise or spiritual self and place of inner wisdom, generating calm and focused energy and the opportunity to center and regroup in times of physical and emotional stress.

The following midline points can be activated to aid in calming and centering:

- Begin with the "Hundred Meeting" point (DU-20 or GV-20), at the crown of the head (see Fig. 15.3).
- Proceed to the "Third Eye" point between the eyebrows (Yintang).
- Press the point at the fulcrum below the nostrils at the place of the upper teeth (CV-26).
- Gently massage the acupressure point in the middle of the breastbone (CV-17).
- Exert gentle pressure at the point right underneath the rib cage (CV-16).
- Do the same at the point three fingers width below the navel (CV-6).
- And finally exert gentle pressure at the point three fingers width above the pubic bone (CV-3).

These "golden points" of the front of the body [2, 3] can be incorporated into a daily routine of centering and breathing to make central energies available for healing and health maintenance.

The organs "Lungs" by the mere act of breathing allow for the exchange of oxygen and carbon dioxide, letting us take in what we need (inhaling natural air), and to let go of what is no longer necessary (exhaling spent air). The "Lung" meridian, connected with the organs "Lungs" (Fig. 15.1), is part of a larger system of meridians that help release and eliminate what is no longer needed in order to make room for the acquisition of what might come in its stead.

The concept of such an exchange refers to both physical and spiritual needs and connects the human being with the larger energies of the Five Elements governing the world and the universe beyond it. Of the Five Elements (Wood, Fire, Earth, Metal, and Water), the Lung meridian is associated with the element "Metal," the element of autumn, harvest, letting go, and taking care of material and spiritual needs [2, 4]. When "Metal" is not balanced, breathing problems can be observed as well as emotional struggles with resolving difficult feelings such as grief and loss, and the inability to grieve fully and appropriately, allowing one to eventually move on. Thus, the Lung meridian is connected with the complex and often intense emotion of grief, which, when unresolved, can cause disease in a person's physical body as well, weakening the immune system and inviting opportunistic diseases, breathing problems, and potentially leading to the dramatic "broken heart syndrome" (Takotsubo cardiomyopathy) [16] after sudden and overwhelming emotional stress and massive release of adrenaline within a short time.

While TCM treatment incorporating Five Elements is complex and cannot be given full justice here, there are acupressure points that can be stimulated in conjunction with other treatment modalities of Western and/or Eastern orientation, in order to aid the overall release of physical and emotional tension related to Lung functioning and to encourage life energies to begin to flow again. LU-1, below the collarbone near the shoulder joint (Fig. 15.1), is a letting-go point, an antidepression point, and helps to deepen breathing. CV-17 in the middle of the sternum will also facilitate the flow of breath. In the case of asthma, these points can be used in conjunction with bronchodilator medication.

Conscious breathing techniques in conjunction with acupressure have to be considered an integral part of the treatment of depleted Lung Qi, whether from organic or emotional causes. Such breathing will help restore immune system functioning and overall energy. It will help to improve sleep and allow for a state of mindfulness indispensable in the emotional work of acknowledging and moving through loss and grief that may accompany breathing difficulties [17].

Breath in Complementary Medicine Approaches

Breathing for Health

Breath constitutes the pivotal mind-body connection. Breath is influenced by both mind and body, and breath influences mind and body, whether consciously or unconsciously. As one of the most basic functions embedded in the autonomic nervous system (ANS), the unconscious breath reacts to every internal or external stimulus. Just a single thought can change the breathing pattern from even and expansive to irregular and tight, depending whether it relates to comfort and affiliation, or whether it constitutes a threat and the need for self-defense.

It is understood that breathing is every individual's own responsibility. In general, we cannot breathe for another person. Therefore, many therapies have the goal of teaching a patient to breathe differently—ultimately engaging that person in the process of moving and changing and unfreezing physical and emotional blockages. This often moves beyond solving any literal breathing problem and extends into problem-solving in the broader context of that person's life. With breath, physical, emotional, and even spiritual stagnation and paralysis can be overcome. Learning how to breathe allows a person to create and be in touch with their own life energy and their possibilities [14, 18] and to overcome stagnated emotions.

It is well understood that one can learn to control emotions through breathing [14, 19]. As fear affects breathing via the activation of the sympathetic nervous system, breathing mindfully can be utilized to reconnect with the parasympathetic system to slow the body down and restore itself. Since unintegrated emotions find their physical manifestation in restricted movement and muscle tensions that negatively impact the available physical and emotional energy for daily living [20], mindful breathing can redirect energy flow to restore "dynamic harmony," and awareness of the actual needs and possibilities of the present moment [15].

All breath training makes use of the fundamentals of the breathing process. The inbreathe or inhale is considered to be the active part of the breath cycle, produced through the contraction of the breathing muscle apparatus. With its tension and willfulness, it is often considered part of the sympathetic nervous system, allowing the breathing person to take in what he or she can. Of course, the transition to exhaling begins at the height of the inhalation, a moment of intense stillness, before we have to let go in order for breath and energy to keep moving. Exhaling occurs without much, if any, effort, counteracting the tension of inhaling in its more passive letting go. As such, it is considered part of the parasympathetic nervous system. At the end of the exhalation is a second moment of stillness, before active inhaling resumes. The rhythmic flow between these two poles creates the desired inner balance of a circle of breathing without beginning and end once it has begun and before it finally ends [18].

Heightening the act of inhaling by rapid chest breathing without complete inhalation (as in asthmatic conditions or in anxiety-related hyperventilation) will of course activate the sympathetic nervous system and the fight-flight-freeze response, while deep abdominal breathing with complete exhalation and slow inhalation will support parasympathetic activity, relaxation, and overall calm. For good reason, breathing well is associated with living a long life [17]. Or as a Hindu proverb puts it: "A person's life is measured in breaths. And you can breathe quickly or slowly."

Conscious breathing to assure the continuous unhindered flow of in and out breath to nourish body mind and spirit, leading to a better physical, emotional, and spiritual life, is considered the goal of all breath work. In order to achieve a greater flow of unhindered energy, it is important to learn how to breathe through physical, emotional, or spiritual blockages [18]. Because of breath's unconscious/autonomic as well as conscious and deliberate aspects, breath is at the interface of the inner/unconscious and the outer/conscious world and can be utilized to connect the two worlds for the greater good of the living being. Many therapeutic approaches make good use of this.

In the **Yogic tradition** of India, "*Prana*" conceptualizes absolute energy, a vital force, life's energy found in all forms of life. Yogic breathing uses all muscles of the breathing apparatus in a controlled and regulated way, in order to extract as much energy from *Prana* as possible. Such energy may then be stored in the cells of the body as well as the brain in order to nourish mind, body, and spirit. At the same time, such breathing gently massages the internal organs, allowing their maximal receptivity to life's energy. Yogic teaching asserts that the body's seven energy centers, *chakras*, are connected through breathing and that breath helps distribute each chakra's available energy for the benefit of mind, body, and spirit.

The *chakra*s correspond to the energy centers known to TCM [21]. For example, the seventh chakra, the *Crown Chakra*, is known as the "Hundred Meeting point" in TCM, signifying connection to inner wisdom, a person's soul, and the spiritual world. The sixth chakra corresponds with TCM's *Third Eye* point, balancing mind and body energetically. The third chakra, the *Solar Plexus Center* (Middle Dantien) with its sympathetic nerves and ganglia connecting it to many parts of the body is considered a central storehouse of *Prana*. There are many breathing exercises, *pranayama*, in Yoga, inviting focus, centeredness, invigoration, and mindful restoration of physical and emotional balance. Here, we will mention several that can be considered essential to emotional and physical self-regulation and anchoring practices.

Foundation Breathing or Three-Part Breath

(1). Sit or lie comfortably, eyes closed, hands in your lap. (2). Notice the ins and outs of your breath without changing anything. (3). Exhale, then inhale deeply through the nose. Exhale and empty your lungs, letting go of any thoughts. (4). Inhale deeply, filling the belly first, then the ribcage, then the upper chest all the way to the collarbone, with air. (5). Hold for a moment. (6). Then exhale, expelling all the air out from your lungs. Draw the navel back toward your spine to make sure that the belly is empty of air. (7). Repeat for five breaths [17].

Six-Second Breath

Inhale for 2 s—hold for 1 s—exhale for 2 s—hold for 1 s—repeat [17].

Alternate Nostril Breathing

(1). Sit comfortably. (2). Bring your thumb to the right side of your nose and your ring finger to the left side. (3). Close off your right nostril with your thumb. (4). Inhale through your left nostril. (5). Close off your left nostril with your ring finger. (6). Open and exhale through your right nostril. (7). Inhale through your right nostril. (8). Close off your right nostril with your thumb. (9). Open and exhale through your left nostril. (10). Inhale through your left nostril. (11). Continue alternating 5–10 times, (http://yoga.about.com/od/breathing/a/nadisodhana.htm)

Qigong and T'aichi, a combination of conscious body movements and breathing methods, encourage the stimulation of the same meridians acupressure uses, in order to allow Qi to circulate more freely. Purposeful breathing is utilized to aid in the generation and movement of Qi to all internal organs and systems via improved lung functioning and decrease in overall muscle tension. This process of mindful movement with breath is believed to aid in transforming stressful emotional states and an overactive sympathetic nervous system into positive inner energy that aids both physical and the emotional rebalancing. Qigong and T'aichi aim to activate the parasympathetic nervous system to harmonize the aggressive and restorative functions, the yang and yin of our nervous system [22]. Lewis [15] remarks that we could learn to fully utilize the 15,000 or more breaths we take each day to support our own inner growth and overall health. Especially in times of stress and narrowed, fear-based focus, when contraction of all muscles is likely, the ability to increase breathing space (instead of increasing breathing frequency) through mindful movement of body and emotions will increase sensory awareness and broaden one's perspective and increase acceptance as well as the potential for problem-solving of existing physical and emotional needs.

In the tradition of **"mindfulness-based stress reduction,"** ***breath awareness*** is a central focus, returning us to the present moment, over and over again (see Chap. 16). Being aware of or observing one's quality of breath without making any deliberate changes is a frequently used mindfulness practice to cultivate mental, emotional, and physical detachment from any interfering problem [17].

Other mindfulness practices involve conscious breathing that is controlled, intentional, and purposeful to achieve a result, such as ***balanced breathing*** (balanced inhalation and exhalation); ***cleansing breath***, which emphasizes exhalation over inhalation; and energizing or ***refreshing breath***, emphasizing inhalation over exhalation [20, 23–28].

Focused breathing in the form of breathing meditations attempts to attain a higher state of consciousness and to reconnect breath with spirit and bring about physical, emotional, and spiritual harmony and balance. Proper postural alignment [28] creates the physical space to, for example, follow the Buddhist invitation to contact one's inner smile through expansive breathing [23, 24]. Mindful breathing can inspire, allow a new focus, and generate new health and growth through stimulation and nourishment that are being drawn into the mind-body system. Thought, feelings, and sensations can move and change through breathing new vitality into every corner of our being, preventing physical or emotional matter from becoming frozen and stale inside [15].

Especially when the respiratory system is already compromised and has become a weak link in the flow of Qi through the body's energy channels, mindful daily breathing practice and a more efficient use of Qi through breath are paramount to supporting overall health. As Lee and Campbell [17] remark, conscious breathing, as a lifeline we can hold on to, does not change the sense of our own mortality, but it changes us. It allows us to live fully and be present for each moment, thus giving us the opportunity to live and therefore eventually die without regret.

Hypnosis

Hypnosis as an established mind-body approach to healing (see Chap. 12) has long focused on conscious breathing to aid in the induction, deepening, and maintenance of a hypnotic trance as well as in the process of realerting [29–33]. Hypnosis pairs breath with imagery and/or cognitive intention to achieve a previously established goal related to physical and/or emotional symptom relief as well as a means to explore the underlying causes of illness. This is true especially in the aftermath of a physical and/or emotional, traumatic, not yet integrated experience that has a somatic memory component, which may significantly contribute to a functional respiratory disorder (see Chap. 1). Notably, Anbar [34, 35] discusses the use of hypnosis in the treatment of respiratory disorders in young people.

We know now that breathing is not just an individual act but that it also creates connection between human beings. Mirror neurons are responsible for our ability to imitate what we observe in others either face to face or through mental practice and imagery. These same mirror neurons allow us to feel another person's emotions and to have empathy for their experience [36–38]. It may well be possible that our mirror neurons allow synchronized breathing in jogging partners as well as groups of people singing together or sitting in meditation together. As those trained in hypnosis know, matching another person's breathing can happen consciously as well as unconsciously, thanks to these mirror neurons, with the net effect of experiencing increased emotional connection and trust—the sense of being "in synch," attuned, physically as well as emotionally. Being in tune with another person often means tracking his or her breathing and, in the case of disordered breathing, slowly, subtly, but deliberately beginning to match it, changing it to a more beneficial rhythm, perhaps thwarting a panic attack through prolonging the exhale [17], or inducing relaxation breathing to cope with acute or chronic breathing difficulties such as in ***quadrant breathing*** (equal inhale—hold—exhale—hold—inhale…; http://breath-mastery.com/principles.htm).

Since breath supports life, any threat to breathing constitutes grounds for physical and emotional alarm, setting in motion an often counterproductive attempt to control breath by tensing and forcing inhalation, rather than letting go and allowing exhalation. In cases of such previously experienced and rehearsed maladaptive breathing, further focus on breathing may be initially contraindicated, as it might induce more anxiety (Anbar, personal communication). As a complementary alternative, the above described acupressure points in conjunction with hypnosis offer themselves as being useful for grounding and methodical slowing down as well as for shifting attention to an action that can be performed. This can help shift the focus and subsequently relax the breathing apparatus enough to provide relief and retrain breathing gradually, eventually allowing the patient to enjoy the inherently soothing, hypnotic quality of slow, satisfying, life-giving breath.

Case Studies

Case 1—Recurring Bronchitis

A 45-year-old woman recently began psychotherapeutic treatment for an adjustment disorder with anxious and depressed mood after she discovered her husband of 20 years was having an affair, which resulted in the rapid dissolution of their marriage 2 years ago. In addition to a host of fleeting physical symptoms such as headaches, stomachaches, and various muscle spasms, she reported low-grade agitation, lack of concentration, and low self-esteem, as well as difficulties falling asleep almost every night. Her third episode of bronchitis in as many months was making matters worse, causing her to rapidly lose stamina and falling behind at work, which only increased her overall anxiety. The various antibiotics prescribed by her primary care physician caused stomach upset and did not seem to truly eradicate the bronchial infection.

It became quickly apparent that the patient continued to feel devastated by the sudden loss of her marriage, experiencing it as a complete shock, with the above reported symptoms of anxiety beginning soon afterward. She reported beginning to seriously doubt herself in all areas of her life, withdrawing socially and experiencing what she called her "midlife existential crisis." She felt "stuck" with intense feelings of sadness, anger, confusion, disbelief, guilt for her perceived shortcomings and failings, and an inordinate amount of anxiety about the chores of daily living—the hallmarks of a complicated grief reaction two years later. Although the recurring bronchitis was taxing, it also afforded her some sympathy at work and legitimate sick days.

The patient's stated treatment goal was to "feel better" about herself. She also was interested in feeling less anxious and overwhelmed. She was amenable to cognitive behavioral therapy interventions and began to recognize different choices she could make toward her stated goals. However, little changed at her weekly presentation, and neither her mood nor her symptoms showed much, if any, improvement. When the therapist proposed to add new treatment modalities, the patient, after much hesitation and anxiety, agreed to explore complementary approaches to see whether these would be beneficial.

The patient was introduced to the concept and philosophy of TCM, and specifically acupressure, and, given her overall anxious presentation, was shown the two hand points (LI-4) on a picture.

She was successful in producing DeQi sensation and began to wonder whether her problem involved, according to TCM, the lack of freely flowing energy, depletion of energy in some areas, and too much "stuck" energy in other areas of her body. Almost imperceptibly, her breathing slowed and became less labored as she was applying those LI-4 points in the web between thumb and forefinger. Her coughing stopped. From there, it was a small step to suggest that she just begin to notice her breathing and enjoying its smooth in and out. She even followed the suggestion to gently increase her exhale, tolerate a little rest before inhaling, and inhaling easily and without strain, holding her breath again for a moment, letting her body become more comfortable with each exhale. She was surprised to notice that her breathing had become less labored, and she was willing to practice on her own during the week, whenever she saw fit.

The following week, the patient reported that she had utilized the LI-4 acupressure points with breathing and the (hypnotic) suggestion to become more comfortable. To her surprise, it had helped her stay calm instead of ruminating at the end of her workday. Next, the patient learned to apply pressure to the two foot points (LR-3), LI-11 at the elbow crease, and ST-36 below the knee to boost her immune system. She expanded her breathing practice, as her bronchitis decreased, to include slow deep abdominal parasympathetic breathing. As she learned to breathe more expansively, some of her anxiety symptoms and overall muscle tension loosened. She agreed to mindfully adjust her posture to allow for more breathing room. She began to attend yoga classes to help her feel more comfortable in her body and in her physical space.

The patient then incorporated specific lung acupressure points (LU-1, underneath collarbones; LU-9, where the thumb joint meets the wrist) into her self-regulation routine and added several midline points (CV-17, middle of breastbone; CV-16, lower end of breastbone) to support the overall balancing of energies.

Lastly, as she began to physically and mentally quiet and began to believe that she had acquired the tools for sustained self-regulation, she was willing and able to enter the necessary grief work which she had so long resisted out of fear of becoming overwhelmed and dysfunctional. She utilized activation of the "Hundred Meeting" point and the "Third Eye" point as a focus for mindful exploration of her thoughts and feelings, and to connect with her own inner wisdom as well as with the wisdom of the universe.

At the end of 6 months of weekly therapy sessions, this patient had not had a recurrence of bronchitis for 3 months, despite the fact that it was in the middle of winter, a time when she typically had symptoms in the past. She felt renewed energy and enjoyed greater clarity of mind and spirit. She no longer felt overwhelmed by grief and had begun to move on. She experienced greater confidence in exploring new opportunities both at work and in her social life. She maintained her daily mindfulness breathing and self-observation practice together with the activation of the basic acupressure points she had come to trust. Through an e-mail follow-up one year later, this patient reported no recurrence of bronchitis or other breathing difficulties. She reported her mood as stable and her outlook on life as generally positive.

Questions:

1. The reason the therapist showed the acupressure points on a picture is
   (a) It is easier to see.
   (b) Touch was not part of this particular therapy setting.
   (c) The patient felt overwhelmed and had already withdrawn from social contact.
   (d) All of the above.
2. The therapist introduced acupressure points in order to
   (a) Facilitate self-regulation
   (b) Unblock energy
   (c) Provide a grounding tool
   (d) All of the above
3. What is the reasoning behind the order in which acupressure points were introduced?
   (a) The order was random.
   (b) The easier to find points come first.
   (c) More general points are introduced first, followed by more specific points.
   (d) The order hinges with whatever the patient can tolerate and is comfortable.

Answers:

1. (d): Especially in a psychotherapist's office, touch is not expected. An anxious and depressed patient deserves a careful and measured approach that gradually increases safety and trust in the therapeutic relationship.

2. (d): Being able to actively participate in one's healing allows a patient to take greater ownership over his or her process. Utilizing self-acupressure regularly promotes unblocking of stuck physical and emotional energies.
3. (d): While it is general practice to begin with the "Five Golden Points," a patient's comfort always comes first.

Case 2—Cough and Chest Pain in Terminal Lung Cancer

A 64-year-old recently retired man entered psychotherapy, in shock after a recent diagnosis of terminal lung cancer and with a life expectancy of no more than 3 months. A nonsmoker all his life, he had been healthy up until this diagnosis and had expected to live long enough to see his young grandchildren get married.

He presented with extreme anxiety and painful sensations around his heart that had been identified as transient due to the release of massive amounts of adrenaline. Other than an incessant cough that bothered him during the day and made sleeping difficult, he did not report any breathing difficulties. His goal for treatment was to help reduce his anxiety, to reduce the stress response in order not to exacerbate physical symptoms, and to die peacefully. He agreed to utilize a combination of hypnosis and acupressure and was willing to invite his wife to learn with him so that she could be of assistance during his final journey if necessary.

Consultation with the treating pulmonologist confirmed that the diagnosis of an inoperable lung carcinoma that at the time of detection (a random chest X-ray for insurance purposes) had grown into the lung walls and adjoining blood vessels and "could burst through the walls at any moment," leading to rapid suffocation and death. No medical interventions were planned other than weekly monitoring with the agreement to keep the patient as comfortable as possible. He was prescribed several medications to stabilize blood pressure and help with sleep. His cough was explained as an attempt to clear mucus and developing bleeding in the lungs.

Under such dramatic circumstances, the patient and his wife were highly motivated to learn what they could do to stabilize both physical and emotional upheaval, in both of them. They learned the Five Golden Points and CV17 (middle of the sternum), and began to practice breath awareness with the suggestion to breathe comfortably and easily, emphasizing open airways and smooth in and out flow of air. As an immediate result, the patient's cough became remarkably less frequent, and he reported that his throat did not feel irritated anymore. Within the first week, his breathing had slowed, his blood pressure had lowered (and the blood pressure medication had to be adjusted accordingly), and he felt more hopeful that he could "learn to die without too much trouble."

The "spiritual points" (crown of head, between the eyebrows) were added and so were extra energy points in the Middle and Lower Dantien. Both he and his wife felt greater calmness and openness, enabling them to review their life together, to grieve the impending loss of their connection, and for the primary patient to grieve the loss of his life and of the opportunities he would have liked to still enjoy. They were able to enter deeper meditative trance states in session, utilizing a combination of acupressure and hypnosis, and allowing themselves to feel a spiritual connection to each other and to "something greater than us," that allowed both of them to eventually move into acceptance of what was going to happen as well as a deep sense of gratitude for what had been.

The patient continued to breathe with relative ease over the last month of his life, to the astonishment of the pulmonologist. He remained calm, appropriately expressed his sadness, grief, and anger about his imminent death and enjoyed what he could every day. When his cough began to produce more sputum with traces of blood, he shared his astonishment because he kept feeling relatively well and had been ambulatory and in decent spirits. At the six-week point, getting up from eating lunch, he collapsed and almost immediately died. The carcinoma had finally broken through the walls of the lung. To the very end, he had been able to maintain his quality of life and had remained at home. He continued to be able to breathe on his own, to say what he had to say to his family, and to maintain his dignity.

Questions:

1. Acupressure was offered to this patient
   (a) To cure his lung cancer
   (b) To extend his life expectancy
   (c) To ameliorate secondary symptoms
   (d) As a distraction
2. Why the combination of acupressure and hypnosis?
   (a) Both modalities acknowledge the mind-body paradigm.
   (b) Both modalities address energy regulation and add to the overall efficacy of treatment.
   (c) In combination, they potentiate self-regulation.
   (d) All of the above.
3. This specific point combination was chosen in order to
   (a) Affect spiritual and physical healing
   (b) Affect emotional and physical healing
   (c) Affect physical comfort, emotional, and spiritual healing
   (d) Give the patient more time to live

Answers:

1 (c): Acupressure in conjunction with standard Western treatment can ameliorate secondary symptoms such as physical and emotional stress and its sequelae.

2 (d): Hypnotically induced trance with suggestions for the movement of energy, for emotional working through, and for spiritual connection and peacefulness of mind and body can support the same goals affected by the activation of acupressure points.

3 (c): In this case, the diagnosis and prognosis were rather clear. Increasing the patient's quality of life and comfort in the dying process seemed to be the appropriate interventions.

Case 3—Asthma

A 13-year-old boy sought acupressure treatment at the recommendation of his parents. He had been diagnosed with asthma at age eight and had been successfully using a bronchodilator as needed, usually no more than a few times per week, and had avoided any emergency interventions. Wheezing was induced by environmental stimuli and physical exertion.

He recently had experienced his first asthma attack playing soccer, and although he was able to avoid the emergency room, this episode scared him and made him hesitant to continue playing. He had just switched from a small elementary school into the seventh grade of a private college preparatory school, and although he had been an academic and athletic star in his elementary school, he found himself to be just one of many talented kids in his new school environment and needed to work much harder just to keep up. He felt himself becoming anxious thinking about school and had started to have trouble falling asleep at night.

His mother reported that she had been quite ill during her pregnancy with unremitting nausea and frequent episodes of "colds." The mother's father had suddenly died 6 weeks before she was giving birth to her son. While her son was born full term and healthy, his APGAR scores were not perfect, and before being diagnosed with asthma, he was prone to frequent colds affecting his ears, nose, and throat, which continues to be the case.

The boy did not want to have needles inserted into his skin, so we agreed on a course of acupressure. He also was interested in learning self-hypnosis skills to reduce his anxiety regarding the academic, athletic, and social aspects of school.

It made sense to him that his overall Qi, but especially his lung Qi, may have been deficient from birth because of his mother's compromised physical and emotional well-being while she was pregnant with him. Because of the overall good care his parents gave him, he was able to generate enough Qi to become strong and capable—but his lungs continued to be affected, and with the first major stressor in his own life, losing his safety net by switching schools and having to fight for position, the lungs signaled problems.

Over a total of five sessions, the youngster had general (Five Golden Points) and specific (CV-17, LU-1, LU-7, DU-20, Yintang) energy points activated via acupressure by the acupuncturist, and, as he learned to find and activate these points on his own body, began to utilize them on his own in between sessions. He had enjoyed a particular hypnotic induction (Spiegel Eye Roll [30]) and had practiced inducing a self-hypnotic trance with it. He favored suggestions of staying calm, focused, and positive in all areas of his current life. He also was amenable to learn several breathing exercises and practiced them daily.

Within the 6 weeks of treatment, the boy had regained his ability to fall asleep, and with this felt more stable during the day. As he utilized acupressure points, self-hypnosis, and mindful breathing to manage his performance anxieties, his ability to perform well academically increased and improved his self-confidence. He was able to reliably breathe again, conscientiously activating acupressure points and deepening his exhale, making room for a smooth inhale, and slowing down his rate of breathing overall. He had greatly reduced the need for his asthma-related medication. Feeling more in control overall, he rejoined the soccer team for a successful season. He also enjoyed the bar and bat mitzvah circuit of seventh grade and reported back to the acupuncturist that so far he did not have to sit out a single dance. No further asthma attacks occurred.

Questions:

1 Why would you consider the prenatal environment in the treatment of a breathing disorder?

(a) You would not.
(b) Because it cannot hurt to get a complete history.
(c) Because a person's Qi at birth is also determined by the parents' contribution.
(d) You would consider it, but in this case, everything was really ok.

2 According to TCM, unresolved grief, loss, and breathing difficulties are connected. How?

(a) The organ lung is governed by the element "Metal," which involves letting go and moving on.
(b) Lung Qi is affected by breathing difficulties in conjunction with unresolved grief.
(c) Breathing difficulties are a sign of deficient Lung Qi.
(d) All of the above.

3 Why would it be important to inform the young patient of the connection between grief, loss, and lung Qi?

(a) He should not have been informed.
(b) Now he can appreciate his condition more fully.
(c) Now he can take better care of himself both emotionally and physically, preventing further depletion of lung Qi and gradually restoring it through complementary approaches.
(d) Now he understands his mother better.

Answers:

1 (c): The mother's compromised immune system alone poses a risk to the amount of Qi transmitted from the mother to the unborn child. Add to this her reduced food intake because of constant nausea and an acute grief reaction because of her

father's sudden death, it can be concluded with certainty following TCM's teachings that the child's Qi would be deficient.

2 (d): TCM proposes that unresolved grief affects Lung Qi. When the Metal element is weak, a person struggles greatly with overcoming loss, and in the process of being "stuck" in grief, available Lung Qi is depleted.

3 (c): Knowing that his Lung Qi will need extra care, and why such care is necessary, this young boy has a chance to implement proper breathing techniques, acupressure support, anxiety management, and emotional awareness of the need to address and work through losses, in order to maintain his Lung Qi.

These three case studies are indicative of the range of possibilities opened by combining the "technologies" of Eastern and Western healing techniques to accomplish a variety of medical outcomes, from life-limiting "physical" problems, to "psychological" problems that inhibit full enjoyment of life, to enhancing the quality of the inevitable end of life.

Conclusions

Breathing disorders can be life-threatening disorders since life itself depends on the availability of breath. Breathing blockages, whether they originate from internal or external disturbances, can be understood as energy blockages, depriving a person of beneficial and smooth flow of physical, emotional, and spiritual life energy. Eastern traditions of healing have long believed in the intricate connection of body, mind, and spirit and have treated all three dimensions following a complex system of energy paradigms. Physical stimulation of acupressure points and precise movements to stretch meridians in combination with conscious breath and mindfulness have been utilized in order to direct healing energy to places of emotional and/or physical injury and have been described as beneficial interventions. With appropriate training, primary health-care practitioners, as well as breathing disorders specialists, will be able to offer acupressure and therapeutic breathing interventions to their patient population.

References

1. Kaptchuk T. The web that has no weaver: understanding Chinese medicine. Chicago, IL: Contemporary Books; 2000.
2. Bauer C. Acupressure for everybody. New York, NY: Henry Holt; 1991.
3. Muenke M, Draeger-Muenke R. Acupressure and hypnosis: healer, heal thyself (and thy patients). Contemp Hypn Integ Therapy. 2011;28(3):224–34.
4. Moss CA. Power of the five elements: the Chinese path to healthy aging and stress resistance. Berkley, CA: North Atlantic Books; 2010.
5. Johnson JA. Chinese medical qigong therapy: a comprehensive clinical text. Pacific Grove, CA: The International Institute of Medical Qigong; 2000.

6. Kenyon J. Acupressure techniques. Rochester, VT: Healing Arts Press; 1988.
7. Gach M. Acupressure's potent points. New York, NY: Bantam Books; 1990.
8. Andrews S, Dempsey B. Acupressure and reflexology for dummies. New York, NY: Wiley; 2007.
9. Kolster B. Heilen durch Fingerdruck [Healing through finger pressure.]. Augsburg, Germany: Weltbild; 2010.
10. Ni M. The yellow emperor's classic of medicine; a new translation of the neijing suwen with commentary. Boston, MA: Shambhala; 1995.
11. Maciocia G. The foundations of Chinese medicine: a comprehensive text for acupuncturists and herbalists. Edinburgh, Great Britain: Churchill Livingstone; 1989.
12. Denmei S. Finding effective acupuncture points. Seattle, WA: Eastland Press; 2003.
13. Lian Y-L, Chen C-Y, Hammes M, Kolster BC. The seirin pictorial atlas of acupuncture, an illustrated manual of acupuncture points. Marburg, Germany: KMV-Verlag; 2000.
14. Middendorf I. The perceptible breath. Paderborn, Germany: Junfermann Verlag; 1990.
15. Lewis D. The tao of natural breathing. Berkeley, CA: Rodmell Press; 2006.
16. Wittstein IS. The broken heart syndrome. Cleve Clin J Med. 2007;74 Suppl 1:S17–22.
17. Lee A, Campbell D. Perfect breathing: transform your life one breath at a time. New York, NY: Sterling Publishing Company; 2009.
18. Dahlke R, Neumann A. Die wunderbare Heilkraft des Atmens [The marvellous healing power of breath.]. Muenchen, Germany: Wilhelm Heyne Verlag; 2000.
19. Schultz JH. Das Autogene Training (Konzentrative Selbstentspannung): Versuch Einer Klinisch-Praktischen Darstellung. [Autogenic Training. Self-Relaxation through Concentration. Attempt of a Clinical-Practical Description.]. Leipzig, Germany: Thieme; 1932.
20. Levine P. Healing trauma. Boulder, CO: Sounds True; 2005.
21. Stux G, Berman B, Pomeranz B. Basics of acupuncture. New York, NY: Springer; 2003.
22. Zi N. The art of breathing. Berkeley, CA: Frog Ltd.; 2000.
23. Thich Nhat Hanh. Dharma Talk. http://here-and-now.org/wwwArticles/breathe.html(1998). Accessed 11 Oct 2011.
24. Thich Nhat Hanh. You are here. Boston, MA: Shambhala, 2001.
25. Kabat-Zinn J. Wherever you go, there you are: mindfulness meditation in everyday life. New York, NY: Hyperion Books; 1994.
26. Kabat-Zinn J. Full catastrophe living: using the wisdom of your body and mind to face stress, pain, and illness. New York, NY: Delta Trade Paperbacks; 1990.
27. Smalley S, Winston D. Fully present: the science, art, and practice of mindfulness. Philadelphia, PA: DaCapo Press; 2010.
28. Kim SH. Power breathing. Santa Fe, NM: Turtle Press; 2008.
29. Cheek DB, LeCron LM. Clinical hypnotherapy. New York, NY: Grune and Stratton; 1968.
30. Hammond DC. Handbook of Hypnotic Suggestions and Metaphors. An American Society of Clinical Hypnosis Book. New York, NY: W.W. Norton and Company; 1999.
31. Phillips M. Finding The energy to heal. New York, NY: Norton and Company; 2000.
32. Daitch C. Affect regulation toolbox. New York, NY: Norton; 2007.
33. Daitch C. Anxiety disorders. New York, NY: Norton; 2009.
34. Anbar RD. Self-hypnosis for anxiety associated with severe asthma: a case report. BMC Pediatr. 2003;3:7.
35. Anbar RD, Hummell KE. Self-hypnosis for pain management in patients with cystic fibrosis. Pediatr Pulmonol. 2004; Suppl 27: 148–149.
36. Rizzolatti G, Craighero L. The mirror-neuron system. Annu Rev Neurosci. 2004;27:169–92.
37. Iacoboni M. Mirroring people: the new science of how we connect with others. New York, NY: Farrar, Straus & Giroux; 2008.
38. Iacoboni M. Imitation, empathy, and mirror neurons. Annu Rev Psychol. 2009;60:653–70.

Chapter 16
Mindfulness Meditation for the Treatment of Functional Respiratory Disorders

Adam S. Elias

Abstract Mindfulness meditation is a powerful and simple tool for helping patients understand and treat their own psychosomatic symptoms. There is initial evidence that mindfulness meditation may be beneficial for patients with some types of functional respiratory disorders. Mindfulness meditation is a skill that can be easily taught to a patient by an experienced clinician and should be practiced over a period of time for maximal benefit. Keys to success in mindfulness meditation are a basic understanding of what it is and how it works, patience, and determination, as well as continual, regular practice over time. Clinicians who have gone through mindfulness meditation training are better able to guide patients through the successful relief of their symptoms using this technique. Neuroscientific evidence for the mechanisms of mindfulness meditation is discussed in this chapter, practical considerations of using mindfulness meditation in the primary care setting are discussed, a sample text of basic instructions on how to teach three techniques of mindfulness meditation is provided, and case studies are presented with accompanying quiz questions and explanatory material regarding patients with chest pain, dyspnea, vocal cord dysfunction, and insomnia.

Keywords Mindfulness meditation • Chest pain • Asthma • Dyspnea • Vocal cord dysfunction • Insomnia

Background

Meditation can be defined as a diverse family of practices and techniques engaged in regulating attention for various ends [1]. The methods of meditation have existed for millennia, but there has been renewed interest in the scientific community

A.S. Elias (✉)
Department of Psychiatry, Cambridge Health Alliance, 1493 Cambridge Street, Cambridge, MA 02139, USA
e-mail: aelias@cha.harvard.edu

R.D. Anbar (ed.), *Functional Respiratory Disorders: When Respiratory Symptoms Do Not Respond to Pulmonary Treatment*, Respiratory Medicine,
DOI 10.1007/978-1-61779-857-3_16, © Springer Science+Business Media, LLC 2012

concerning the physiological and neurophysiological changes that occur as a result of meditation and the particular clinical applications. One current model of meditation appears to have relevance to both modern neuroscientific and older meditation traditions. This model divides meditation types into two broad categories based upon differing aspects of employing attention: focused attention and open monitoring [1]. Focused attention meditation refers to various concentration techniques wherein an individual places and maintains attention on one object, while open monitoring meditation refers to various techniques where one openly and nonreactively attends to whatever object arises in the practitioner's awareness. This framework is both flexible and broad enough to encompass many meditation techniques. Specific examples of meditation techniques that fit into one or both categories include mindfulness meditation, verbalization meditation, visualization meditation, compassion meditation, and analytic meditation.

Mindfulness meditation, commonly referred to as Vipassana, or Insight meditation, is the process of directing attention to present-moment experience using a nonjudgmental attitude [2–4]. Attention can be directed toward any aspect of experience, including one's thoughts, emotions, sensations, or mental states [5]. Mindfulness meditation uses aspects of both focused attention and open monitoring because during a given session, the practitioner focuses on one primary object, often the breath or body sensations, but also nonreactively attends to other thoughts and feelings as they automatically arise in one's awareness. The non-evaluative attitude that is developed in mindfulness helps to cultivate acceptance with pleasant or unpleasant experiences of the patient. The popularity of mindfulness meditation has increased significantly over the past few decades, and it can effectively address numerous mental and physical problems. It can be introduced to a patient quickly, over the course of one session, and has been shown to improve symptoms in as short a time as 1 week [6].

Neuroscientific Evidence of Mindfulness Meditation

There have been a growing number of neuroscientific studies elucidating the effects and mechanisms of mindfulness meditation. Since the brain is plastic and is able to change as a result of training, mindfulness meditation is thought to be a type of mental training activity which produces certain changes in the brain that can be studied using modern neuroimaging and other methods.

From neuroimaging studies, mindfulness meditation has been shown to activate the medial and lateral prefrontal cortex, the insula, the somatosensory cortex, the inferior parietal lobes, the cingulate cortex, and the amygdala among other brain regions [7–16]. Mindfulness meditation is involved in a wide range of mental processes, and the types of mental training for which mindfulness meditation may be used are possibly diverse. For example, the prefrontal cortex is involved in executive decision-making as well as the regulation of attention; the insula is involved in interoception, which is related to awareness of internal states; the somatosensory cortex is involved in bodily sensation; the parietal lobes are involved in spatial awareness; the cingulate cortex is involved in the regulation of attention as well as positive and negative emotion; and the amygdala is involved in the processing and regulation of fear, anger, and other negative emotional states. Specifically, it is now thought that mindfulness meditation may have a role in wide-ranging areas such as attention, bodily awareness, and emotion.

In line with the role of meditation as mental training, recent investigations have focused on particular brain changes as a result of meditation, after both short-term and long-term practice. One study demonstrated that an 8-week program of mindfulness meditation training produced changes in activation in the dorsomedial prefrontal cortex, ventromedial prefrontal cortex, lateral prefrontal cortex, the insula, and the inferior parietal lobule, where pre- and post-fMRI imaging was employed [7]. Areas that were associated with the ability to focus on present moment-to-moment awareness, such as the lateral prefrontal cortex, insula, and inferior parietal lobe, showed increased activation, while areas associated with past and future narrative thinking, such as the medial prefrontal cortex, showed decreased activation. Present-moment awareness is an important skill in mindfulness meditation because among other things, it allows participants to disengage from automatic, negative patterns of past and future thinking.

Another study showed a difference in gray matter density between long-term meditators and controls in the left inferior temporal gyrus, the right anterior insula, and the right hippocampus, where long-term meditators showed increased cortical density in these regions [8]. Since mental training has been found to increase gray matter in regions of the brain that are responsible for the respective skill or task, the implication is that mindfulness meditation training increases neuronal function associated with mindfulness skills to such an extent that the actual structure of the brain changes and becomes more dense. In this study, the insula, which is involved in interoception; the hippocampus, which is involved in cortical activation as well as learning; and the temporal lobe, which has been reported to be involved in various spiritual experiences, all showed increased density.

A longitudinal study by Lazar et al. [9] showed that long-term mindfulness meditation experience was associated with increased cortical density in the prefrontal cortex and insula. Increased cortical thickness, if it is a result of mental training, was hypothesized to occur either from greater neuronal arborization, increased glial volume, or increased vasculature, all of which are evidence of increased neuronal functioning and could be reflective of increased awareness of internal states and increased attention regulation.

Mindfulness meditation has also been reported to increase emotional well-being, and it is thought that this is achieved through changes in the brain that are involved with affect regulation [10]. Hölzel et al. demonstrated that after 8 weeks of mindfulness meditation training, decreases in gray matter density in the amygdala were associated with reports of decreased stress [11]. The amygdala has been repeatedly shown to be involved in responses characterized by stress and fear and is thought to be one of the most important brain structures involved in anxiety disorders. Since the decreased stress as a result of mindfulness meditation was shown to be highly correlated with the decreased density of the amygdala, this is strong evidence that demonstrates how a clinical intervention with positive clinical findings can be correlated with precise neuroanatomic changes.

In addition, a prospective study using 8 weeks of mindfulness meditation training was shown to increase gray matter density in the left hippocampus, posterior cingulate cortex, temporoparietal junction, and the cerebellum compared to matched controls [12]. The hippocampus is known to be an important region for memory and learning processes, as well as the regulation of emotional control. The posterior cingulate cortex has been suggested to be involved in the integration of stimuli into one's sense of self as a whole person [13]. Thus, mindfulness meditation has implications that not only affect attention and emotion but also influence memory, learning, and the sense of oneself. This could have implications in a therapeutic context by guiding the patient to train in new ways of relating to oneself that are characterized by emotional well-being and positivity.

Other forms of meditation in addition to mindfulness include compassion and loving-kindness meditation, verbalization meditation, visualization meditation, contemplation, and analytic meditation. Compassion meditation, which involves the cultivation of the mental state of desiring the relief of suffering of others, has been shown to involve increased activity in the amygdala, insula, and anterior cingulated gyrus, all important structures involved in the processing of emotion [14]. Consistent with the model of meditation as a type of mental training, meditators who were very experienced with compassion meditation were better able to regulate the amygdala and anterior cingulate gyrus during compassion meditation compared to controls [14]. Verbalization meditation involves the use of specific words said either internally or out loud that are employed as the object of meditation. Studies have shown increased activity during verbalization meditation in the right temporal and posterior cingulated gyrus, the dorsolateral prefrontal and parietal cortices, hippocampus and parahippocampus, temporal lobe, pregenual anterior cingulate cortex, striatum and pre- and postcentral gyri, the left parietal, inferior parietal, and inferior frontal areas [15–18]. Visualization meditation is defined as the use of internalized mental imagery as the object of meditation. Studies have shown increased activity in the occipital cortex, as well as the cingulated gyrus, inferior and orbital frontal cortex, dorsolateral prefrontal cortex (DLPFC), and thalamus [17, 19, 20]. We are not aware of any studies investigating analytic meditation, which is the process of understanding an object through the use of intellect, or reasoning.

As the neuroscientific study of meditation is still in its infancy, the exact relationship for the activity patterns described above and specific clinical outcomes needs to be further elucidated. Furthermore, there has been little research to date comparing different types of meditation for specific diseases [21, 22]. This chapter will concentrate on mindfulness meditation because of the wide range of problems for which it is known to be clinically effective. Other forms of meditation also may be beneficial for functional respiratory disorders, and thus, it is suggested that future research compare various forms of meditation for their relative efficacy in treating those disorders.

Evidence for the Efficacy of Mindfulness Meditation for Respiratory Disorders

There have been multiple studies investigating the use of mindfulness meditation for insomnia. One randomized controlled trial investigated the efficacy of mindfulness-based stress reduction (MBSR) with thirty adults with primary chronic insomnia, which consisted of 8 weekly 2.5-h classes, a day-long meditation retreat, and ongoing home meditation practice. The study found significant improvements for sleep-onset latency, insomnia severity, and sleep quality comparable in magnitude to the control group given eszopiclone (Lunesta) [23]. A pilot study using mindfulness-based cognitive therapy (MBCT) treating insomnia in 19 patients with anxiety disorders showed significant improvement in the Pittsburgh Sleep Quality Index as well as a variety of anxiety-related questionnaires [24]. A study that was not randomized or controlled combined mindfulness meditation with cognitive behavior therapy for insomnia and found statistical improvements in presleep arousal, sleep effort, and dysfunctional sleep-related cognitions [25].

There are published studies for treating asthma using types of meditation other than mindfulness. One controlled study used yoga asanas (postures) integrated with verbalization meditation and breathing techniques for 53 patients matched for age, sex, and type and severity of asthma who used medication treatment as usual and found significant improvement in the yoga and meditation group in number of weekly asthma attacks and peak expiratory flow rate [26]. Additionally, a double-blind, randomized, controlled trial used Sahaja Yoga meditation, which uses affirmations in order to achieve a state of mind free from mental elaboration, for the treatment of asthma in 30 patients. The study found statistically significant improvement in airway hyperresponsiveness to methacholine greater in the yoga group compared to controls, although asthma-related quality-of-life differences were not statistically significant nor were changes between the yoga group and controls at 2 months follow-up [27]. These studies provide initial preliminary evidence that there may be a role for meditation and yoga in the treatment of asthma, but studies need to be completed to determine whether mindfulness meditation in particular has a role.

For the treatment of chest pain, Kabat-Zinn [28] evaluated the use of mindfulness meditation for 51 patients with chronic pain, including noncoronary chest pain, and found that 65% of patients had a reduction in the mean total Pain Rating Index of at least 33%, and 50% of patients showed a reduction of at least 50%. Furthermore, there is a strong body of evidence which shows that meditation is associated with decreased sensitivity to pain in general, as well as decreased ratings of experimentally induced pain [29–32]. A recent study showed that healthy subjects who were taught focused attention meditation over four 20-min classes and then were exposed to thermal stimuli showed an average of 40% reduction in pain intensity and a 57% reduction in pain unpleasantness, as well as associated decreases in somatosensory activation using arterial spin labeling MRI [33]. However, the author is not aware of any studies that limited the scope of study to chest pain, and therefore, studies in this area should be pursued.

Mindfulness meditation has also been shown to improve symptoms of other functional medical problems. An open pilot study showed improvements in IBS symptoms with mindfulness meditation, and a controlled study showed that relaxation response meditation showed improvements for IBS [34, 35]. The relaxation response is a set of physiological changes that occur as a result of meditation, such as decreased respiratory rate and decreased blood pressure [36]. The type of meditation most often associated with the relaxation response is a simple verbalization meditation where the word "one" is silently repeated during each exhalation [36]. There were no studies found that investigated the efficacy of mindfulness meditation for dyspnea or vocal cord dysfunction. However, since contributing factors for dyspnea and vocal cord dysfunction often involve anxiety, and since mindfulness meditation has been shown in meta-analysis to have a moderate effect size for treating anxiety, it is proposed that more studies evaluate the efficacy of mindfulness meditation for dyspnea and vocal cord dysfunction where anxiety plays a contributing role [21, 37, 38].

Practical Application

The possibility of using mindfulness meditation may be introduced during a regular office visit when a patient presents with a symptom that may be addressed with this therapy. There are several important points to communicate with patients so that they may receive the most benefit possible from this intervention. An overview of a mindfulness meditation teaching session can be found in Table 16.1. Patients should first be told that mindfulness meditation is the practice of attending to present-moment experience with a nonjudgmental attitude. They should be told that learning the skills of mindfulness meditation may help them have increased awareness of their thoughts, feelings, and sensations and help them feel less of their physical and mental symptoms.

Second, patients should be told that an essential skill of mindfulness meditation is changing the perspective they have toward their own respiratory symptoms. They can learn a new way to understand their symptoms; instead of regarding them as problems that must be eliminated, they can be regarded as opportunities from which the patient can learn.

Third, it is important to communicate to patients that there is no one "right way" of practicing mindfulness. One should not be concerned whether one is "good" or "bad" at meditation. As long as one is making the effort, or intention, one is practicing effectively. Moreover, if one only feels unpleasant emotions or negative thoughts during meditation, this also does not mean that one is practicing "badly." It should be communicated to the patient that the point is to observe whatever he is thinking or feeling with acceptance, even if it is very unpleasant or painful. In this way, real nonjudgmental awareness of experience can be embraced.

Fourth, it should be emphasized that regular, routine practice is essential in order to experience the benefits of meditation. Although the exact amount of time to dedicate

Table 16.1 Instructions for mindfulness meditation

Breathing meditation

- The patient is instructed that mindfulness meditation is the practice of attending to present-moment experience with a nonjudgmental attitude. He is told that learning the skills of mindfulness meditation may help him have increased awareness of his thoughts, feelings, and sensations and help him feel less of his physical symptoms
- He is instructed that usually during mindfulness meditation, attention is placed on one object, such as the breath, or body sensations, and one attempts to bring and keep attention on this object. Initially, it is suggested that the primary object of attention would be his breathing at his abdomen. Every time the patient inhales and the abdomen rises up, he is instructed to internally note "rising." Every time the patient exhales and abdomen falls, he is instructed to internally note "falling." For each and every breath, the patient is instructed to note "rising, falling, rising, falling," continuously, as long as the patient is able to sustain his attention [39]
- The patient is instructed to become aware of when his mind starts to drift or wander from the primary object of attention. When this begins to happen, he is told to note "wandering, wandering." He is then told to simply observe nonreactively whatever he is thinking, feeling, or sensing, which caused his mind to wander. After observing for a moment, he is told to gently return his attention back to the rising and falling of the abdomen. Alternatively, the patient may note the type of thoughts he is having, such as "remembering," "hoping," "analyzing," or "criticizing," for any thought brings the mind away from the breath [39]
- Whenever a strong emotion, such as anger, worry, confusion, or fear, arises in the patient and distracts him from keeping the attention on the abdomen, the patient is instructed to silently note that emotion, internally saying "anger, anger, anger," or "worry, worry, worry," until the patient is able to return to the breath. The noting of these emotions is considered to be an important part of the mindfulness meditation. The patient is also instructed to note sensations, such as pain, numbness, tingling, pressure, etc., in the same manner. Using this method, all aspects of experience become part of mindfulness meditation

Body scan

- The patient can be taught a second form of mindfulness meditation, the body scan. The patient is instructed to slowly move attention from his head to his feet, becoming aware of the sensations in each body part [2]. When he finishes, he is instructed to return to his head and go back down again, each time becoming more and more immersed in the sensations he is feeling. Whenever the patient's mind starts to wander from the sensations in his body, he may use the same technique described above and simply note the emotions or thoughts gently and without judgment, and then return to the given area of the body

Loving-kindness meditation

- The patient is instructed to choose a person to whom he wishes to direct kind and loving thoughts. Once that person is chosen, he is instructed to imagine that person in front of him and internally say the following words: "May you be happy. May you be healthy. May you be free from harm. May you lead a joyous life." These instructions are repeated twice, and then the patient stays in that state of mind for a short period of time. Afterward, the patient is told that whenever he wishes to end the meditation, he may simply open his eyes

to practice will differ from person to person, this author recommends practicing at least three to four times a week for at least half an hour. Finally, it should be explained to the patient that the power of meditation lies in the patient's ability to use it for self empowerment, not in something that is done to him/her by the clinician. This distinction is important as it leads the patient to greater growth and independence through the practice of meditation itself.

Commonly, when mindfulness meditation is practiced, the patient places and attempts to maintain attention on one "object." There are a multitude of primary objects a patient can use, such as the breath, various body sensations, sounds, or even images. However, because of the nature of the symptoms of patients with functional respiratory problems, it is suggested that the breath is a very good place to begin. The sensations associated with breathing can be observed around the nostrils, chest, or abdomen. The patient may choose the area to focus upon, but once the location is decided, attention should not move from that area. The patient then simply observes the sensations without attempting any cognitive elaboration, using bare attention to note the sensations as they arise and pass. If the patient chooses to place attention on the area around the nostrils and the upper lip, then he may observe the touch of the incoming and outgoing breath as the air moves in and out. If the patient decides to observe the breath at the abdomen, then he may watch the rise and the fall of the abdomen with each inhale and exhale.

For every breath, the patient would continuously note "rising" when the abdomen rises and "falling" when the abdomen falls, for as long as the patient is able to sustain attention [39]. Wandering thoughts or emotions that bring the attention away from the breath also should be considered part of mindfulness meditation, not extraneous to it. They should be noted with acceptance, and then the attention should gently return to the breath. Mindfulness meditation can also be practiced using the body scan or using loving-kindness meditation (Table 16.1).

Integrating Mindfulness with Hypnosis

Meditation may be integrated with other forms of therapy to achieve an optimal response in the patient. Recently, hypnosis was successfully integrated with mindfulness meditation for the treatment of anxiety in an adolescent [6]. It has been proposed that mindfulness and hypnosis might work well in tandem for multiple reasons. First, the mechanisms behind the efficacy of mindfulness and hypnosis in therapy are both thought to lie in their ability to deautomatize maladaptive response sets and create new, adaptive response sets, wherein response sets are thought of as "conditioned patterns of associations composed of expectancies, intentions, and cognitive-representations or constructions of the self [40]." Mindfulness meditation can deautomatize negative response sets by making the patient more aware of his/her negative thought patterns and thus creating the space for the introduction of positive response sets. Hypnosis, with the use of suggestions, can also facilitate the actual development of new response sets [40].

Furthermore, both mindfulness and hypnosis are used to promote the therapeutic goals of acceptance and lessening avoidance. It has been proposed that since hypnosis enhances the effectiveness of both psychodynamic and cognitive-behavioral psychotherapies, there may be corresponding enhanced effectiveness with mindfulness as well [40]. By using hypnotic suggestions, the skill of mindfulness may be cultivated more readily.

The Benefits of Training in Mindfulness Meditation

In order for a clinician to use mindfulness meditation effectively with patients, it is essential to be properly trained, as is the case with many other therapeutic methods. Trainings include professional programs in mindfulness, such as MBSR, MBCT, or active participation in mindfulness meditation retreats.

Proper training in mindfulness meditation involves knowledge about mindfulness meditation as well as proficiency in its actual practice. Therefore, becoming a skilled practitioner of meditation is essential in becoming a proficient teacher of mindfulness meditation to patients. The framework of mindfulness meditation highly emphasizes the value of experience. There are multiple reasons for this approach. First, if one speaks from personal experience rather than mere intellectual knowledge, the patient may be more likely to listen to and benefit from the clinician's instructions. For example, if someone wanted to learn how to play a sport, they would choose someone who excels at playing that sport. Similarly, if one wanted to learn meditation properly, that person would choose someone skilled at meditation. Second, by going through the practice of mindfulness meditation, a clinician can more easily understand the problems and difficulties that arise when the patient practices. Additionally, an important part of receiving maximum benefit from mindfulness meditation comes from practice that is regular and routine over a period of time. When the clinician has gone through the process of this committed practice, it will be easier to guide and motivate the patient using the clinician's own training.

Questions and Case Studies

The following case studies represent scenarios that highlight key elements of teaching mindfulness meditation to patients with functional respiratory disorders. Such interventions will need to be conducted with multiple patients to validate whether these techniques typically are efficacious in each situation.

Case 1: Chest Pain

A 25-year-old woman with no history of medical problems complains of chronic, substernal chest pain for the past year. The pain occurs more frequently when the patient is anxious or during especially stressful periods. The patient states that over the past year, she has had increased pressure at work and is increasingly arguing with her housemates. Her chest pain does not radiate and is not associated with dizziness, nausea or vomiting, or with eating certain types of foods. There is no associated shortness of breath. The patient is not taking oral contraceptives, does not smoke or use any other drugs, and has no family history of heart disease. An EKG is normal.

The chest pain is interpreted to be functional, and mindfulness meditation is suggested to the patient as a way of managing her stress and related symptoms. The patient is interested in learning the technique. She is instructed to place one hand on her abdomen and watch the rising and falling of her hand each time she inhales and exhales. She is to maintain her attention on her breath and gently return her attention to her abdomen when she notices her mind wandering. If she begins to feel pain in her chest, and the sensations are sufficiently distracting, she is instructed to note the sensations and label them by internally saying "discomfort, discomfort, discomfort" until the sensations decrease in intensity. When she is able to disengage her mind from the unpleasant sensations, she can return to the silent noting of her breath. She is told that it does not matter how long she stays noting her chest discomfort; as long as she is observing the sensations nonreactively, she would be successful.

The patient meditates for 5 min during the first session with the therapist. She is then instructed to meditate by herself at home for 15 min four times for the first week. She can either sit cross-legged on the floor or in a chair. If she is inclined, she can continue with her hand on her abdomen or she can place them in her lap or on her knees. During those 15 min, she is instructed to meditate silently, slowly and gently moving her body when necessary. During the next session a week later, the patient discusses her initial impressions of the usefulness of meditation with the therapist. She is then instructed to increase her time meditating to 30 min four times weekly.

Questions:

1. Why was it suggested that the patient place her hand on her abdomen?
   (a) Her hand should always be placed where she is noticing sensations.
   (b) By pressing on her abdomen, she can forget about the pain in her chest.
   (c) The patient may more easily notice the abdomen's movement using her hand.
   (d) (a) and (c).
   (e) None of the above.
2. Why was the patient instructed to meditate in silence?
   (a) Silence helps her collect her thoughts.
   (b) Silence aids in developing concentration.
   (c) Silence allows her to access insights concerning the triggers of her chest pain.
   (d) Silence promotes a more relaxed, calm mood in the patient.
   (e) All of the above.
3. What was the purpose of internally noting the sensations of discomfort during meditation?
   (a) If the patient gets bored of following the breath, she can switch to something more interesting.
   (b) By making a verbal note of the discomfort, it allows her to more directly acknowledge her present-moment experience.
   (c) Simply noting the experience without judging it as good or bad allows her to develop nonreactivity.

(d) (b) and (c).
(e) All of the above.

Answers:

1. (c): Placing the hand on the abdomen is completely optional and may help beginners notice their breathing at the abdomen. If the hand is not on the abdomen, both hands can be placed in the lap or on both knees. The patient may be seated in a chair while practicing mindfulness or on the floor in a cross-legged position. In either case, the back should be straight. Effort should be made to move as little as possible during meditation without causing undue pain. However, that effort should be secondary to the primary goals of watching the breath and cultivating a nonreactive attitude toward experience. Patients should be kind to themselves and listen to their bodies when they are in a physical posture that is too uncomfortable.
2. (e): Silence has traditionally been an essential component of many meditative methods, including mindfulness. When the patient is first learning meditation, clear instructions during meditation should be given. However, they should be interspersed with silence to help the patient achieve calm and tranquility. As the patient becomes more skilled in mindfulness meditation, silence should be used more frequently during sessions. At home, the patient should meditate in complete silence.
3. (d): Mental noting of experience is one common method of mindfulness meditation [35]. This noting can be of the sensations associated with the presenting complaint, in this case, the chest tightness, or it can be of any experiences that the patient is having, whether they be thoughts, emotions, other sensations, or mental states. For example, if the patient is worrying about the future, she can note, "worrying, worrying," or if the patient is angry during meditation, she can note "anger, anger, anger." All types of experiences can be noted in this way, which allows her to become more fully aware of her experiences and develop a non-identified perspective at the same time. The patient can learn that she is not her anger, worry, or chest tightness; these experiences do not need to define who she is.

Case 2: Dyspnea

A 13-year-old adolescent male with a history of anxiety and obsessive-compulsive disorder complains of shortness of breath while thinking about possible catastrophic events in family members. The patient reports that his dyspnea started 2 weeks ago when his older sister was using the barbeque and the patient was fearful that she would be seriously hurt. He states that it is difficult to get air into his lungs, and then he becomes even more anxious and starts to breathe faster. He also reports tightness in his throat. The patient has worried excessively about his family for over a year, but before this episode, there was no associated dyspnea. He denies any wheezing, coughing, or stridor. He was not recently sick, does not take any medications, and has no allergies.

Mindfulness meditation of breathing is explained and taught to the patient as described above. In addition, a mindful body scan is taught. The patient is instructed to bring his attention to various body parts, starting from the head and moving to the feet. In each body location, he is instructed to become aware of the associated sensations. When he reaches his throat and his chest, he is instructed to become aware of whether he is feeling tight or relaxed, and he is to simply note that sensation, without trying to change it. If his throat is feeling tight, he is to note "tight, tight, tight" until the sensation reduces. Furthermore, he is instructed to maintain calmness of mind even if his throat feels tight in order to develop nonreactive acceptance of his body. During the meditation, he is encouraged to explore his feelings of anxiety toward his family members. While actively watching his thoughts, he is told to become aware of any wisdom arising from inside that could help him think in less catastrophic ways.

Questions:

1. Why is the patient instructed to simply observe the sensations of tightness in his throat rather than use a method to relax the tightness?
   (a) The tig.htness will never go away, so there is no point in using any method.
   (b) Mindfulness meditation cultivates an attitude of acceptance for even unpleasant experiences such as throat tightness.
   (c) By simply developing nonreactive awareness of the sensations in his throat, the patient may notice that his throat eventually will relax on its own.
   (d) (b) and (c).
   (e) All of the above.
2. How would mindfulness meditation help the patient discover his own solutions to his anxiety-related dyspnea?
   (a) Taking slow, deep breaths counteracts his rapid breathing.
   (b) Watching his thoughts as an observer during meditation can provide self-directed insight into the nature of his anxiety.
   (c) It is more effective if the patient makes his own connections during meditation rather than receiving instructions from someone else.
   (d) He will become more aware of associated triggers.
   (e) (b), (c), and (d).
3. What is the difference between mindful breathing and a body scan?
   (a) During mindful breathing, attention stays on the breath, while during a body scan, attention moves systematically to various sensations in different parts of the body.
   (b) Mindfulness can only be applied when attending to one object.
   (c) A body scan helps one become aware of tensions and pain in various parts of the body, of which one may not be aware with mindful breathing.
   (d) (a) and (c).
   (e) All of the above.

Answers:

1. (d): Mindfulness meditation can be effective on two levels for this anxiety-related dyspnea and other related functional problems. On the first level, mindfulness meditation changes the relationship of the patient to his complaint. Doing this reduces the psychological intolerability of the dyspnea because the patient is no longer bothered as much by it. On the second level, the dyspnea itself actually may decrease because since the problem is mind-body related, it is at least partly intensified by the anxiety itself.
2. (e): By becoming more aware of his experiences, and learning to relate to them in a direct way, the patient is empowered to see the problems and solutions for himself. Therefore, any insights that arise will be more important for him, and he may be more apt to recognize in the future any triggers he discovers. For choice (a), although it is true that deep breathing can help counteract rapid, shallow breathing seen in anxiety, by itself it will not give him insight to discover his own solutions.
3. (d): Mindfulness can be applied whether or not one is keeping the attention in one place or moving the attention to different areas. During the body scan, areas of discomfort in the body are localized, and greater awareness of the differences in how various parts of the body feel can lead to a new feeling of wholeness in the body, as well as an increased ability to know what the body feels without experiencing increased unpleasantness.

Case 3: Vocal Cord Dysfunction

An 18-year-old female athlete presents with difficulty with inhalation and associated stridor that developed a few minutes after beginning competitive field hockey as a college freshman. She reports that it feels as if her throat constricts when she develops her symptoms. The symptoms do not occur during practice. The patient needs to stop her participation in the games in order to rest for a few moments until her symptoms resolve. Pulmonary function tests are normal. She had tried various asthma medications with no improvement. She is diagnosed as having vocal cord dysfunction.

The patient is instructed in mindfulness meditation as described previously. After being instructed regarding her airway anatomy, she is instructed to pay particular attention to the specific details of the sensations of her vocal cords and overall neck region both while she is and is not experiencing respiratory distress. She is asked to pay attention to what she is thinking about just before the throat constriction occurs, as well how her sensations change over time and how long it takes for one sensation in her vocal cords to change into another sensation. She is instructed to keep the attitude that no one sensation is "better" or "worse" than another sensation, and each and every sensation deserves her open curiosity and acceptance. The patient is motivated in learning meditation and wants to practice 30 min 4 days a week. It is also suggested that if she is interested, she can write down her thoughts and insights each time she ends a mindfulness meditation session.

Questions:

1. Why did this patient start with 30 min of mindfulness meditation while other patients began with less?
   (a) Each patient's personal motivations and capabilities should be taken into account when deciding upon the amount of meditation to practice.
   (b) The amount of time given to meditation has no effect on the results.
   (c) If the patient is willing to practice more, he or she may experience benefits more quickly.
   (d) (a) and (c).
   (e) All of the above.
2. Why was the patient encouraged to pay attention to the changing nature of her sensations around her vocal cords and the beginning, middle, and end of each sensation?
   (a) Curiously paying attention more carefully to her sensations helps to prevent her from being emotionally overcome by the spasms.
   (b) Understanding her sensations as temporary and constantly changing helps her to develop a healthy perspective toward her discomfort.
   (c) By paying closer attention to how the sensations change, she can understand what causes her throat constriction to start and stop.
   (d) All of the above.
   (e) None of the above.
3. What was one purpose of writing her reflections after the session of mindfulness meditation?
   (a) To re-create her previous experience.
   (b) To review and consolidate what she learned about herself.
   (c) To capture what she experienced forever on paper.
   (d) To show to other people.
   (e) None of the above.

Answers:

1. (d): It is important for the provider to keep in mind the individual patient's needs and abilities when formulating an amount of meditation to recommend. Some patients will be ready early on to dedicate much time to practicing mindfulness meditation, while others will be ready for less time. Younger children especially should start with less time each session than older adolescents and adults. Thus, the time and frequency of practicing mindfulness meditation should be determined on a case-by-case basis.
2. (d): Much emphasis in mindfulness practice is dedicated to observing how sensations change over time and can be applied in this patient's case to her

vocal cord dysfunction. The advantages of paying attention to the impermanence of unpleasant sensations are numerous and are described in all of the answer choices.

3. (b): It is not necessary to do any writing after mindfulness practice, but sometimes it may be helpful gathering one's thoughts together after a session. Patients may find that their thoughts and ideas are much clearer after a sit because they have already let their mind settle and become calm. Thus, any reflections afterward may be even more valuable.

Case 4: Insomnia

A 17-year-old female reports a 1-year history of difficulty falling asleep, as it takes her approximately 1–1.5 h to fall asleep each night. Once she is asleep, she states she sleeps deeply and does not recall waking up in the middle of the night. She reports that after lying down in bed, she immediately starts worrying about her family problems, since her father and mother are in the middle of a divorce. She then becomes upset that it is taking her so long to fall asleep, and this causes her to stay up even longer. She has already changed some of her habits to improve sleep hygiene. She goes to bed at the same time nightly, avoids caffeine, and does not watch television while in bed.

The patient is taught mindfulness meditation to help her sleep better. She is instructed to focus on her abdominal breathing as she lies in bed. She notices that it is easier to feel the rise and fall of her abdomen when she is lying down. She also is instructed to regard all of her worried thoughts about her family as clouds passing by in the sky. They appear and disappear, and she does not need to identify with any of them. She is told to regard the rise and fall of her abdomen as waves rising and falling in the sea. Also, she is encouraged to view her time meditating in bed before going to sleep as very valuable, since it is a time for her to learn about herself and become more in tune with her inner self. Therefore, it does not matter how long she is awake, watching her thoughts as clouds and her abdomen as waves. She is told to practice this technique every night before going to sleep, until she actually falls asleep, whether it is 5 min or 2 h.

Questions:

1. What was the purpose of encouraging the patient to not worry how long it took for her to go to sleep?
   (a) Part of her inability to fall asleep arose from her worry about not being able to fall asleep.
   (b) Her concern was not valid.

(c) The time before sleep can be valuable by viewing it as an opportunity to collect one's thoughts and practice mindfulness.
(d) (a) and (c).
(e) All of the above.

2. Why were the metaphors of clouds in the sky and waves in the sea used for this patient?

   (a) The patient will not practice correctly unless metaphors are used.
   (b) Metaphors help to clarify instructions for the patient.
   (c) Imagery can help to strengthen the meditative experience if the patient is consumed by her thoughts.
   (d) (a) and (b).
   (e) (b) and (c).

3. What should the patient do if her worried thoughts caused her to completely forget to practice mindfulness of her breath?

   (a) If she is practicing correctly, this will not happen.
   (b) She should blame herself because it is her fault that she cannot focus on her breath.
   (c) She can let her thoughts take their course, and when they run out of steam, she can gently return her attention to breathing.
   (d) She should stop trying to meditate because she is not good at it.
   (e) None of the above.

Answers:

1. (d): As seen in other cases, mindfulness meditation can serve multiple purposes at once. By relating to her insomnia differently, she can learn to worry less about how long it takes to fall asleep. Instead, she can learn to regard her time in bed as valuable, since it allows her to collect her thoughts about the next day and give her time to meditate. This change in attitude by itself will help her feel more comfortable when she does not fall asleep immediately. Also, focusing on her breath allows her to disengage from her worried thoughts, which are preventing her from relaxing and falling asleep.
2. (e): Metaphors are often very useful to help patients use their imaginations to understand the instructions more fully. During the actual practice of meditation, the patient may use the metaphor to help them concentrate on the meditation object, such as their breath. However, using this technique, emphasis should be place primarily on the sensations themselves. In this way, mindfulness meditation is different from other forms of mental imagery.
3. (c): It is very common for beginners to become frustrated and think that they are not good at meditation so they should not practice. This misconception is problematic because it may cause beginners to stop practicing. First, as explained

previously, there is no such thing as being "good" or "bad" at meditation, since the idea is to give up judgmental feelings of "good" or "bad." Even feelings of frustration, inadequacy, and doubt can be objects of meditation, and the meditator can observe those experiences nonjudgmentally as well, noting "doubt," "frustration," "impatience," or "feeling inadequate." This is often very fruitful, when one begins to simply note these very unpleasant states of mind. Second, in the beginning of training, the mind wanders very frequently, and since this is extremely common, patients should not feel that anything out of the ordinary is happening. Third, it should be emphasized that progress can always be made, even with someone whose worried mind wanders constantly. Therefore, satisfaction is gained through the improvement one makes, wherever the baseline may be. With this attitude, any patient may benefit.

Conclusions

Mindfulness meditation may be a useful and effective tool to engage patients with functional respiratory disorders, including those with chest pain, dyspnea, vocal cord dysfunction, and insomnia. Mindfulness meditation allows patients to develop a new perspective and attitude toward their symptoms that enable them to become more aware and accept their symptoms. The practice of mindfulness meditation may decrease the severity of the symptoms themselves. There is initial evidence that mindfulness meditation is effective for various types of psychosomatic problems. More studies of mindfulness meditation for functional respiratory disorders are needed in order to further evaluate its efficacy in this setting.

References

1. Lutz A, Slagter HA, Dunne JD, Davidson RJ. Attention regulation and monitoring in meditation. Trends Cognit Sci. 2008;12(4):163–9.
2. Kabat-Zinn J. Full catastrophe living: using the wisdom of your body and mind to face stress, pain, and illness. New York, NY: Bantam Dell, Delta Publishing; 2005.
3. Kabat-Zinn J. Mindfulness-based interventions in context: past, present, and future. Clin Psychol Sci Pract. 2003;10(2):144–58.
4. Cahn BR, Polich J. Meditation states and traits: EEG, ERP, and neuroimaging studies. Psychol Bull. 2006;132(2):180–211.
5. Gunaratana BH. Mindfulness in plain english. Somerville, MA: Wisdom Publications; 2002.
6. Elias AS, Anbar RD. Integrating mindfulness and hypnosis: a case report. American Society of Clinical Hypnosis annual meeting. Las Vegas, NV; 2011.
7. Farb NA, Segal ZV, Mayberg H, et al. Attending to the present: mindfulness meditation reveals distinct neural modes of self-reference. Soc Cognit Affect Neurosci. 2007;2(4):313–22.
8. Hölzel BK, Ott U, Gard T, et al. Investigation of mindfulness meditation practitioners with voxel-based morphometry. Soc Cognit Affect Neurosci. 2008;3(1):55–61.
9. Lazar SW, Kerr C, Wasserman RH, et al. Meditation experience is associated with increased cortical thickness. Neuroreport. 2005;16(17):1893–7.

10. Brown KW, Ryan RM. The benefits of being present: mindfulness and its role in psychological well-being. J Pers Soc Psychol. 2003;84(4):822–48.
11. Hölzel BK, Carmody J, Evans KC, et al. Stress reduction correlates with structural changes in the amygdala. Soc Cognit Affect Neurosci. 2010;5(1):11–7.
12. Hölzel BK, Carmody J, Vangela M, et al. Mindfulness practice leads to increases in regional brain gray matter density. Psychiatr Res. 2010;191(1):36–43.
13. Northoff G, Bermpohl F. Cortical midline structures and the self. Trends Cognit Sci. 2004;8(3):102–7.
14. Lutz A, Brefczynski-Lewis J, Johnstone T, Davidson RJ. Regulation of the neural circuitry of emotion by compassion meditation: effects of meditative expertise. PLoS One. 2008;3(3): e1897.
15. Khalsa DS, Amen D, Hanks C, Money N, Newberg A. Cerebral blood flow changes during chanting meditation. Nucl Med Comm. 2009;30(12):956–61.
16. Lazar SW, Bush G, Gollub RL, Fricchione GL, Khalsa G, Benson H. Functional brain mapping of the relaxation response and meditation. Neuroreport. 2000;11(7):1581–5.
17. Lehmann D, Faber PL, Achermann P, Jeanmonod D, Gianotti LR, Pizzagalli D. Brain sources of EEG gamma frequency during volitionally meditation-induced, altered states of consciousness, and experience of the self. Psychiatr Res. 2001;108(2):111–21.
18. Newberg A, Pourdehnad M, Alavi A, d'Aquili EG. Cerebral blood flow during meditative prayer: preliminary findings and methodological issues. Percept Mot Skills. 2003; 97(2):625–30.
19. Lou HC, Kjaer TW, Friberg L, Wildschiodtz G, Holm S, Nowak M. A 15O-H2O PET study of meditation and the resting state of normal consciousness. Hum Brain Mapp. 1999;7(2): 98–105.
20. Newberg A, Alavi A, Baime M, Pourdehnad M, Santanna J, d'Aquili E. The measurement of regional cerebral blood flow during the complex cognitive task of meditation: a preliminary SPECT study. Psychiatr Res. 2001;106(2):113–22.
21. Hofmann SG, Sawyer AT, Witt AA, Oh D. The effect of mindfulness-based therapy on anxiety and depression: a meta-analytic review. J Consult Clin Psychol. 2010;78(2):169–83.
22. Ospina MB, Bond K, Karkhaneh M, et al. Meditation practices for health: state of the research. Evid Rep Tech Assess. 2007;155:1–263.
23. Gross CR, Kreitzer MJ, Reilly-Spong M, et al. Mindfulness-based stress reduction versus pharmacotherapy for chronic primary insomnia: a randomized controlled clinical trial. Explore (NY). 2011;7(2):76–87.
24. Yook K, Lee SH, Ryu M, et al. Usefulness of mindfulness-based cognitive therapy for treating insomnia in patients with anxiety disorders: a pilot study. J Nerv Ment Dis. 2008;196(6): 501–3.
25. Ong JC, Shapiro SL, Manber R. Combining mindfulness meditation with cognitive-behavior therapy for insomnia: a treatment-development study. Behav Ther. 2008;39(2):171–82.
26. Nagarathna R, Nagendra HR. Yoga for bronchial asthma: a controlled study. Br Med J(Clin Res Ed). 1985;291(6502):1077–9.
27. Manocha R, Marks GB, Kenchington P, Peters D, Salome CM. Sahaja yoga in the management of moderate to severe asthma: a randomised controlled trial. Thorax. 2002;57(2):110–5.
28. Kabat-Zinn J. An outpatient program in behavioral medicine for chronic pain patients based on the practice of mindfulness meditation: theoretical considerations and preliminary results. Gen Hosp Psychiatr. 1982;4(1):33–47.
29. Perlman DM, Salomons TV, Davidson RJ, Lutz A. Differential effects on pain intensity and unpleasantness of two meditation practices. Emotion. 2010;10(1):65–71.
30. Zeidan F, Gordon NS, Merchant J, Goolkasian P. The effects of brief mindfulness meditation training on experimentally induced pain. J Pain. 2010;11(3):199–209.
31. Grant JA, Rainville P. Pain sensitivity and analgesic effects of mindful states in Zen meditators: a cross-sectional study. Psychosom Med. 2009;71(1):106–14.
32. Rosenzweig S, Greeson JM, Reibel DK, Green JS, Jasser SA, Beasley D. Mindfulness-based stress reduction for chronic pain conditions: variation in treatment outcomes and role of home meditation practice. J Psychosom Res. 2010;68(1):29–36.

33. Zeidan F, Martucci KT, Kraft RA, Gordon NS, McHaffie JG, Coghill RC. Brain mechanisms supporting the modulation of pain by mindfulness meditation. J Neurosci. 2011;31(14): 5540–8.
34. Ljótsson B, Andréewitch S, Hedman E, Rück C, Andersson G, Lindefors N. Exposure and mindfulness based therapy for irritable bowel syndrome—an open pilot study. J Behav Ther Exp Psychiatr. 2010;41(3):185–90.
35. Keefer L, Blanchard EB. The effects of relaxation response meditation on the symptoms of irritable bowel syndrome: results of a controlled treatment study. Behav Res Ther. 2001;39(7):801–11.
36. Benson H. The relaxation response. New York, NY: William Morrow and Company; 1975.
37. Dietrich M, Verdolini-Abbott K, Gartner-Schmidt J, Rosen CA. The frequency of perceived stress, anxiety, and depression in patients with common pathologies affecting voice. J Voice. 2008;22(4):472–88.
38. Han JN, Zhu YJ, Li SW, et al. Medically unexplained dyspnea: psychophysiological characteristics and role of breathing therapy. Chin Med J. 2004;117(1):6–13.
39. Sayadaw M. Practical insight meditation: basic and progressive stages. Kandy, Sri Lanka: Buddhist Publication Society; 1971.
40. Jay Lynn S, Surya Das L, Hallquist MN, Williams JC. Mindfulness, acceptance, and hypnosis: cognitive and clinical perspectives. Int J Clin Exp Hypn. 2006;54(2):143–66.

Appendix

Resources Regarding Treatment of Functional Respiratory Disorders

This appendix provides information regarding resources for health-care professionals who are interested in learning more about some of the treatments described in this book.

Chapter 9: Cognitive Behavioral Therapy

For more information about cognitive behavioral therapy and training opportunities, clinicians can consult:

National Association of Cognitive Behavioral Therapists (NACBT)
Website: http://www.nacbt.org
Training opportunities: http://www.nacbt.org/cognitive-behavioral-seminars.htm

The Beck Institute
Website: http://www.beckinstitute.org
Training: http://www.beckinstitute.org/cbt-training-application/

Chapter 10: Heart Rate Variability Biofeedback

Competence in biofeedback is assured by the clinician's attainment of certification by the Biofeedback Certification Institute of America (BCIA) (www.bcia.org). Certification is available for unlicensed technicians, who must practice under supervision of the physician; for licensed health-care providers, often a nurse, social worker, or psychologist, who can work within a physician's practice; and for

R.D. Anbar (ed.), *Functional Respiratory Disorders: When Respiratory Symptoms Do Not Respond to Pulmonary Treatment*, Respiratory Medicine,
DOI 10.1007/978-1-61779-857-3, © Springer Science+Business Media, LLC 2012

academicians who primarily use biofeedback in research and education. Some physicians obtain BCIA certification and offer biofeedback treatment themselves. This ordinarily requires taking a course in biofeedback and having a required number of hours of supervised practice with the technique. The specific blueprint of training requirements is available at www.bcia.org. Forty-eight hours of didactic biofeedback and psychophysiology training are required, most of which will already have been obtained by medical education. Additionally, 20 contact hours with a BCIA-approved mentor are required to review 10 sessions of personal biofeedback demonstrating self-regulation, 50 sessions of patient/client treatment, and 10 h of case conference presentations.

The Association for Applied Psychophysiology and Biofeedback (www.aapb.org) offers periodic BCIA-approved workshops throughout the country.

Chapter 11: Breathing Techniques

Teaching breathing techniques can be undertaken in a variety of ways. Several studies used a physiotherapist with skills and knowledge in breathing training, specifically teaching diaphragmatic breathing, nasal route of breathing, and prolonged exhalation as well as good posture and relaxation. Other studies have used video teaching that patients watch in their own time, including at home, and which enables them to access a real-life demonstration of the necessary maneuvers and encourages them to practice these on a daily basis. At least one of these videos is available as a free download on the Cooperative Research Centre (CRC) for Asthma website: www.asthmacrc.org.au or www.woolcock.org.au. This DVD provides accessible free information to patients and also enables practitioners to learn the evidence as well as the skills in order to teach them effectively.

Primary care physicians may not have time to teach these techniques, but the availability of videos and DVDs enables practice nurses and physiotherapists to acquire the expertise. Several studies enabled patients to contact the physiotherapist throughout the study or an investigator to discuss the techniques to ensure they were following them appropriately. This is probably an important component and should be made available in practices where these techniques are promoted.

Chapter 12: Hypnosis

Clinical hypnosis is best learned through active participation in hypnosis workshops sponsored or endorsed by medical hypnosis organizations. Hypnosis instruction is appropriate and encouraged for various staff members who might be employed at a primary care practice or respiratory specialty centers including physicians, fellows, residents, physician's assistants, nurse practitioners, master's level nurses, psychologists, respiratory therapists, physical therapists, child life specialists, and master's level social workers.

Basic-level workshops typically are taught over 3–4 days and provide at least 20 h of training, including at least 6 h of supervised skill development in small-group hypnosis practice sessions of workshop participants. Following such an initial introductory course, the health-care provider can be ready to start employing hypnosis successfully with patients who have common diagnoses that tend to respond well to hypnosis such as vocal cord dysfunction and habit cough. Follow-up intermediate- and advanced-level hypnosis courses often are helpful.

Training for clinicians caring for children and adults is offered several times a year around the United States by the American Society of Clinical Hypnosis.
Website: www.asch.net
Telephone number: (630) 980-4740

Training for clinicians caring for children and adults is offered annually in the United States by the Society for Clinical and Experimental Hypnosis.
Website: www.sceh.us
Telephone number: (617) 469-1981

Training for clinicians caring for children is offered annually in Minnesota, USA, by the National Pediatric Hypnosis Training Institute.
Website: www.nphti.org
Telephone number: (800) 776-8636

Training for clinicians caring for children and adults is offered every 3 years around the world by the International Society of Hypnosis.
Website: www.ish-hypnosis.org
Telephone number: +39 06 854 8205

Training for clinicians caring for children and adults is offered several times a year throughout Europe by the European Society of Hypnosis.
Website: www.esh-hypnosis.eu
Telephone number: +44 114 248 8917

Training for clinicians caring for children and adults is offered several times a year throughout Australia by the Australian Society of Hypnosis.
Website: www.ozhypnosis.com.au
Telephone number: +61 2 9747 4691

Chapter 13: Speech Therapy

Training on the speech therapy techniques for the treatment of vocal cord dysfunction (VCD), cough, breathing disorders, and/or voice disorders is recommended. Professional workshops are an appropriate course to pursue and should be approved by professional medical or speech-language pathology governing agencies. Such training can be pursued by the interested primary care physician, orolaryngologist, allergist, pulmonologist, gastroenterologist, psychologist/psychiatrist, neurologist, or speech-language pathologist.

Typically, training for VCD and cough control programs occurs over a 1- to 2-day course, with 8–12 contact hours provided. Some such courses will include training on vocal care and/or means for remediating dysphonia. More specialized training on dysphonia treatment may include additional 1- to 2-day workshops. More rarely, a speech-language pathologist specializing in VCD, cough, and dyspnea, such as those on the team at National Jewish Health, may provide observation opportunities for visiting medical staff.

Training for clinicians treating adult and pediatric populations may be found via The Association for Speech-Language and Hearing Association (ASHA).
Website: www.asha.org
Telephone number:
Members: 800-498-2071; Nonmember: 800-638-8255

Sites frequently offering these in-person or webinar workshops include:
National Jewish Health
Website: http://www.njhealth.org/cme

Contact information for the ProEd Office:
The Office of Professional Education
National Jewish Health
1400 Jackson Street
Denver, Colorado 80206
303-398-1000
Email: ProEd@njhealth.org

University of Pittsburgh Medical Center
Website: www.upmc.com
Telephone number: (412) 648-6304

Chapter 15: Traditional Chinese Medicine and Acupressure

There are many ways to formally train in traditional Chinese medicine and acupressure. For those health-care professionals who would like to pursue training that will allow to practice with a state license, it is recommended to consult the following websites:

For physicians: American Board of Medical Acupuncture (http://www.dabma.org/)

For nonphysician health-care providers: The Accreditation Commission for Acupuncture and Oriental Medicine (http://www.acaom.org/)

Chapter 16: Mindfulness Meditation

Mindfulness meditation is best learned from those with extensive experience in the practice and teaching of meditation and through one's own active practice over time. The following are a list of resources to gain further experience in mindfulness meditation.

The mindfulness-based stress reduction (MBSR) program created and popularized by Jon Kabat-Zinn has been found to be especially useful for clinicians and researchers of mindfulness meditation.

MBSR programs are offered at the Center for Mindfulness in Medicine, Health Care, and Society at the University of Massachusetts Medical School, as well as worldwide.
Website: http://www.umassmed.edu/cfm/stress/index.aspx
Telephone number: (508) 856-2656

Trainings in mindfulness-based cognitive therapy (MBCT), which integrates mindfulness meditation and cognitive behavioral therapy, are offered through the Oxford Cognitive Therapy Centre.
Website: http://www.octc.co.uk/index.asp?ID=5&PageID=11
Telephone number: +44 (0)1865 738816

Mindfulness meditation retreats are an excellent opportunity to train in mindfulness meditation from highly skilled teachers within a more intensive environment and are given at the following centers. Retreats can last anywhere from 1 or 2 days to months or longer and typically involve the silent practice of mindfulness meditation throughout the day, with specific instructions from teachers.

Insight Meditation Society, Barre MA
Website: http://www.dharma.org/
Telephone number: (978) 355-4378

Spirit Rock Meditation Center, Woodacre, CA
Website: http://www.spiritrock.org/
Telephone number: (415) 488-0164

Bhavana Society
Website: http://www.bhavanasociety.org/about/
Telephone number: 304-856-3241

There are a large number of other mindfulness meditation training opportunities, both in the United States and abroad. Some of these resources can be found through the Insight Meditation Society's website (http://www.dharma.org/), under "outside resources."

Index

R.D. Anbar (ed.), *Functional Respiratory Disorders: When Respiratory Symptoms Do Not Respond to Pulmonary Treatment*, Respiratory Medicine, DOI 10.1007/978-1-61779-857-3, © Springer Science+Business Media, LLC 2012